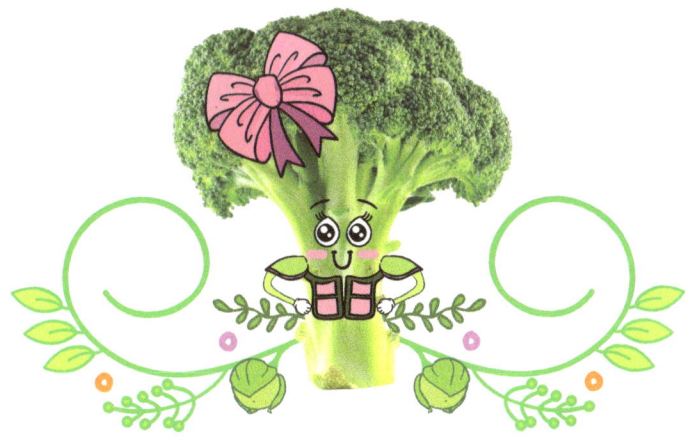

This book belongs to:

_____

experience delicious

Experience Delicious LLC

All Rights Reserved. This book or any portion thereof may not be reproduced or used in any manner whatsoever without the express written permission of the publisher except for the use of brief quotations in a book review.

Copyright 2018 Experience Delicious, LLC.
ISBN: 978-1-947001-14-5
www.experiencedeliciousnow.com

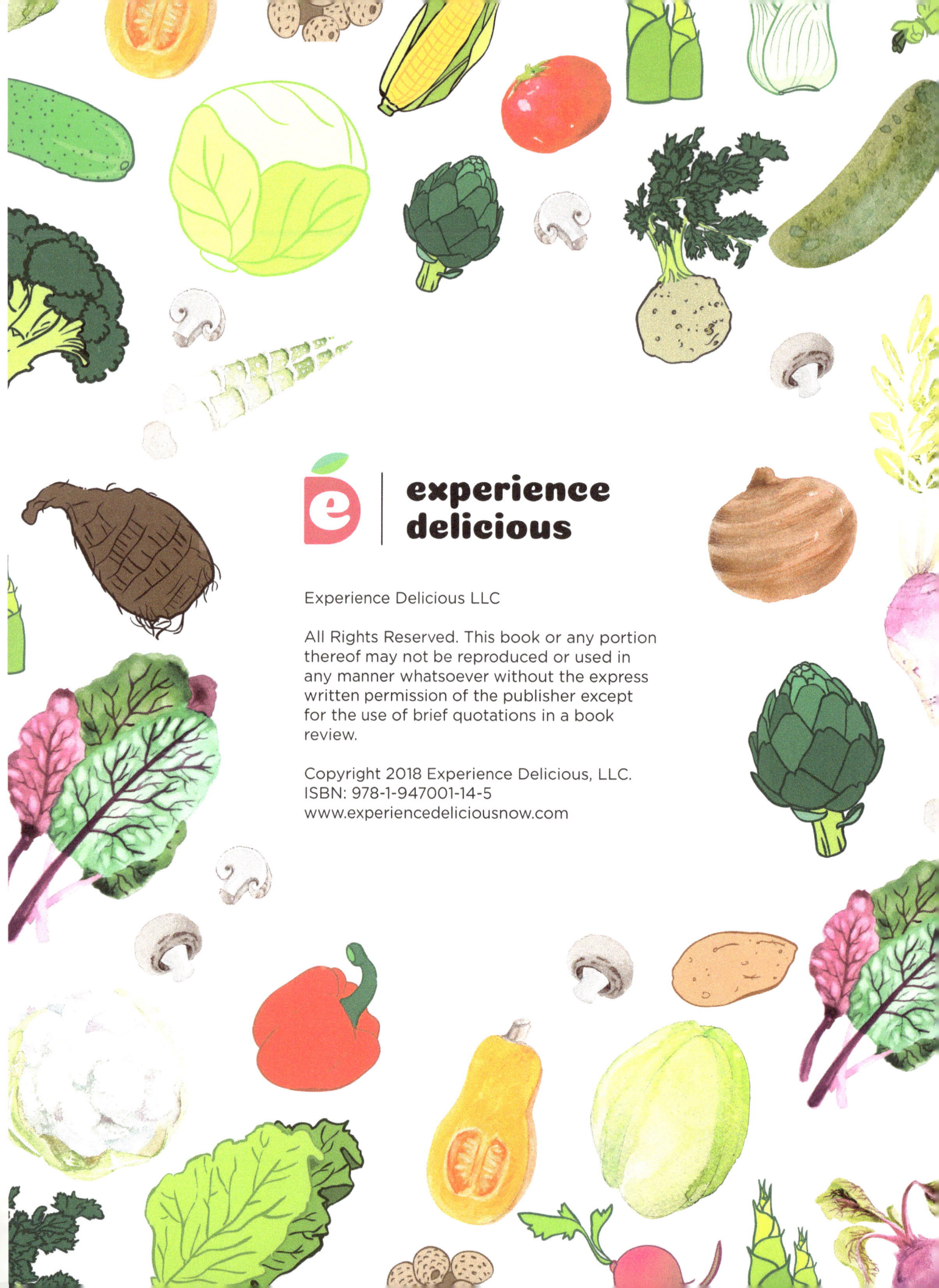

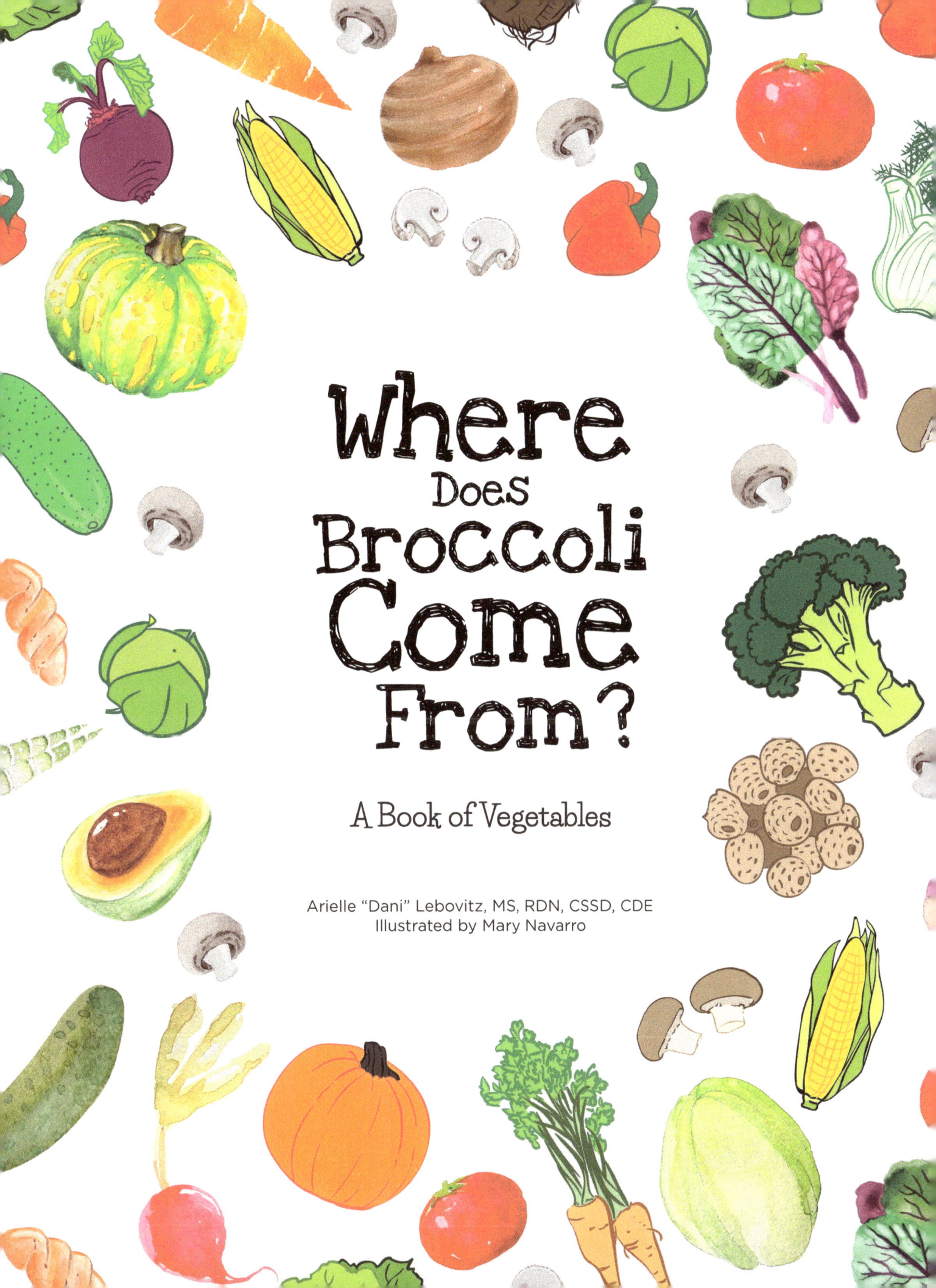
Where Does Broccoli Come From?

A Book of Vegetables

Arielle "Dani" Lebovitz, MS, RDN, CSSD, CDE
Illustrated by Mary Navarro

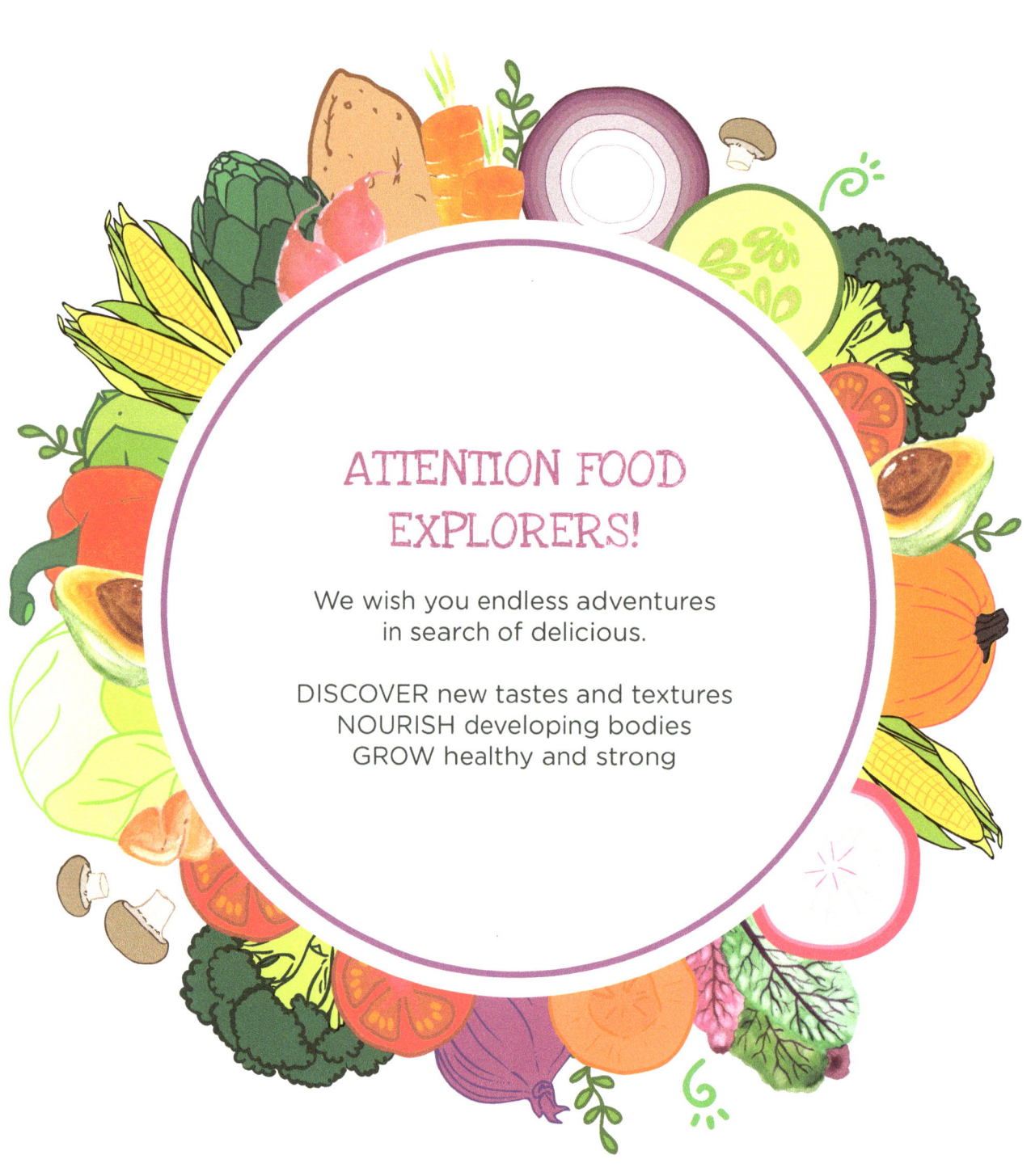

ATTENTION FOOD EXPLORERS!

We wish you endless adventures in search of delicious.

DISCOVER new tastes and textures
NOURISH developing bodies
GROW healthy and strong

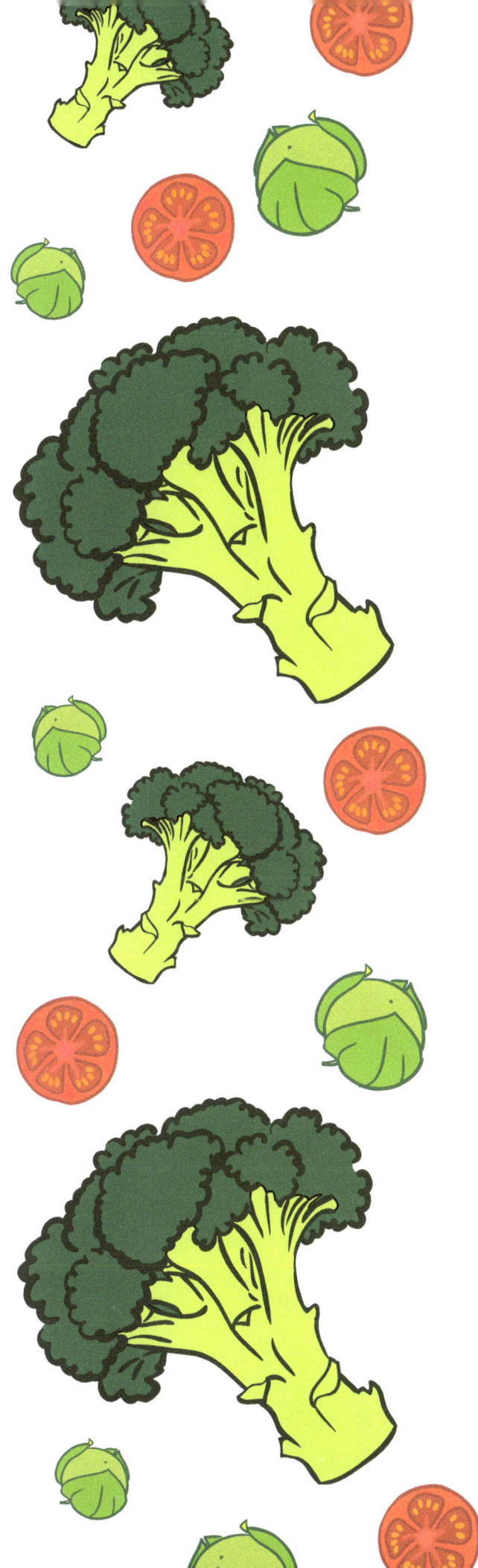

ACKNOWLEDGEMENTS

This book and series is truly a labor of love, a passion for change, and a mission to improve the health of our youth. Food nourishes. Food heals. Food is love.

To my best friend and husband Michael: You Are Everything.

To my daughter Shiloh: Your taste for adventurous foods from around the world and connoisseur-like palate inspires even a seasoned foodie to experiment outside of their comfort zone. You remind me every day why I dedicate my time to improve the health of our future and you make mealtime 1000% more fun.

To my siester Brette: Life is better with a sister. Thank you for being there every step of the way.

To the extraordinary Mary Navarro: My life has been endlessly blessed since the day I met you. Thank you for sharing my passion and for your partnership as we make whole foods fun and approachable for the entire family.

To my family, friends, and the kiddos who helped make this dream come true: Thank you for your time and feedback. Your excitement, observations, and experiences continuously improve our efforts and provide constant inspiration for pursuing our mission.

With gratitude and love,
Arielle Dani

TELL ME AND I FORGET.
TEACH ME AND I REMEMBER.
INVOLVE ME AND I LEARN.

Benjamin Franklin

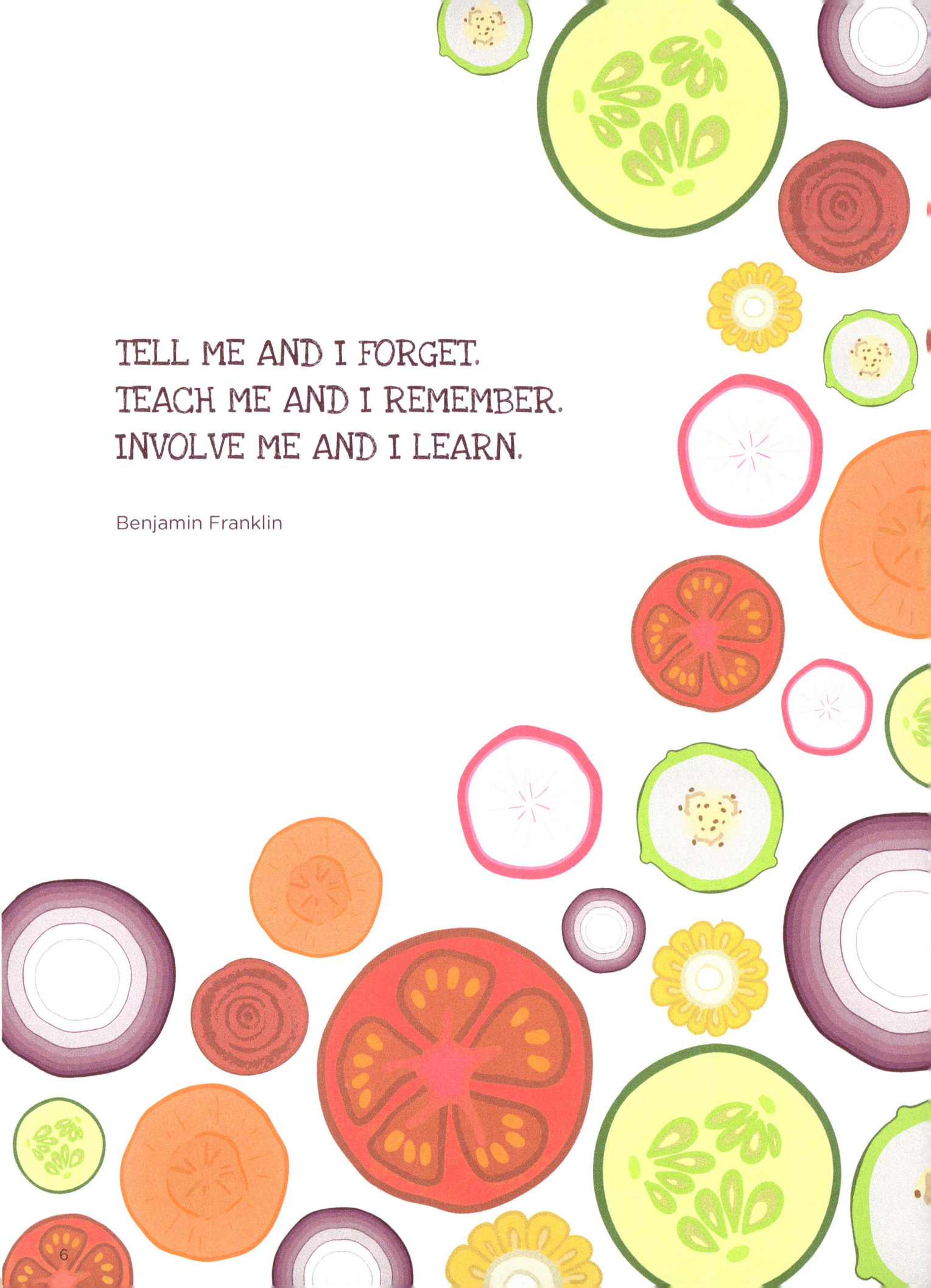

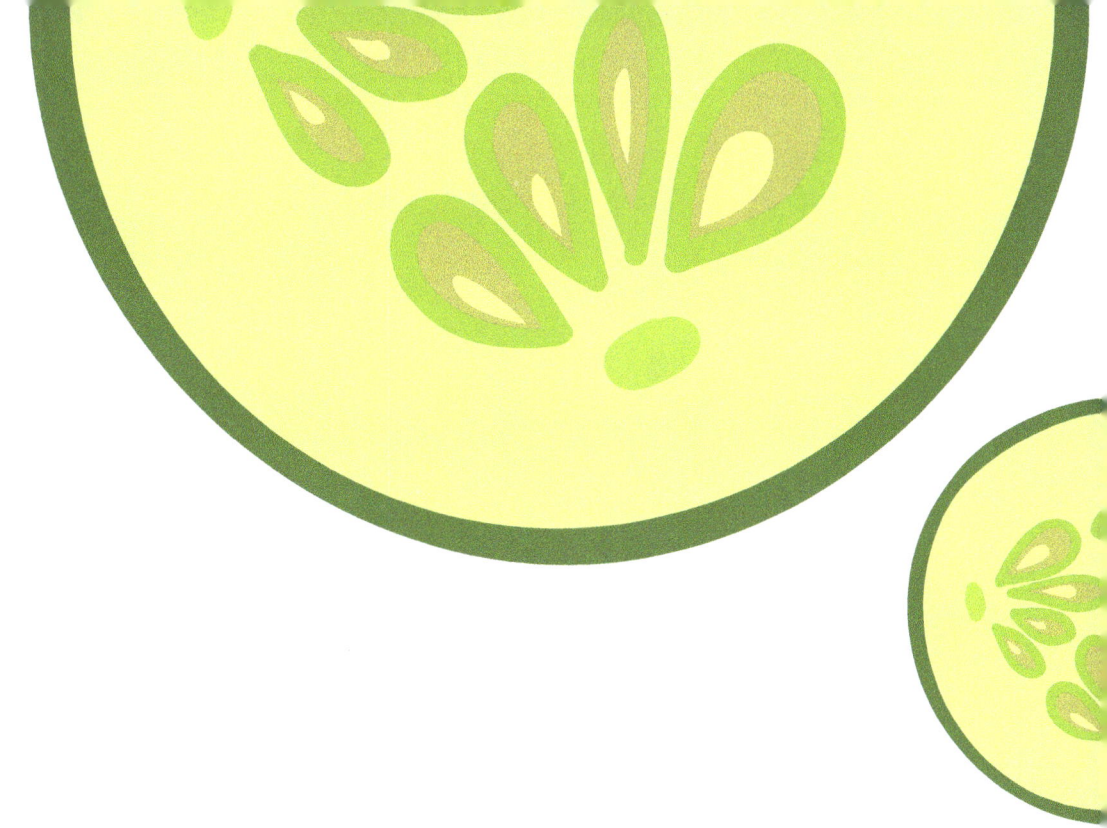

DEDICATION

To parents, grandparents, caregivers, and teachers:

Children's palates are based on senses and experiences. Early feeding, cultural background, taste-bud memory, visual presentation, knowledge, and preconception all influence taste and beliefs about food. This book series is intended to delight, inspire, and foster an interest in real food. A useful resource for children and adults alike, this book creates positive associations with mealtime.

Experiment with food. Conduct your own taste tests with new vegetables or old favorites prepared in different ways. Visit a farm. Pick local produce. Plan and grow a garden. Get kids involved in picking, storing, and cooking. Engage with kids, make food fun, and transform young palates.
Create memories – they will last a lifetime!

Now put your Food Explorer hats on and get ready for adventures in food.

Experience Delicious,
Discover – Nourish – Grow

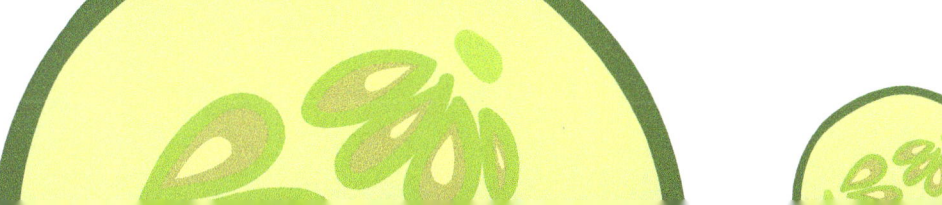

How To Read This Book

Review this page before reading the book for the best experience on your adventures with vegetables. This book is designed to be easy to read so you can experiment and explore new foods!

Vegetable
Veggie name(s) and how to pronounce them.

Descriptive Words
These words will help you describe the veggie on the page using sensory words. Check out page 158 to learn definitions for each word.

Good For My Body Nutrients
These symbols are the Good for My Body Nutrients and tell you how each veggie helps your growing body. Check out page 22 to learn more!

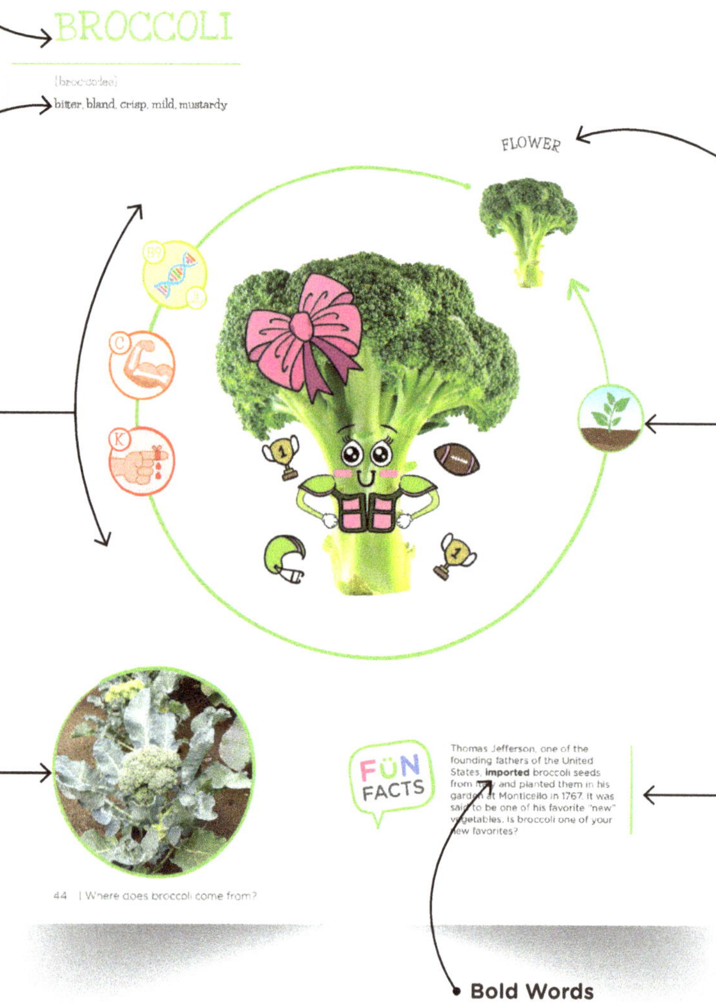

Type of Veggie
This label tells you the type of veggie or the part of the plant that you eat.

Where Veggies Grow
This symbol shows you how the veggie grows: above ground, below ground, above and below ground, or below or near water.

Veggie Plant
Each veggie plant looks different. These photos are of the plants from which a vegetable grows so you can recognize them when you see them.

Fun Facts
Learn fun facts about each veggie here!

Bold Words
Anytime you see a **BOLD** word, it means the term is defined in the Glossary on page 160.

WHERE VEGGIES GROW

Veggies can grow above ground, below ground, or above and below ground. Other veggies **flourish** below water and some near water. These **symbols** show you where a veggie grows.

 Above Ground
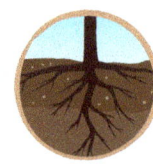 Below Ground
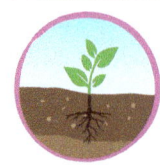 Above and Below Ground
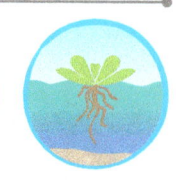 Below or Near Water

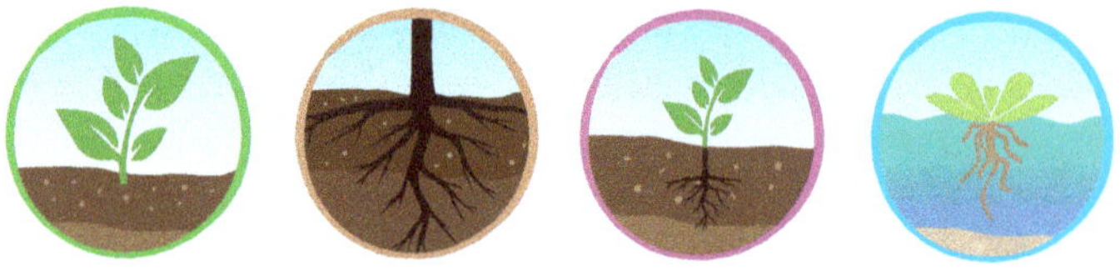

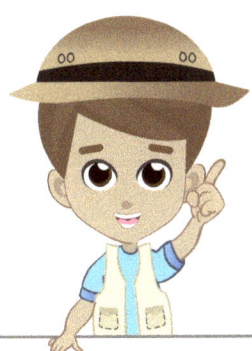

VEGGIE VARIETIES

Many veggies have several **varieties** of the same type of vegetable that we love to eat! The veggie varieties pages introduce you to some of the commonly consumed veggie varieties with interesting facts, how to recognize them, or details about flavor and **texture**.

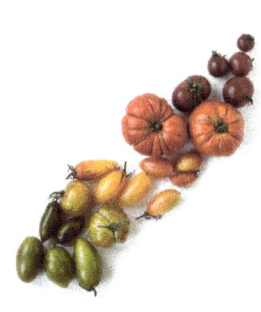

Pick
Learn how to PICK the perfectly delicious veggie here!

PICK
Pick dark green to bluish-green **florets** with firm, compact buds, and firm stems that feel heavy for their size. Avoid broccoli with open buds, yellowing in color, or soft **wilted** stems.

Seasonality
A vegetable may be in-season locally when the months are filled with color.

Peak Season
October-April

Store
Learn how to STORE your veggies and keep them fresh until you are ready to eat them.

STORE
Refrigerate unwashed, raw broccoli in an open plastic bag for up to 5 days. Refrigerate cooked broccoli in an airtight container for 3-5 days.

Peak Season
The lighter colored sections with small triangles tell you when a veggie is in peak season which means it is fresh, yummy, less expensive, and easier to find!

Veggie Preparation
These photos show you ways the veggie is often prepared.

EAT
Clean the skin, cut the florets off the stem, and chop florets and stems into uniform sized pieces.

Steamed Broccoli
Steam florets and stems for 5 to 7 minutes. Broccoli is ready to eat when the pieces are tender.

BROCCOLI TIDBITS

The part of the broccoli you eat are actually baby flowers that haven't opened yet!

Veggies Tidbits
Learn extra information about each veggie from interesting facts to preparation methods.

Cooking Methods
These symbols highlight ways to cook or prepare each vegetable and give you ideas for different ways to try them. Check out page 28 to learn more!

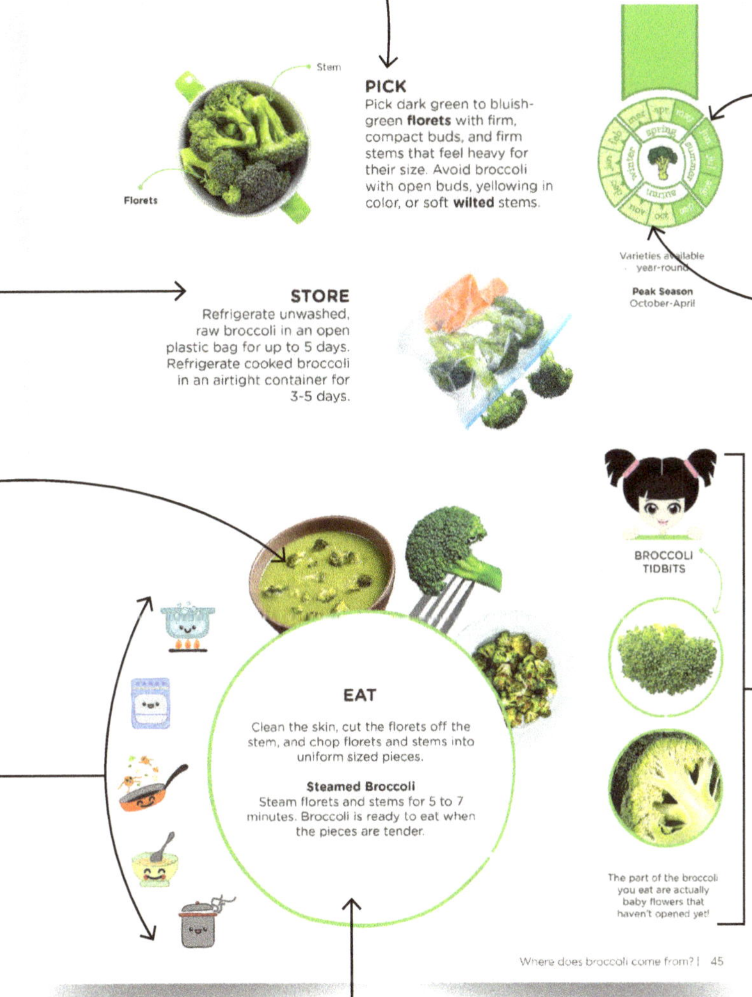

Where does broccoli come from? | 45

Eat
Learn how to EAT each veggie from whole vegetable to cooked and ready for taste-testing. Try the simple recipe, then explore the flavors and textures using your 5 senses!

MY 5 SENSES

This book is all about veggie exploration! Learn how to use your 5 senses on page 24. Become a Food Explorer by picking a vegetable to try and using your senses to experience it. Record your observations on the "My 5 Senses Worksheet" found on page 25 or print them from our website for FREE! (www.experiencedeliciousnow.com)

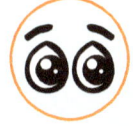 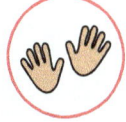  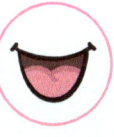 

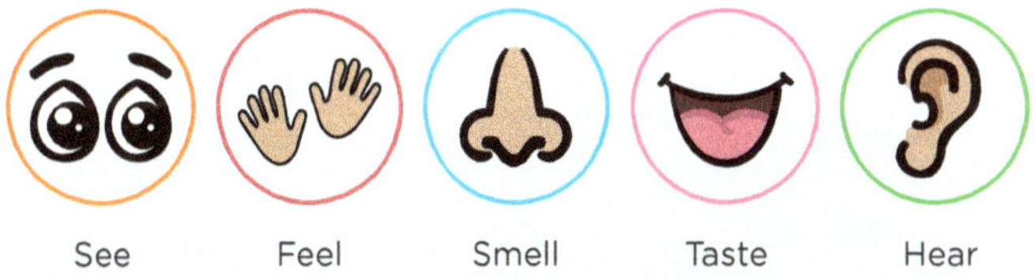

See   Feel   Smell   Taste   Hear

Table of Contents

What Are Veggies?	12-13
How Do Veggies Grow?	14
Edible Parts of a Plant	15
Types of Veggies: Bulb and Corm	16
Types of Veggies: Tuber and Root	17
Types of Veggies: Stem and Leaves	18
Types of Veggies: Flower and Fruit	19
Mushrooms, Sea Vegetables, Sprouts and Shoots	20
When Do Veggies Grow?	21
Good for My Body Nutrients	22-23
Using Your 5 Senses	24-25
My 5 Senses Worksheet	26-27
Cooking Methods	28-29
Origin Map: North America	30
Origin Map: South America	31
Origin Map: Asia	32
Origin Map: Africa	33
Veggies	34-157
Descriptive Words	158-159
Glossary Words	160-163

Welcome! We are the Food Explorers in search of delicious!

Join us as we discover new tastes and textures on an adventure into the wonderful world of vegetables.

Over the following pages, we hope to enhance your experience with fun facts and interesting tidbits about our favorite veggies.

Let's dig in!

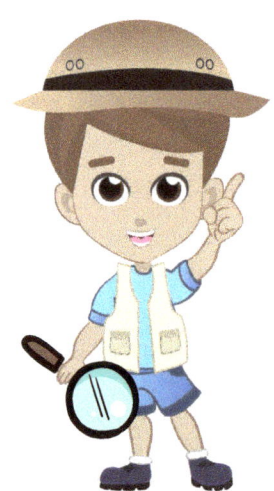
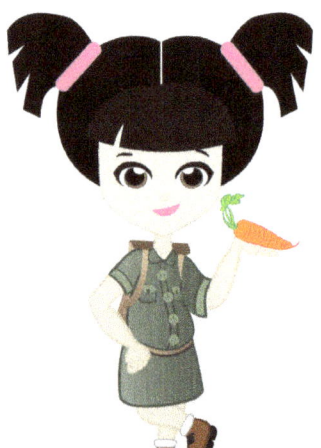
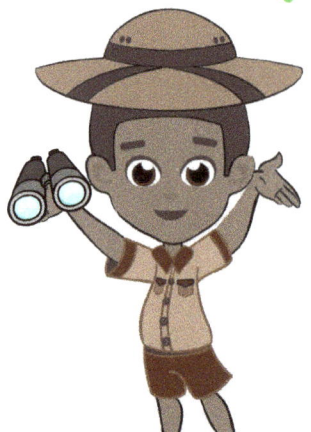
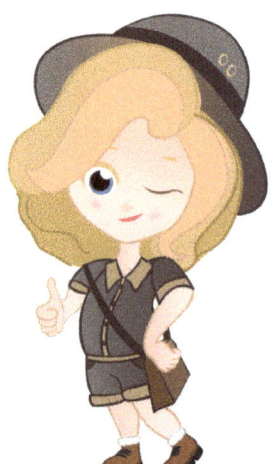

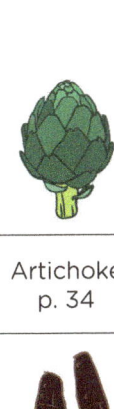	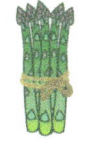	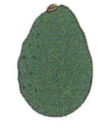	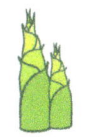	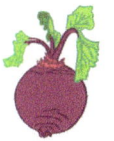	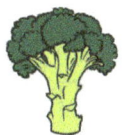	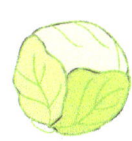	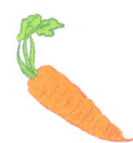
Artichoke p. 34	Asparagus p. 36	Avocado p. 38	Bamboo Shoot p. 40	Beet and Greens p. 42	Broccoli p. 44	Cabbage Varieties p. 46	Carrot and Greens p. 50
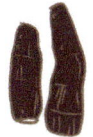	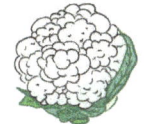	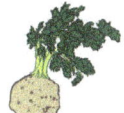		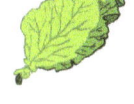	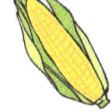	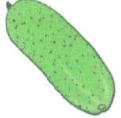	
Cassava p. 52	Cauliflower p. 54	Celeriac p. 56	Celery p. 58	Collard Greens p. 60	Corn p. 62	Cucumber p. 64	Daikon and Greens p. 66
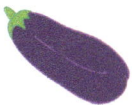	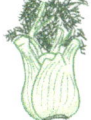		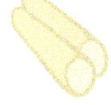	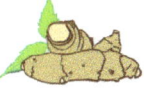	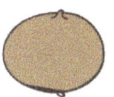	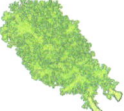	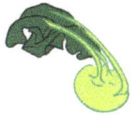
Eggplant p. 68	Fennel p. 70	Fiddlehead Fern p. 72	Hearts of Palm p. 74	Jerusalem Artichoke p. 76	Jicama p. 78	Kale p. 80	Kohlrabi and Greens p. 82
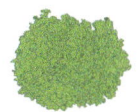	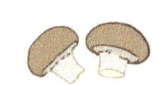	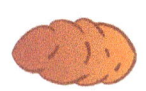	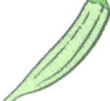	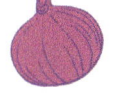	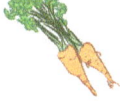	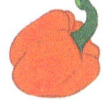	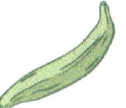
Lettuce Varieties p. 84	Mushroom Varieties p. 88	Oca p. 92	Okra p. 94	Onion Varieties p. 96	Parsnip p. 100	Pepper p. 102	Plantain p. 104
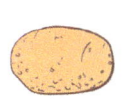	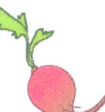	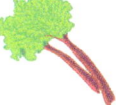	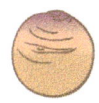	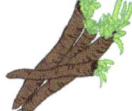	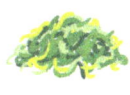	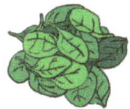	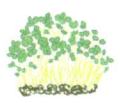
Potato Varieties p. 106	Radish and Greens p. 110	Rhubarb p. 112	Rutabaga p. 114	Salsify p. 116	Sea Vegetable Varieties p. 118	Spinach p. 122	Sprout Varieties p. 124
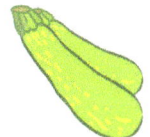	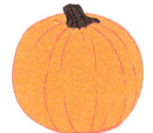	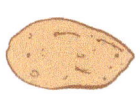	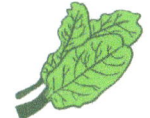	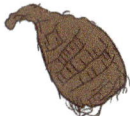	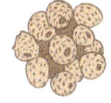	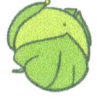	
Squash, Summer Varieties p. 128	Squash, Winter Varieties p. 132	Sweet Potato p. 136	Swiss Chard p. 138	Taro p. 140	Tiger Nut p. 142	Tomatillo p. 144	Tomato Varieties p. 146
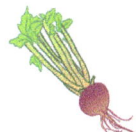			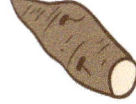				
Turnip and Greens p. 150	Water Chestnut p. 152	Watercress p. 154	Yam p. 156				

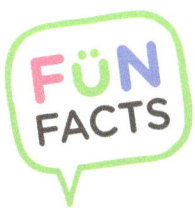

Horticulture is the science of growing **fruits**, **vegetables**, and **flowers**.

What Are Veggies?

A vegetable or veggie is the part of a plant that is **edible** – meaning the part that is safe to eat. Vegetables come from different parts of plants, but not all parts of every plant can be eaten.

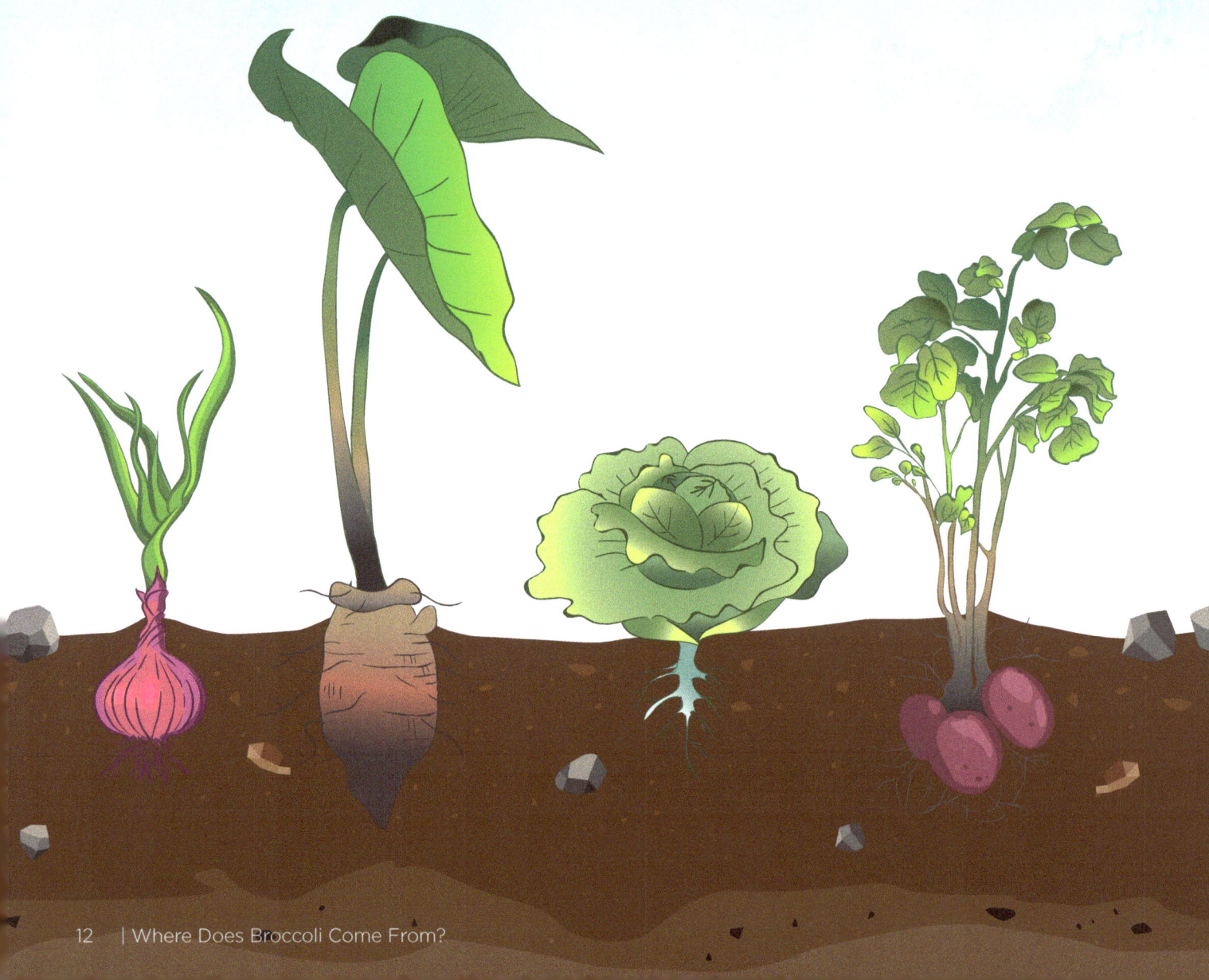

Vegetable Classification

Vegetables are **classified** or grouped based on how we eat them. Vegetables come in all different shapes, sizes, and colors. There are many different parts of plants to eat too!

From **bulbs** to **flowers** and **roots** to **leaves**, vegetables are truly **diverse**. For some veggies, such as beets, you can eat the entire plant including the root and the leaves! For other veggies, such as bulb onions, you must remove the dry outer leaves before eating them.

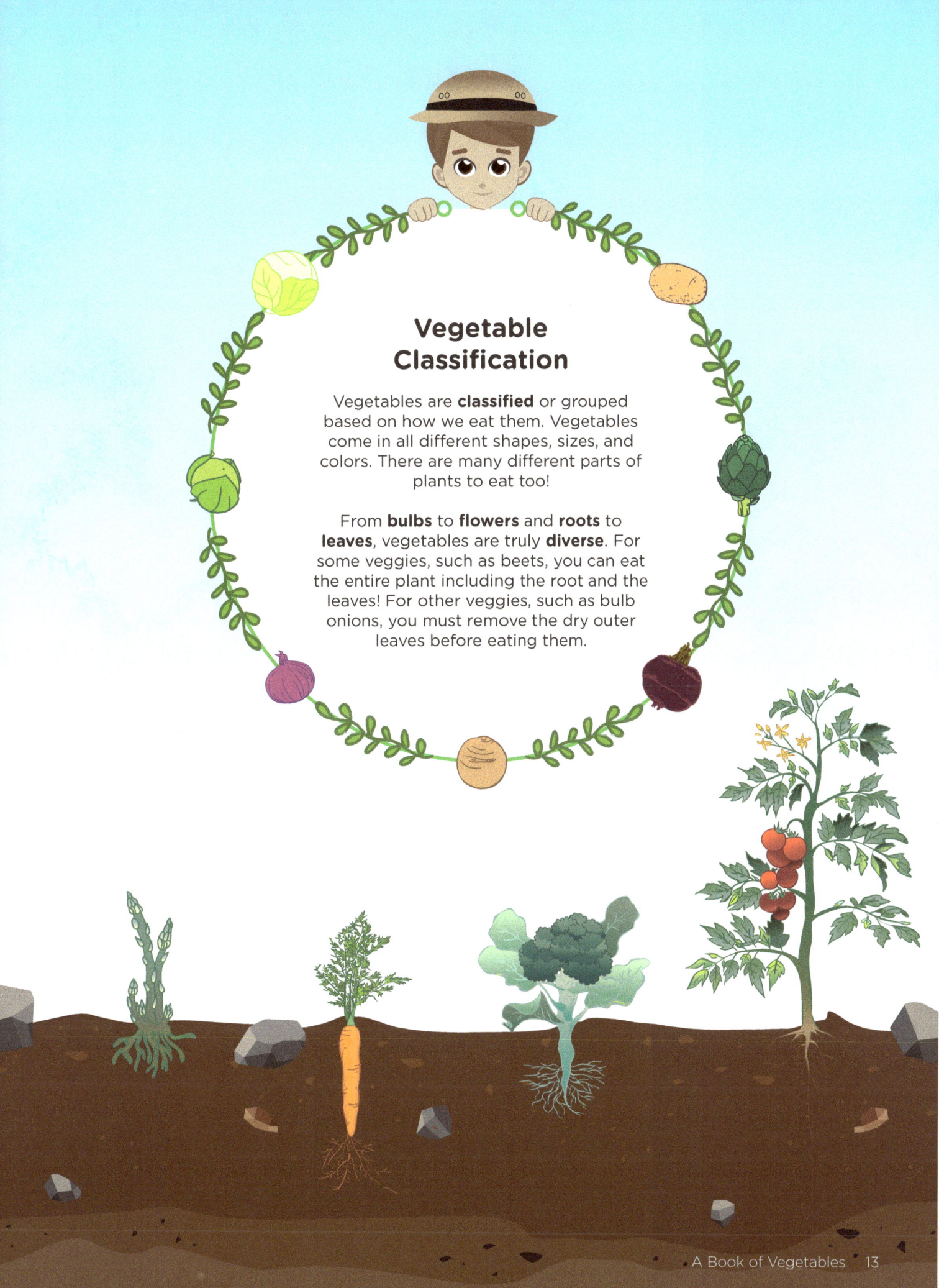

How Do Veggies Grow?

Plants make their own food through **photosynthesis**. They take water and **nutrients** from the soil, **carbon dioxide** from the air, and light from the sun and transform it into **oxygen** and **energy**.

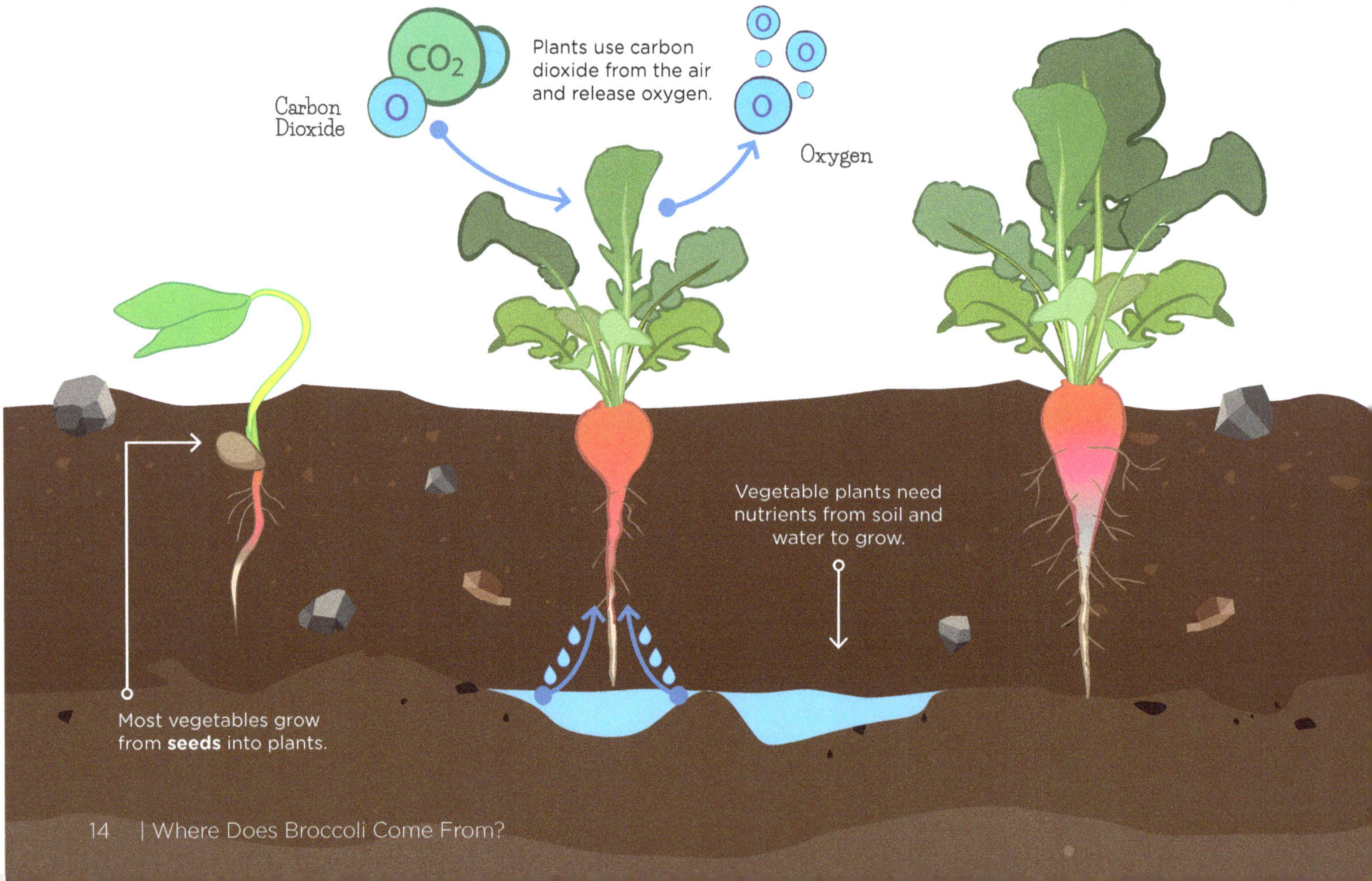

Some vegetable plants need lots of sunlight while others grow in the shade

Many vegetables **thrive** or grow in warm weather and others **flourish** or grow in cold weather

Carbon Dioxide

Plants use carbon dioxide from the air and release oxygen.

Oxygen

Vegetable plants need nutrients from soil and water to grow.

Most vegetables grow from **seeds** into plants.

14 | Where Does Broccoli Come From?

Edible Parts of a Plant

Edible parts of plants include **bulbs**, **corms**, **tubers**, **roots**, **stems**, **leaves**, **flowers**, and even some **fruits**.

Some fruits are **classified** as vegetables because of how we eat them! This includes avocado, cucumber, eggplant, pepper, squash, and tomato.

Below is a made-up veggie plant to show you the parts that are edible.

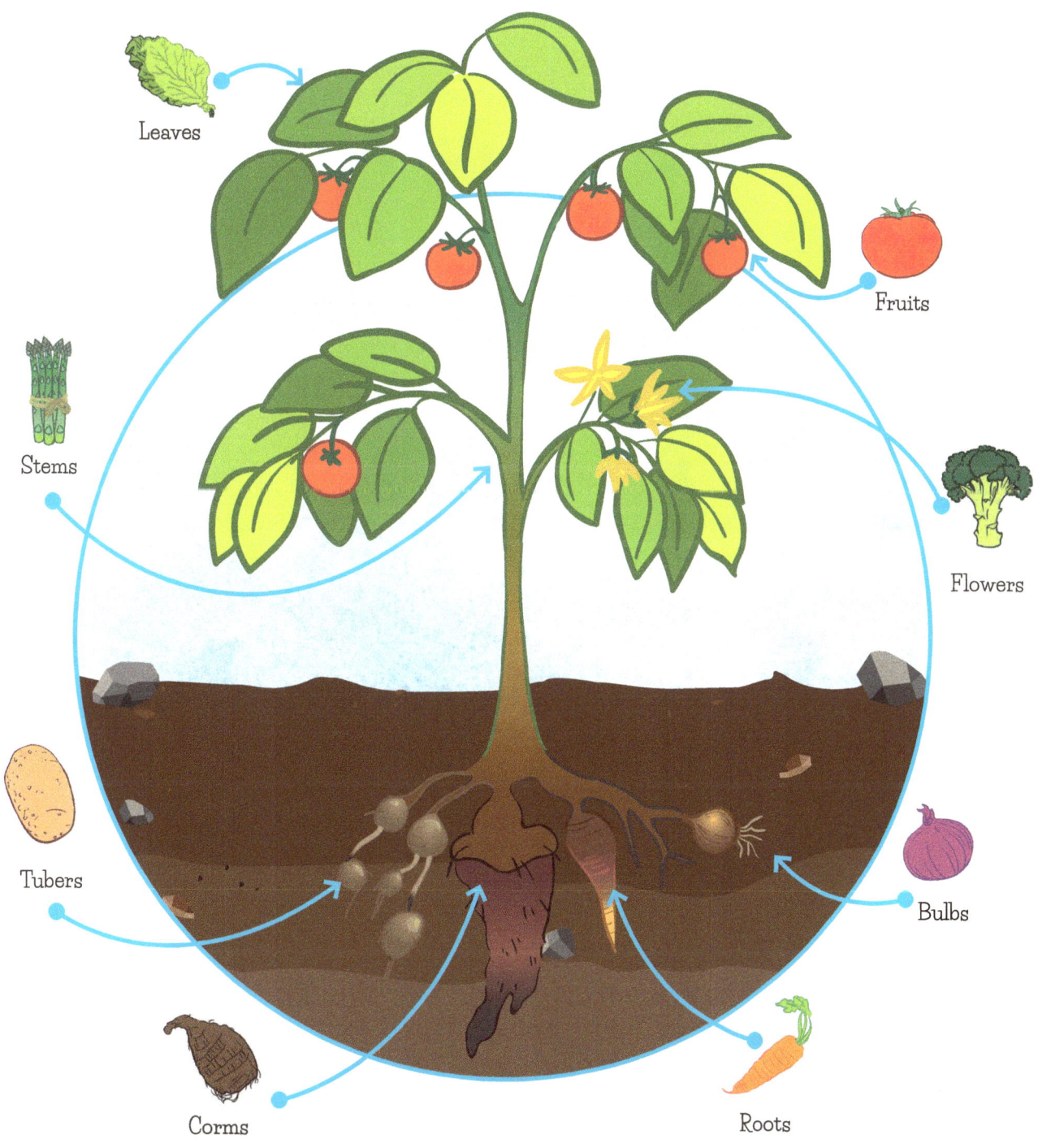

A Book of Vegetables 15

Types of Veggies

Each veggie, or **edible** part of a plant, grows in their own special way and are **classified** by how they develop into the different parts of the plant that we eat.

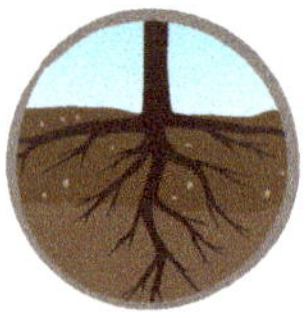

Bulb

Layers of overlapping **fleshy leaves** surround a short **stem** that grows just below the surface of the ground.

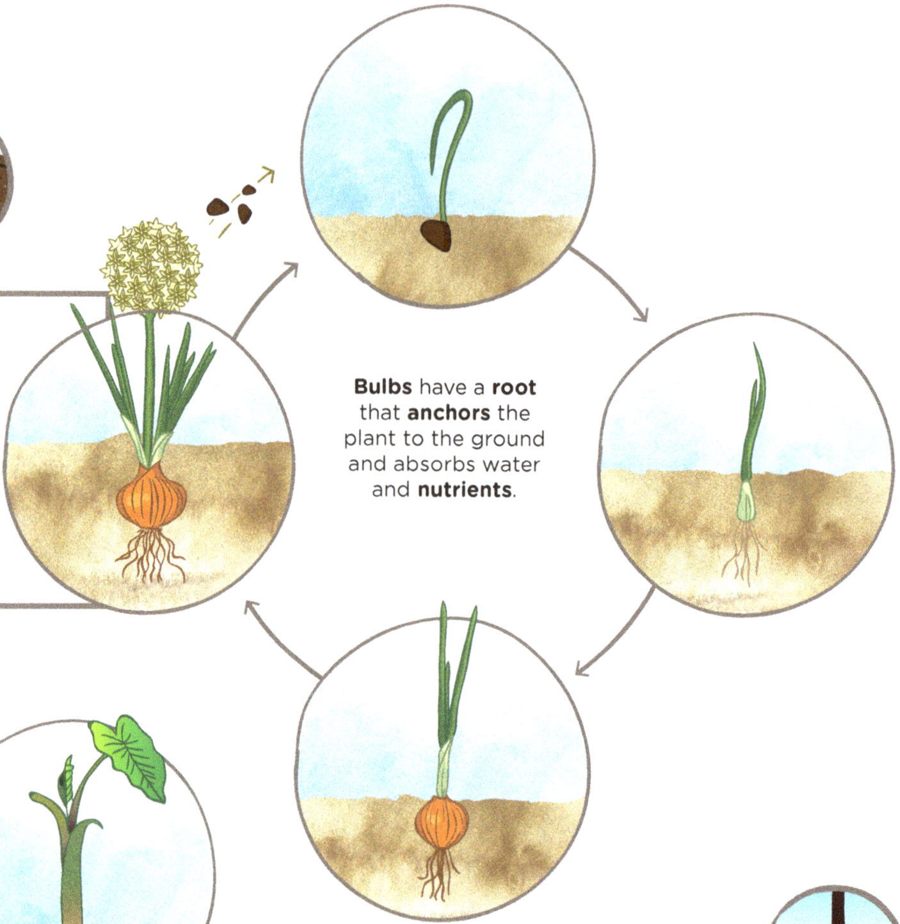

Bulbs have a **root** that **anchors** the plant to the ground and absorbs water and **nutrients**.

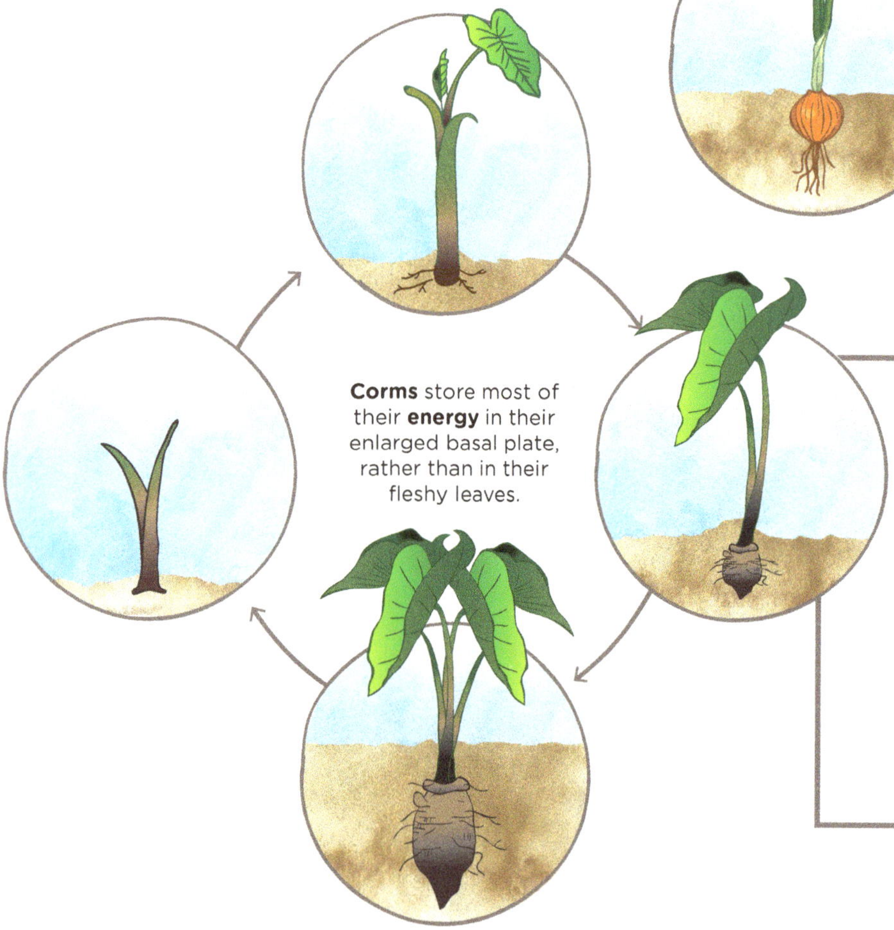

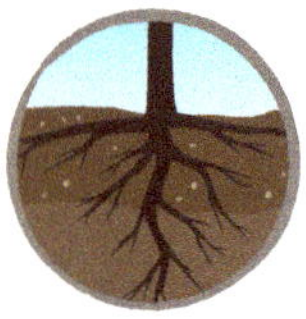

Corm

Large, dense, scaly leaves, and **buds** or eyes that can grow new plants above ground and have underground stems with a solid **basal plate**. Basal plates are the bottom of bulbs where roots grow.

Corms store most of their **energy** in their enlarged basal plate, rather than in their fleshy leaves.

16 | Where Does Broccoli Come From?

Types of Veggies

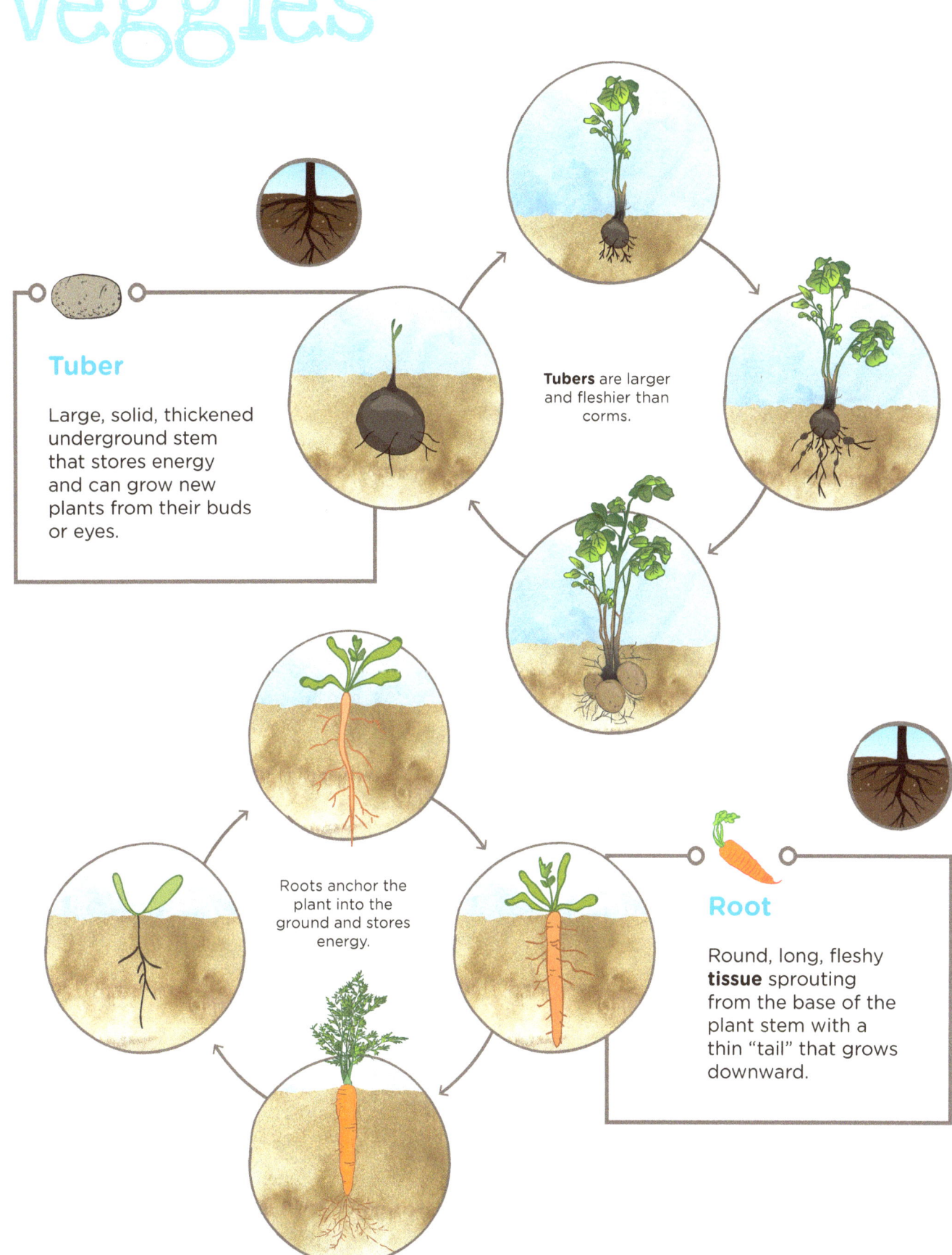

Tuber

Large, solid, thickened underground stem that stores energy and can grow new plants from their buds or eyes.

Tubers are larger and fleshier than corms.

Roots anchor the plant into the ground and stores energy.

Root

Round, long, fleshy **tissue** sprouting from the base of the plant stem with a thin "tail" that grows downward.

A Book of Vegetables 17

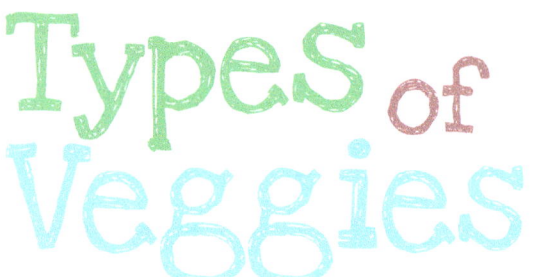

Types of Veggies

Each veggie, or **edible** part of a plant, grows in their own special way and are **classified** by how they develop into the different parts of the plant that we eat.

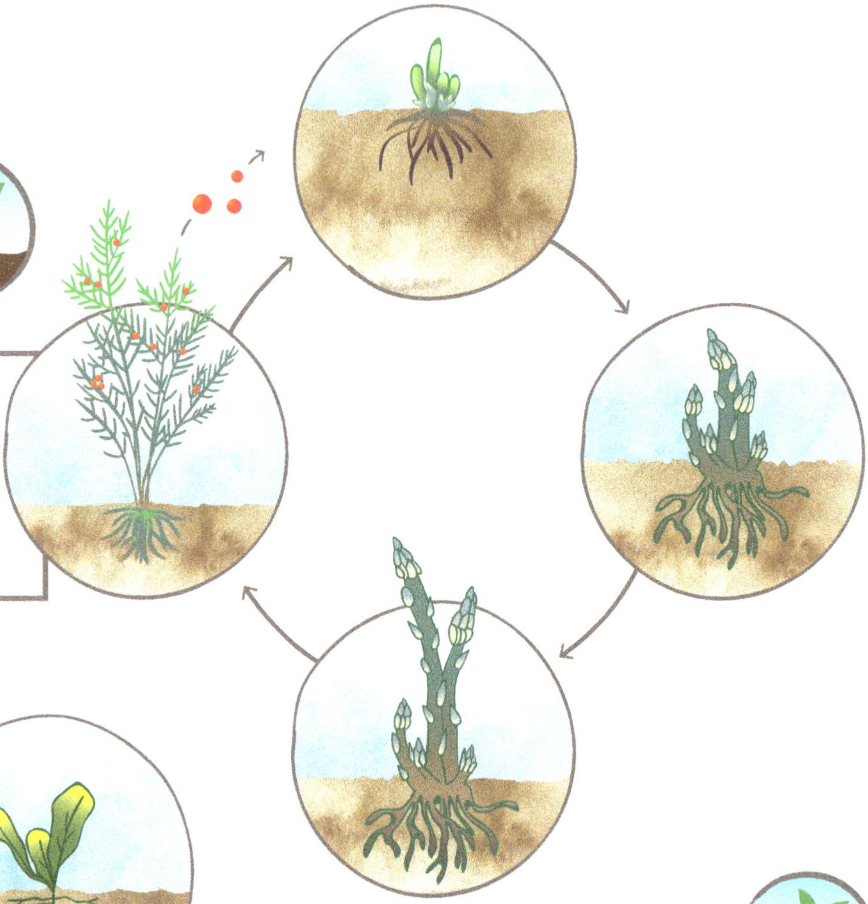

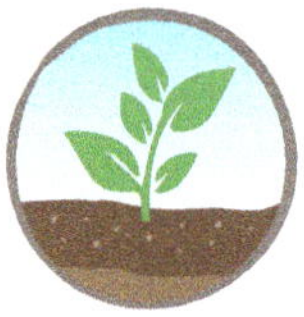

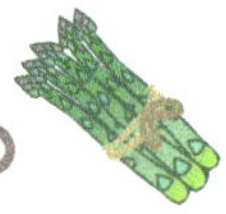

Stem

Main part of a plant that supports **leaves** and flowers also known as a **stalk**.

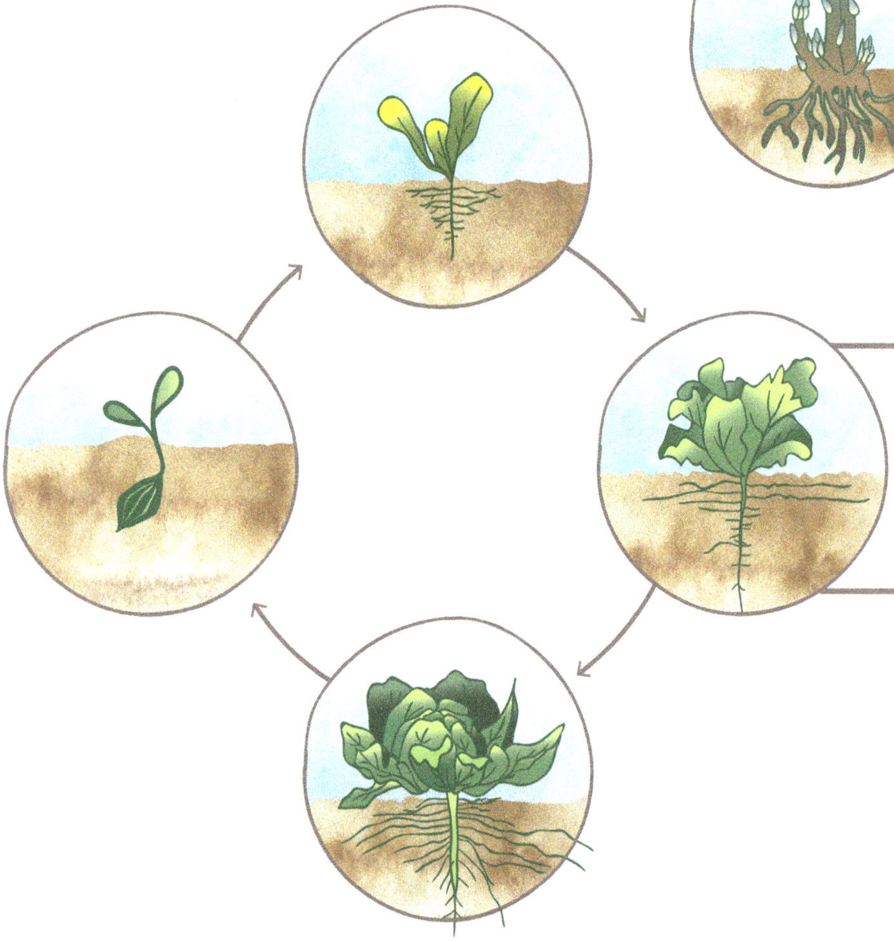

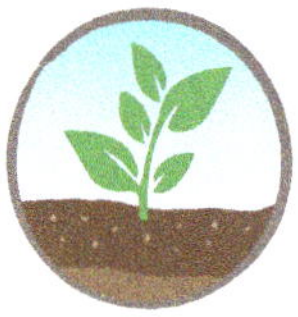

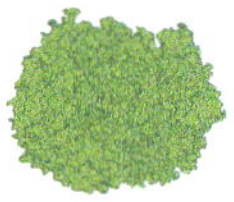

Leaves

Edible part of the plant that grows from the **stem**.

Types of Veggies

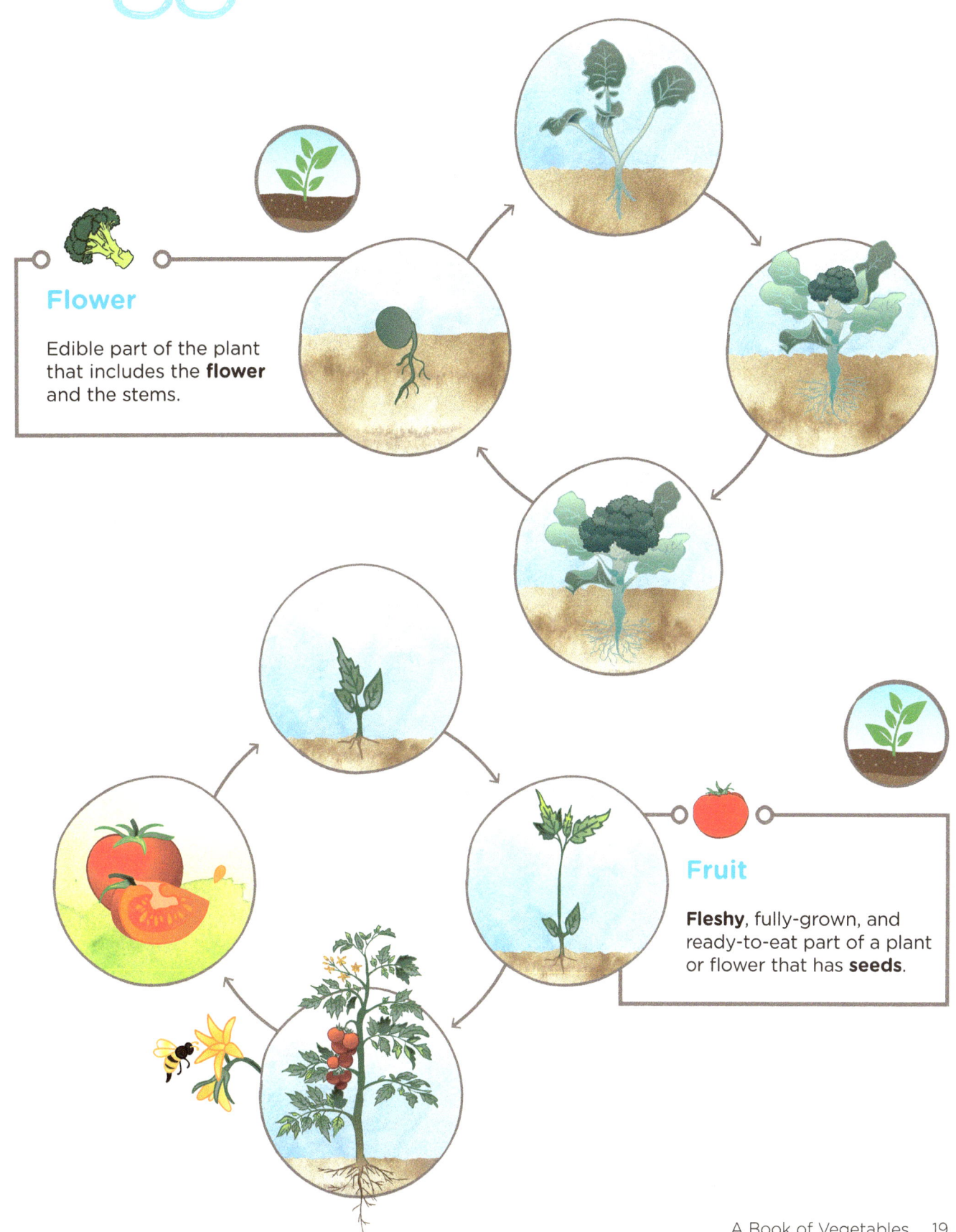

Flower

Edible part of the plant that includes the **flower** and the stems.

Fruit

Fleshy, fully-grown, and ready-to-eat part of a plant or flower that has **seeds**.

A Book of Vegetables

Mushrooms
Sea Vegetables
Sprouts and Shoots

Some vegetables are not **classified** as vegetables but are considered vegetables because of how we eat them.

Mushrooms
A form of fungi that typically **reproduce** from **spores** and lack **seeds**, **roots**, **leaves**, and **flowers**.

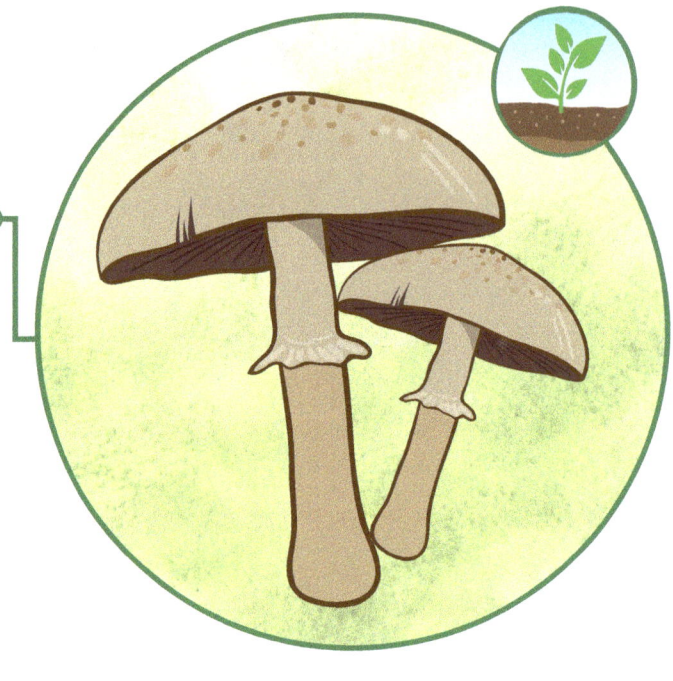

Sea Vegetables
Edible plants grown in the sea that lack true roots, **stems**, or leaves. They are classified as marine **algae**.

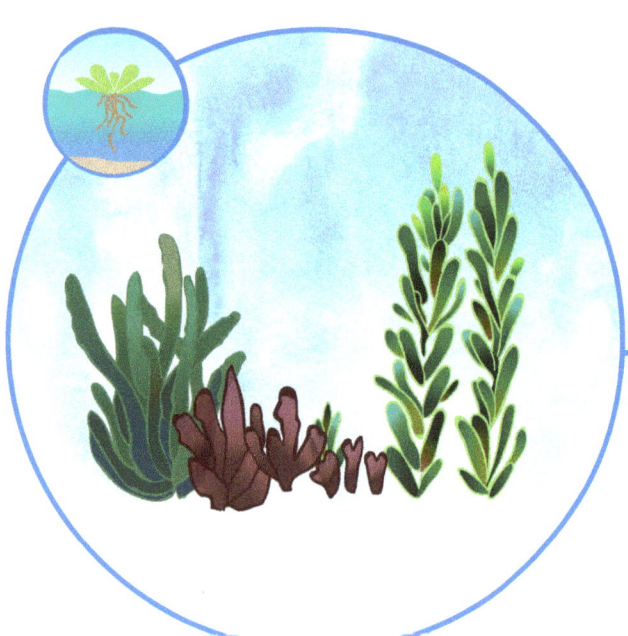

Sprouts and Shoots
The tender, first stems after seeds grow. **Sprouts** are seeds and tiny leaves. **Shoots** are grown a little longer than sprouts and have more developed stems and small leaves.

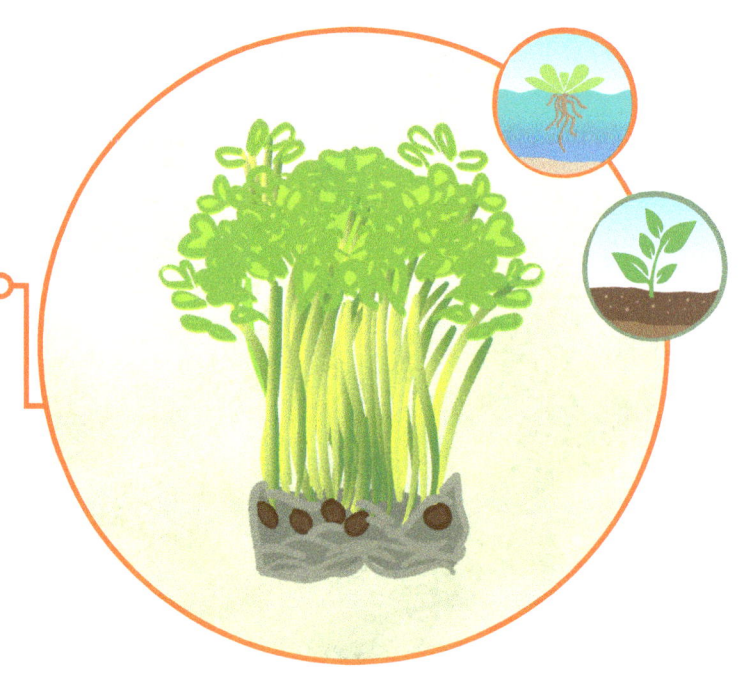

20 | Where Does Broccoli Come From?

When Do Veggies Grow?

Vegetables are **seasonal** which means they are grown and **harvested** based on the time of year and location. Varying **climates** mean that **fruits** and vegetables may only be available locally at certain times of the year and can differ from state to state. Visit your local farmer's market to see what produce is in season near you!

When vegetables are in season they are fresh, yummy, less expensive, and easier to find!

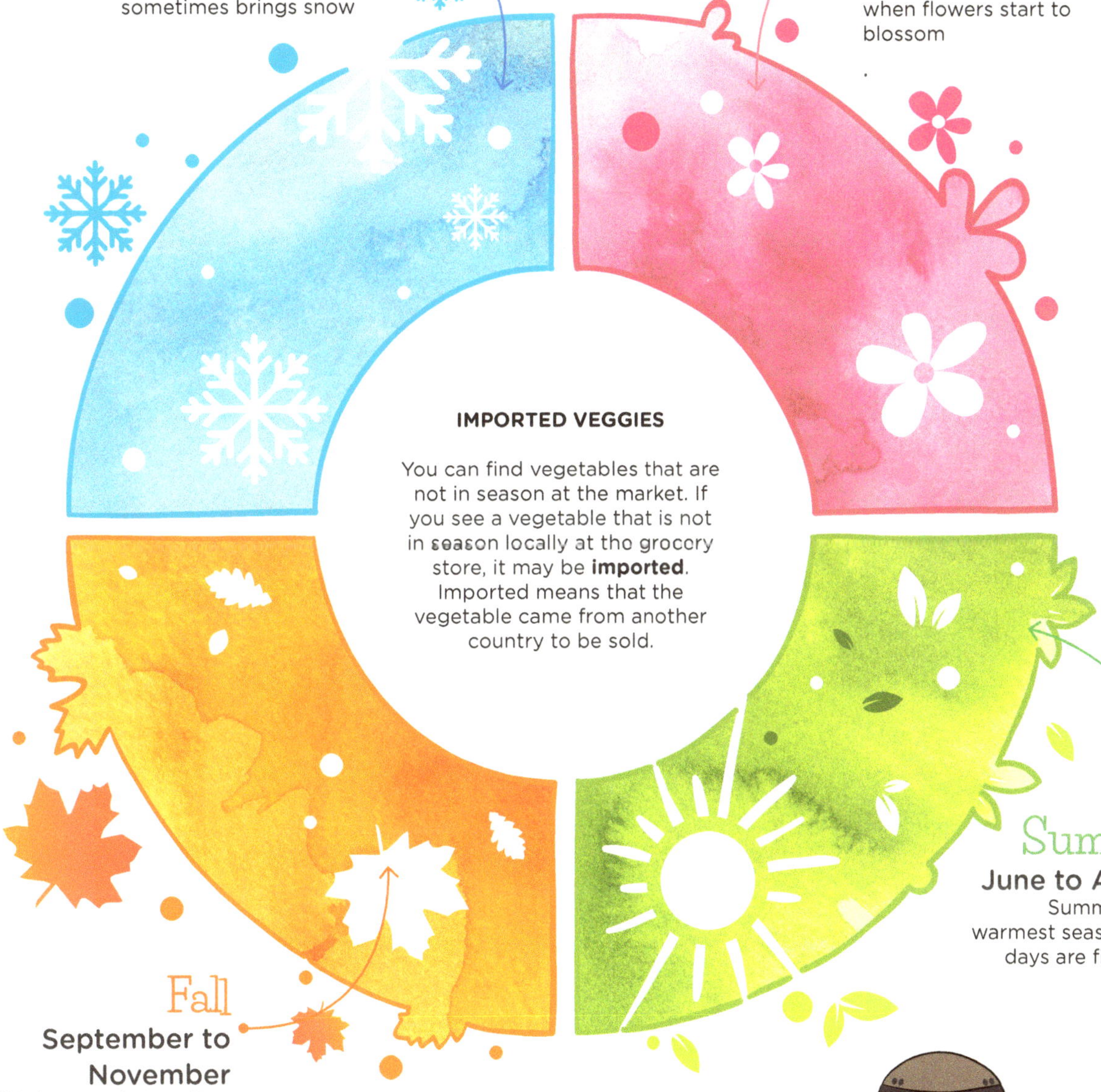

Winter
December to February
Winter is the coldest season and sometimes brings snow

Spring
March to May
Spring is the rainy season when flowers start to blossom

Summer
June to August
Summer is the warmest season when days are filled with sunshine

Fall
September to November
Fall brings cooler weather and leaves start to drop from trees

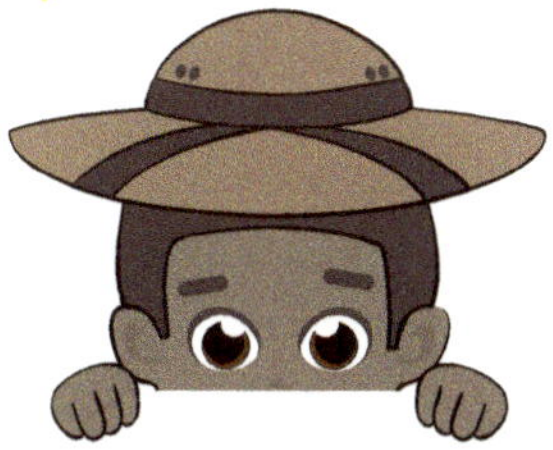

IMPORTED VEGGIES

You can find vegetables that are not in season at the market. If you see a vegetable that is not in season locally at the grocery store, it may be **imported**. Imported means that the vegetable came from another country to be sold.

Seasonality in this book is based on availability in North America.

A Book of Vegetables 21

Good for my Body Nutrients

Vegetables are important to keep our bodies healthy because they are filled with **nutrients**. Nutrients are the part of food that help our bodies function or work their best.

Each vegetable contains many different nutrients such as **vitamins**, **minerals**, **antioxidants**, and **phytonutrients**. These nutrients work together in the body to help us grow healthy and strong, learn our best in school, play sports, and fight off sickness.

We call vitamins, minerals, and antioxidants Good for My Body Nutrients (GFMBN)!

*When you see these **symbols** along with a vegetable you will know how they help your growing body.*

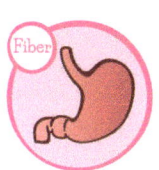 **FIBER [fahy-ber]**
helps keep your heart healthy, your insides clean by moving food through your **digestive system**, and makes your tummy feel full. **Digestion** is how your body gets nutrients and **energy** from the food you eat.

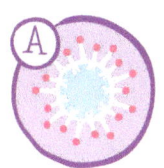 **VITAMIN A**
supports a healthy immune system, your body's defense to fight sickness. Vitamin A also helps with eyesight especially at night, as well as with growth, development, and healthy skin.

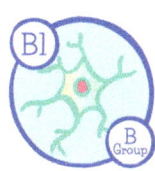 **VITAMIN B1 (Thiamin) [thi-a-min]**
supports your body's **nervous system**, the body's super highway that controls how your body works. Vitamin B1 also helps your body use energy from the food you eat.

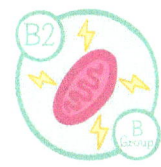 **VITAMIN B2 (Riboflavin) [ri-bo-flay-vin]**
helps your body use energy from the food you eat so your body works at its best. Vitamin B2 also assists other vitamins to do their jobs in the body which helps keep you healthy and active!

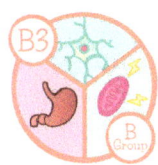 **VITAMIN B3 (Niacin) [ni-a-cin]**
supports many functions in the body from assisting with digestive health, to supporting your body's nervous system, and using energy from the food you eat. Vitamin B3 also helps with growth and healthy skin.

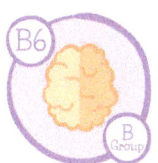 **VITAMIN B6 (Pyridoxine) [pyr-i-dox-ine]**
supports brain function and helps your body make red blood cells that carry **oxygen** throughout your body. Vitamin B6 also helps your body use energy from the food you eat and supports a healthy immune system.

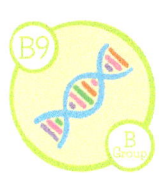 **VITAMIN B9 (Folate) [foll-ate]**
helps make **DNA**, the instruction manual for your body. Vitamin B9 also helps your body make red blood **cells** that carry oxygen throughout your body so you can run and play.

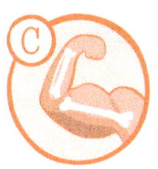 **VITAMIN C**
promotes strong muscles and bones so you can be active and play your favorite sports. Vitamin C also supports healthy skin, teeth, brain cells, and helps heal cuts when you get a scrape.

 **VITAMIN E**
an antioxidant that defends the cells and **tissues** in your body against damage. Vitamin E also boosts your **immune system** to keep you healthy and active.

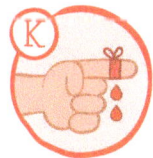 **VITAMIN K**
helps blood to **clot** or stop bleeding when you get cuts and scrapes.

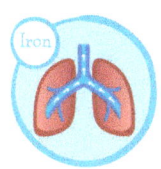 **IRON [ahy-ern]**
is a mineral that works like a big yellow school bus transporting oxygen from your lungs to your whole body and keeps you moving.

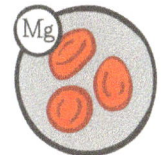 **MAGNESIUM [mag-nes-c-um]**
is a mineral used by every cell in your body. Magnesium helps turn the food we eat into energy, and supports healthy bones, muscles, and nerves.

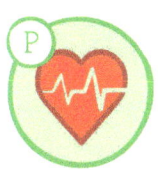 **POTASSIUM [po-tas-c-um]**
is a mineral that helps your heart and muscles function. Potassium aids in maintaining the balance of water and **electrolytes** in your body so you can feel good and play sports longer!

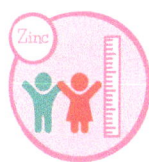 **ZINC [zingk]**
is a mineral important for growing up healthy. Zinc helps your **immune system** fight off sickness, and heals cuts and scrapes. Zinc also supports your sense of smell for tasting new foods!

Good for My Body Nutrients (GFMBN) are based on data from a 1 cup serving, recommended serving from the United States Department of Agriculture (USDA) nutrient database, or accessible research studies. GFMBN are defined as a "good source" based on the Recommended Dietary Allowances (RDAs) providing at least 10% of the percent Daily Value (% DV) of the Reference Daily Intakes (RDIs) with Daily Reference Values (DRVs) established by the Food and Drug Administration (FDA).

Using Your 5 Senses

Broccoli, you've probably seen it on your plate, but have you explored it?

Do you like broccoli? What do you like about it? How do you like to eat it? Do you eat broccoli raw dipped in ranch dressing or steamed with shredded cheese on top?

Exploring foods with our 5 senses is fun and can help us discover and engage with what we eat. Learning and using descriptive words is a tool that helps us identify unique qualities about foods and explain what we like or dislike about something.

When you sit down for a meal or snack, take a moment to think about how it looks, how it smells, how it sounds, how it feels in your mouth, and how it tastes using your 5 senses.

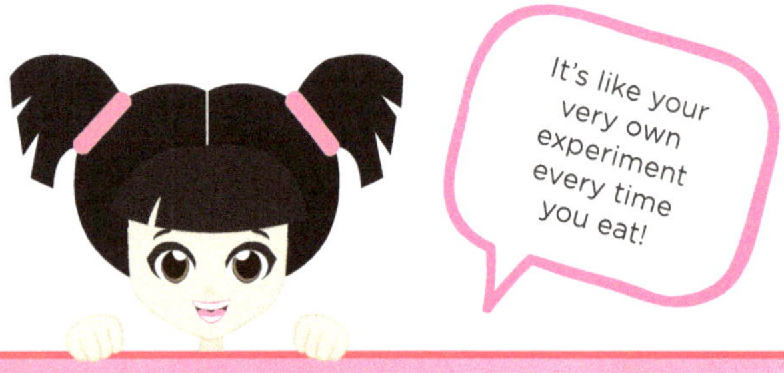

It's like your very own experiment every time you eat!

5 Senses

Can you describe broccoli? Each preparation method can change the experience. We can use our 5 senses to discover things we never knew we liked about a food!

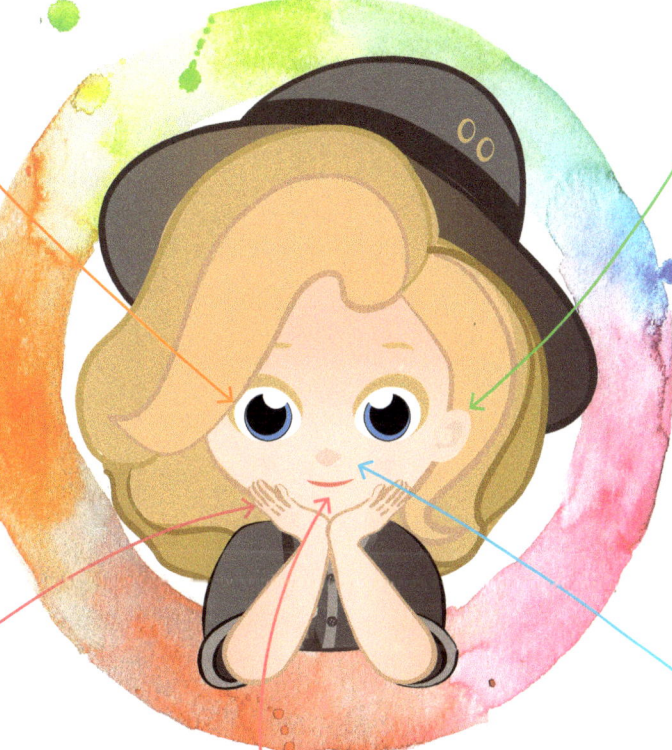

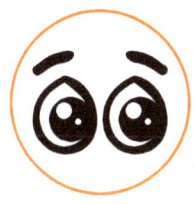

See

Let's take a closer look at broccoli! What colors and **textures** do you SEE? Does broccoli remind you of anything? A lot of people say that broccoli **florets** look like miniature trees. Do you agree? Can you see the **stem** and **leaves** of a tree?

Hear

What sound do you HEAR when you run your fingers over raw broccoli? Is it squeaky or silent? Now take a bite. Did you HEAR anything? Keep chewing. Are there any sounds? Is each bite a loud crunch or a quiet chew?

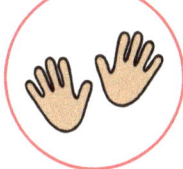

Feel

How does broccoli FEEL in your hands? Is the texture bumpy, smooth, or both? What about when you take a bite? What does the texture FEEL like? Is it crisp or tender? Does it make a hard snap each time you chew or is each bite soft and tender? Try this with raw broccoli and cooked broccoli!

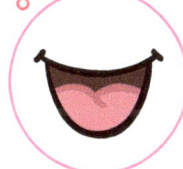

Taste

How does broccoli TASTE? What is the flavor? Can you describe it? Is it bitter or mustardy? Does it have a flavor at all? Does it TASTE different when it is raw than when it is cooked? Which do you like better and why?

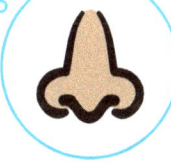

Smell

Have you ever sniffed broccoli!? That might sound silly, but SMELLING food is a big part of tasting! Hold a piece of broccoli up to your nose and take a good whiff. What does broccoli SMELL like? Does it SMELL like rotten eggs? Does it have a scent at all?

My 5 Senses

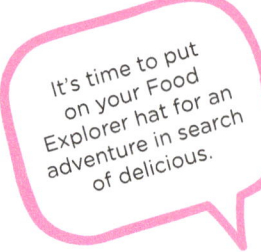
It's time to put on your Food Explorer hat for an adventure in search of delicious.

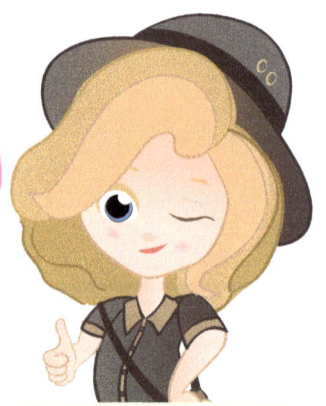

Pick a vegetable and use your senses to experience it!

Notice the colors and shapes of the vegetable. Feel the vegetable in your fingers and listen for any sounds. Lift the vegetable to your nose and give it a smell. Now take a bite. How does it taste? What does the **texture** feel like in your mouth? Does it make funny sounds when you chew it? How was it **prepared**? Was it raw, steamed, or roasted?

Download the "My 5 Senses Worksheet" for FREE on our website.

www.experiencedeliciousnow.com

Fill out the worksheet for each vegetable and the different ways you experience them. Write down as many descriptive words as you can! Use the Descriptive Words table on pages 158-159 to help you!

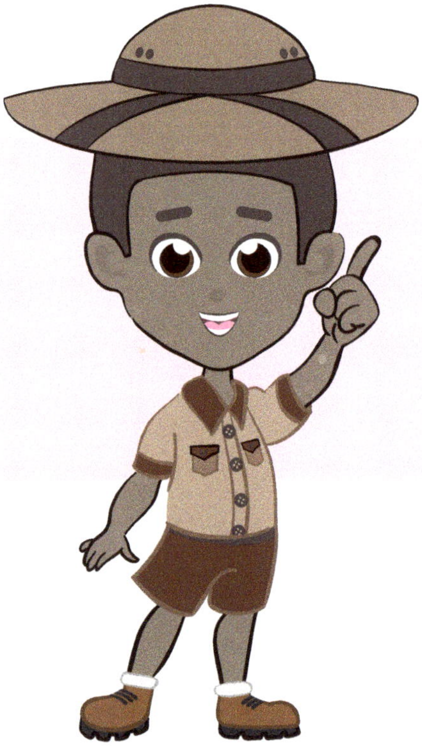

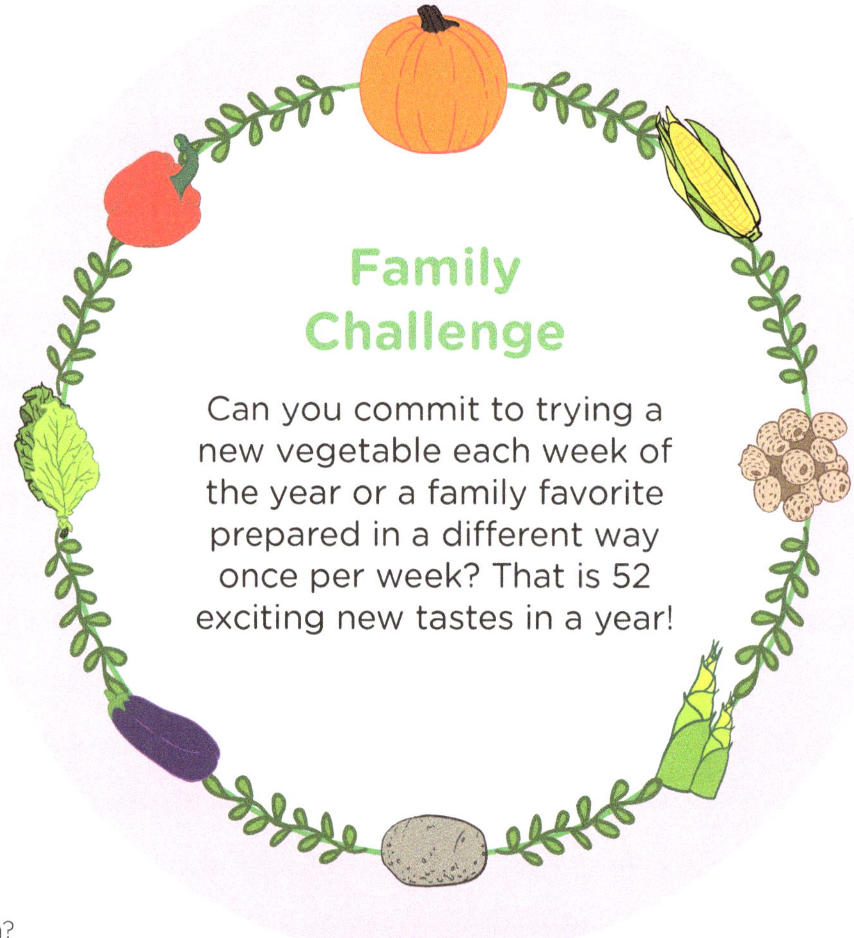

Family Challenge

Can you commit to trying a new vegetable each week of the year or a family favorite prepared in a different way once per week? That is 52 exciting new tastes in a year!

| Where Does Broccoli Come From?

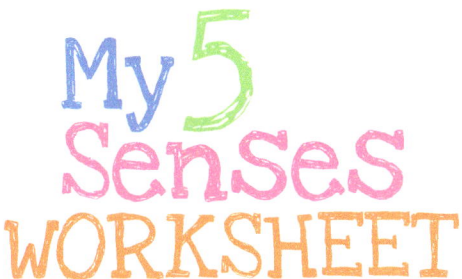
My 5 Senses WORKSHEET

Veggie Name _____

Preparation Method _____

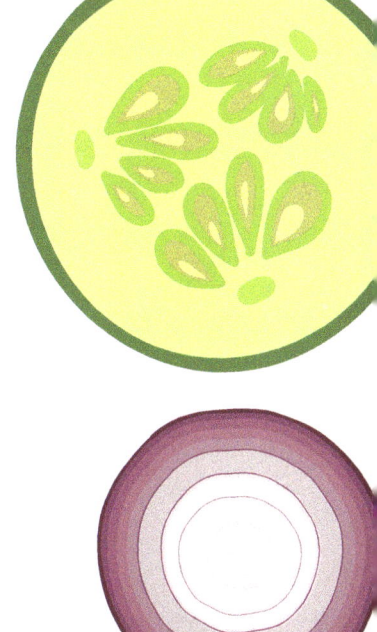
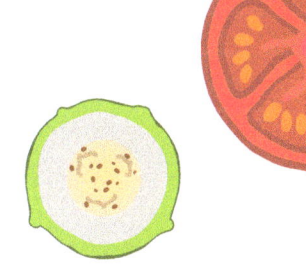
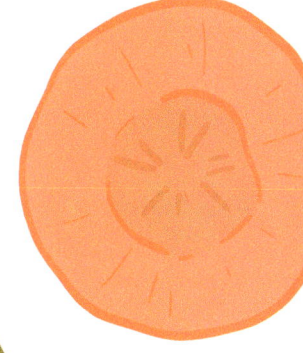

Did you like this vegetable?

  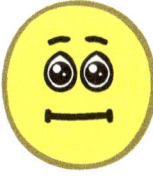   

Cooking Methods

There are so many wonderful and delicious ways to **prepare** vegetables! In this book you will see **symbols** that give you ideas for how to try a new vegetable. Below are a few explanations of common cooking methods to get you started.

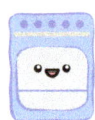
Bake or Roast
Cook with dry heat typically in an oven.

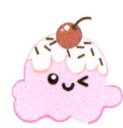
Dessert
Sweet foods such as cakes, cookies, ice cream, pies, and pudding. Desserts are typically served at the end of a meal.

Boil, Blanch, or Simmer
To boil vegetables, cook with hot water at boiling point, which is when the surface of the water has big active bubbles. Blanching vegetables involves briefly dipping them in water at boiling point. To simmer vegetables, cook with water that is gently bubbling below the boiling point.

Garnish
A food that is meant to be eaten as a topping or as an addition to other foods. Garnishes add flavor, texture, or decoration.

Dip, Dressing, or Sauce
Foods prepared to be eaten as a topping or as an addition to other foods. They are available in many consistencies or **textures** from liquid, to semi-liquid, to thick, to chunky.

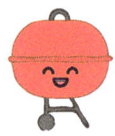
Grill or Barbeque
Cook foods with direct, dry heat from fire on a grated surface with thin, parallel, metal bars.

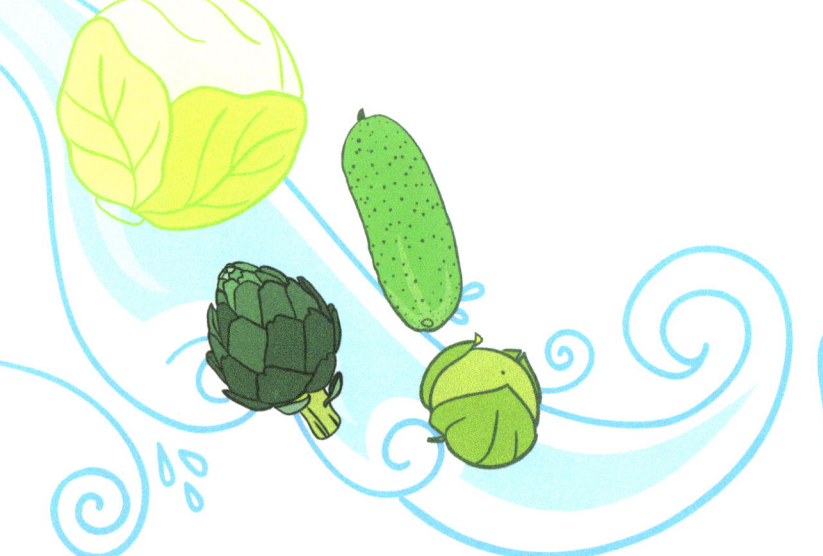

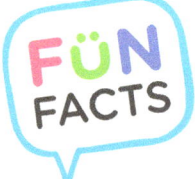

Clean all veggies under cool, running water before eating them. This prevents harmful bacteria on the outside from getting on the inside of the vegetable. Harmful bacteria can come from your hands, knives, or other surfaces they come in contact with and make you sick!

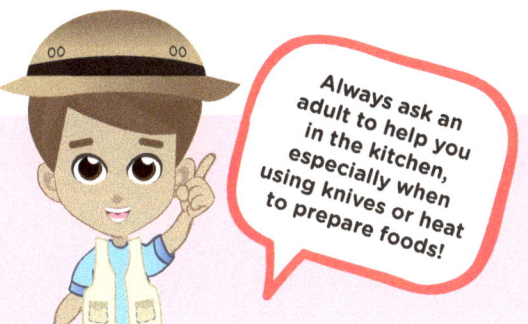

Always ask an adult to help you in the kitchen, especially when using knives or heat to prepare foods!

Temperature is a measurement that indicates how hot or cold something is and can be measured using a thermometer in degrees **Fahrenheit** or degrees **Celsius**. Fahrenheit is labeled as degrees F in this book.

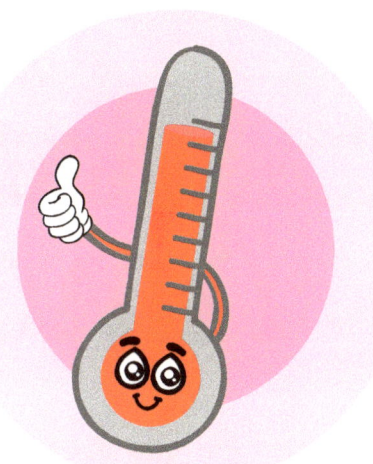

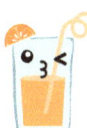
Juice or Smoothie
A preparation method of **fruits** and vegetables that transforms them into a liquid ready to drink. Juicing removes the liquid from a food and smoothies blend food into a liquid.

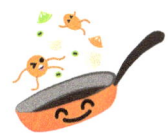
Sauté [saw-tey] or Stir-Fry
To sauté, heat food in a small amount of fat (e.g. butter or oil) in a pan or wok on top of a stove or heat source. Preparing stir-fry is similar to sautéing food; however, stir-frying is typically at a higher **temperature** and the food is consistently moved when being cooked.

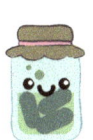
Pickle or Ferment [fur-ment]
Food storage and preparation methods that may include vinegar, **brine**, or helpful **bacteria**, also known as **probiotics**. Helpful bacteria support **digestion** and fight harmful bacteria.

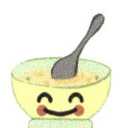
Soup or Stew [stoo]
A preparation method when liquids are boiled or simmered with ingredients such as meats, beans, and vegetables. Stews typically have less liquid than soups and are a thicker texture.

Raw
Raw food is when something is eaten in its natural, uncooked form.

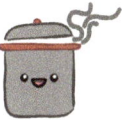
Steam [steem]
Cook foods with moist heat in the form of water. Steam is created when water is boiled and creates a **gas**.

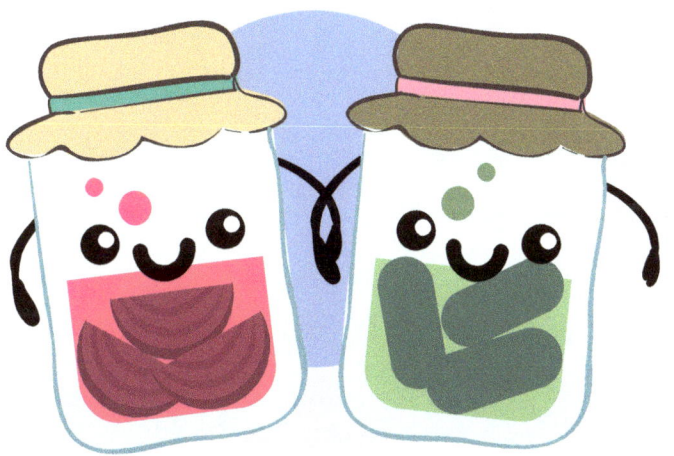

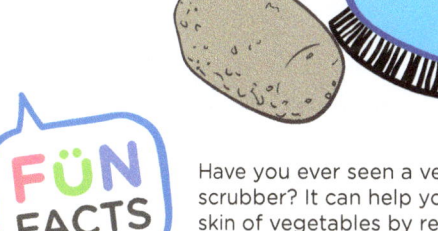

FUN FACTS

Have you ever seen a vegetable scrubber? It can help you clean the skin of vegetables by removing dirt and sand.

North America

Have you ever wondered where people first discovered the veggies you eat? These maps of the world will show you where early Food Explorers are thought to have originally tasted the veggies in this book!

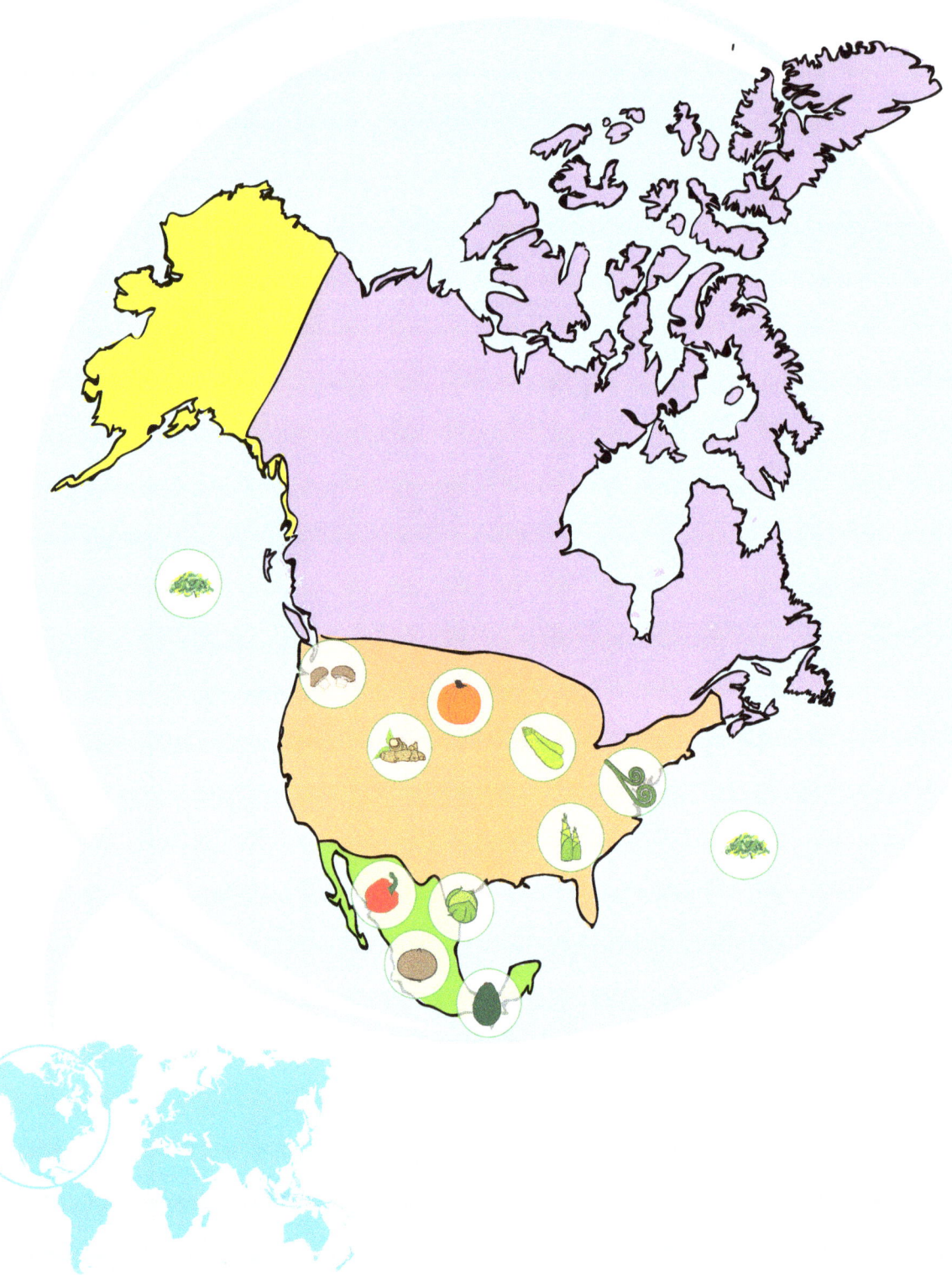

30 | Where Does Broccoli Come From?

South America

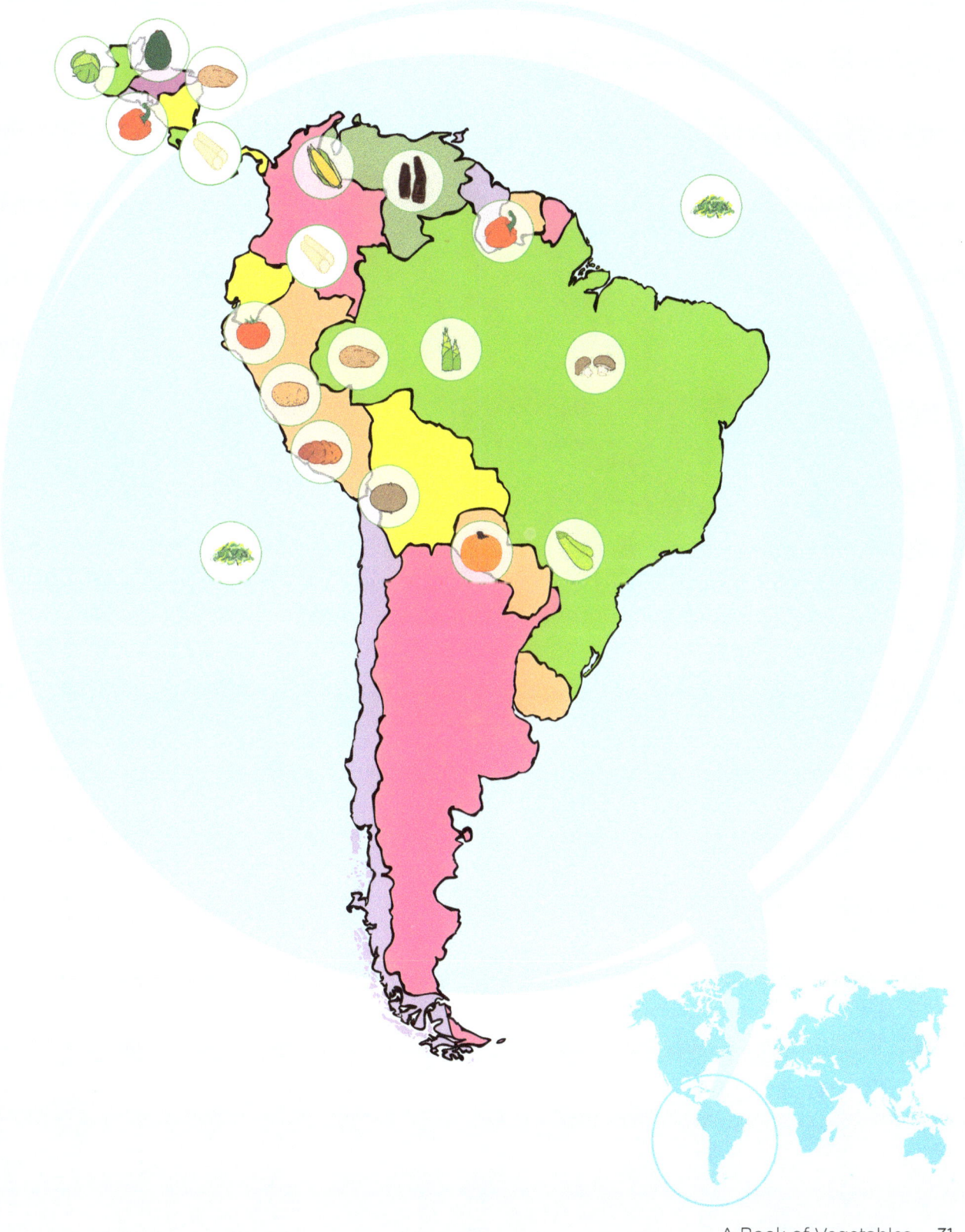

A Book of Vegetables

Asia

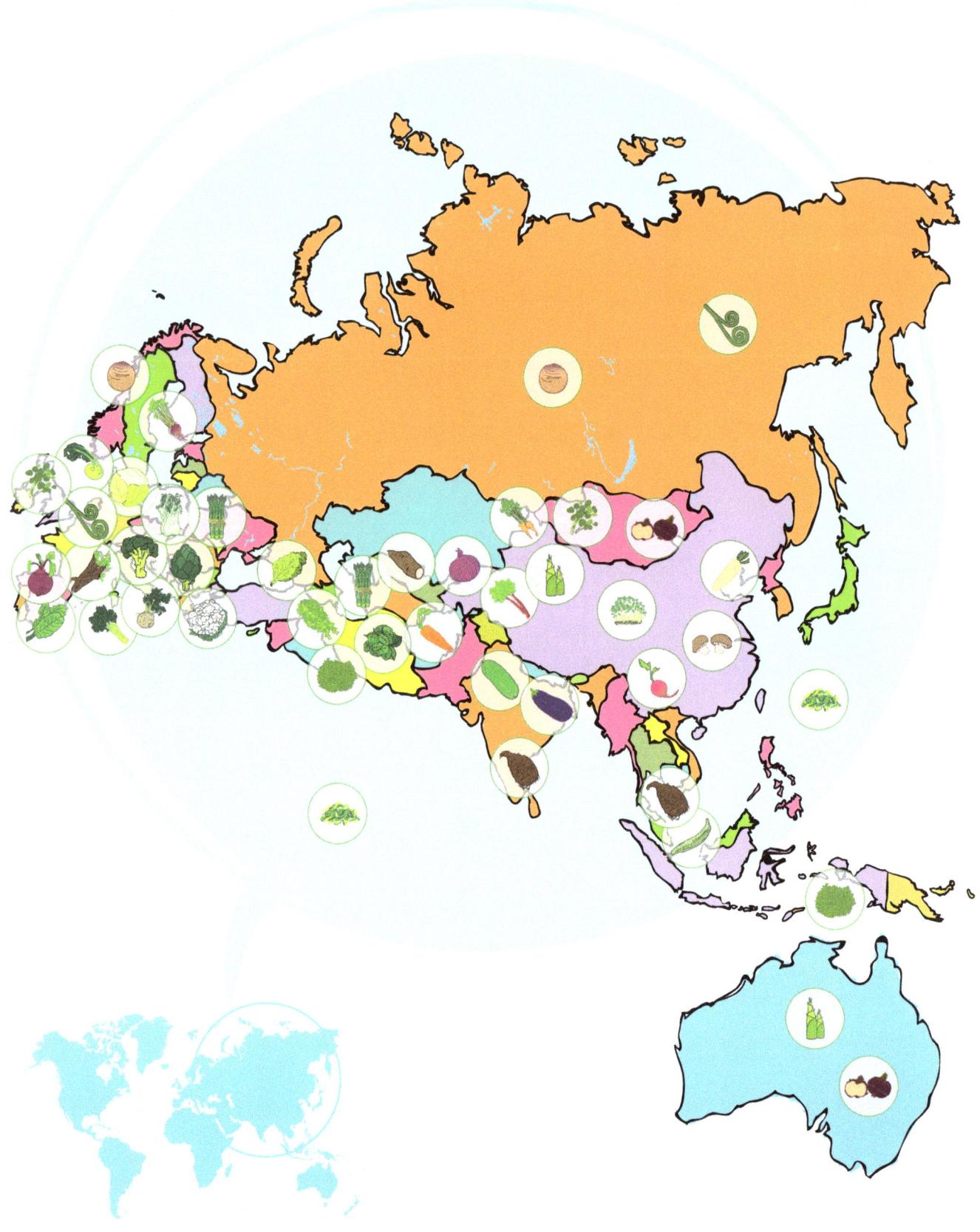

32 | Where Does Broccoli Come From?

Africa

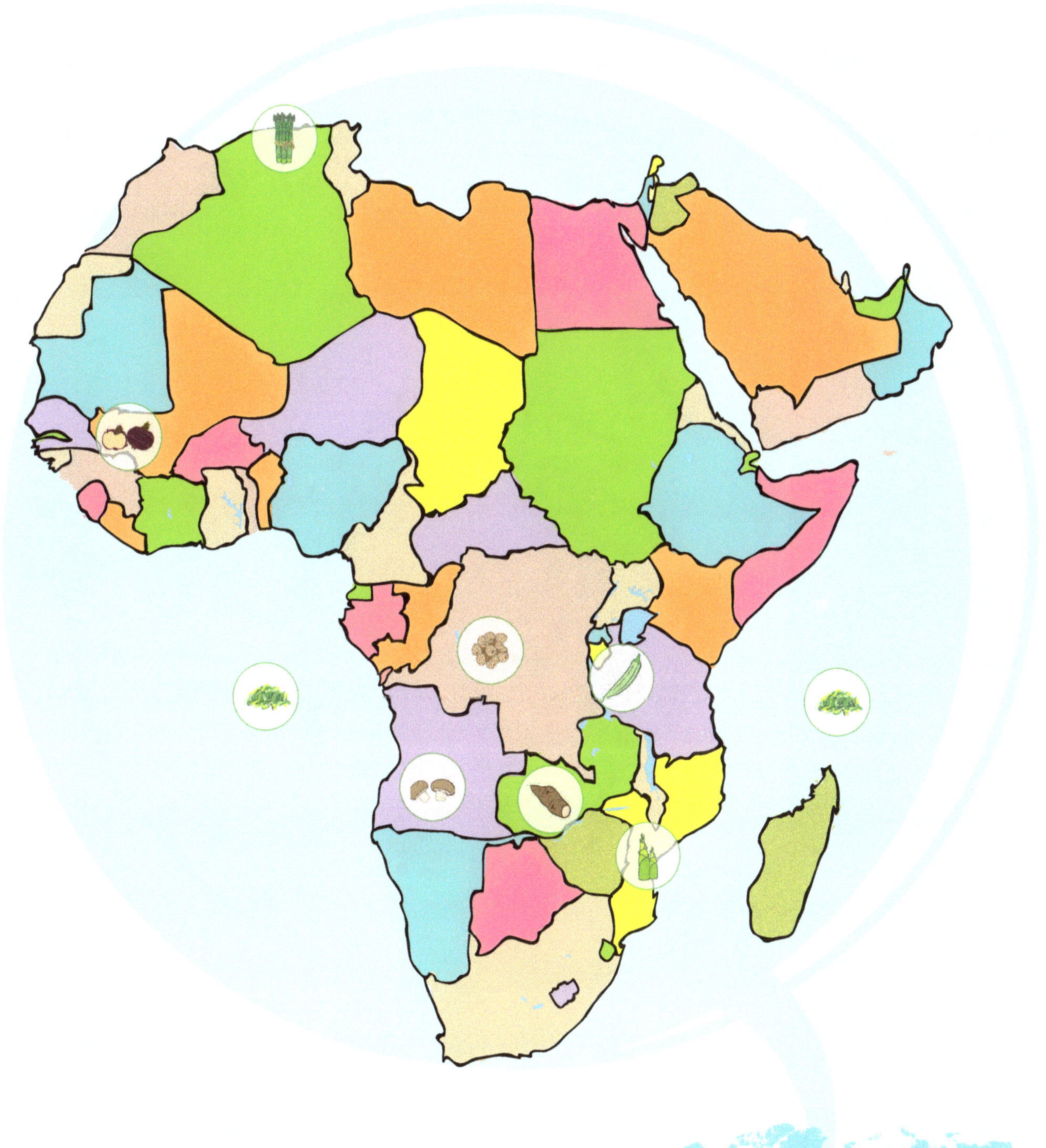

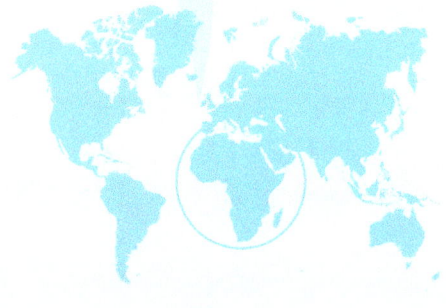

A Book of Vegetables 33

ARTICHOKE

[ar-ti-choke]

earthy, nutty, sweet, tender, velvety

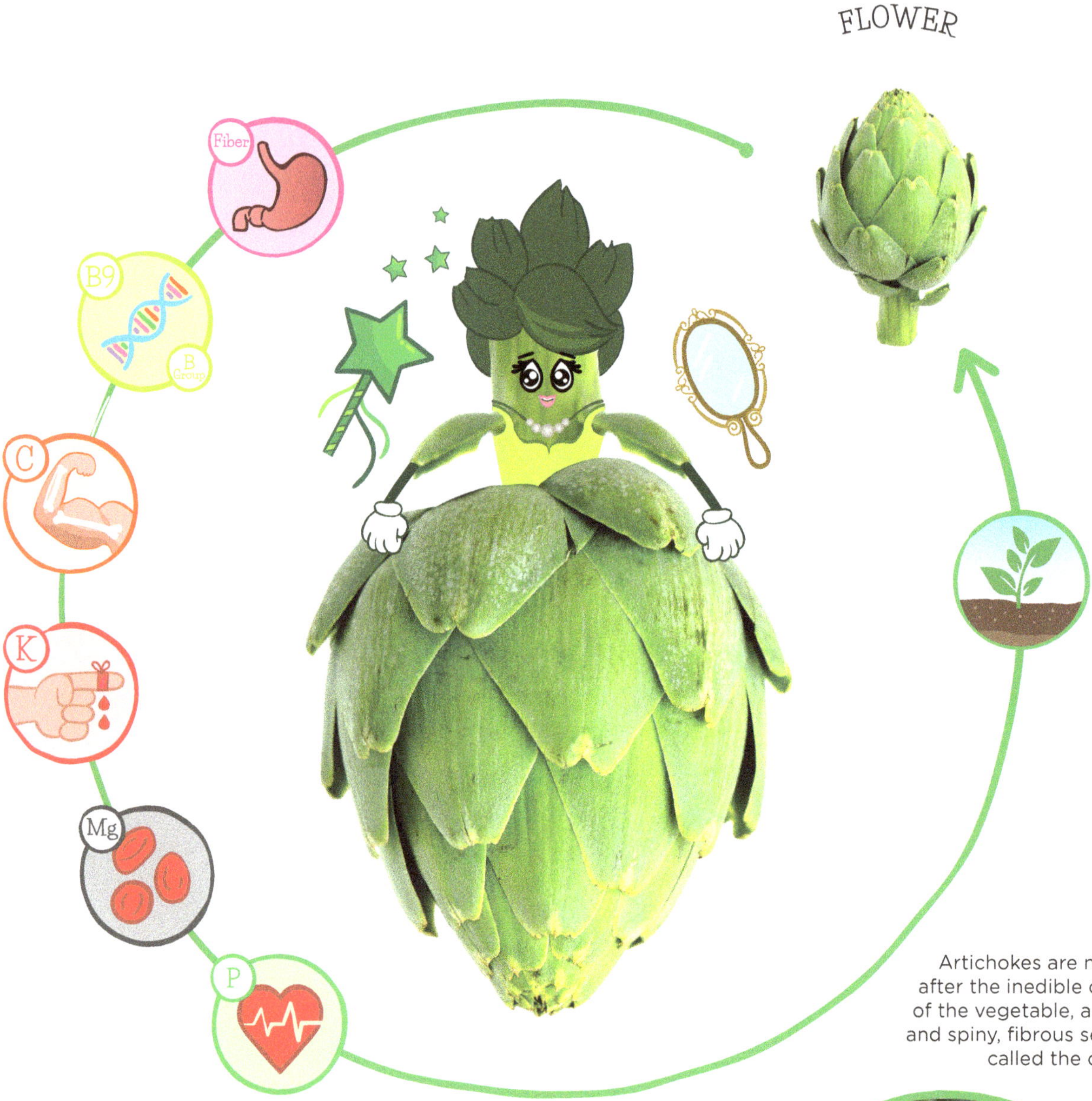

FLOWER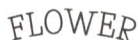

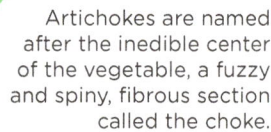

Artichokes are named after the inedible center of the vegetable, a fuzzy and spiny, fibrous section called the choke.

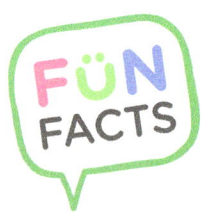 A sip of water may taste sweet after eating an artichoke because of a natural acid that coats your mouth called **cynarin**. Try a bite of an artichoke and take a sip of water. Does it taste sweet?

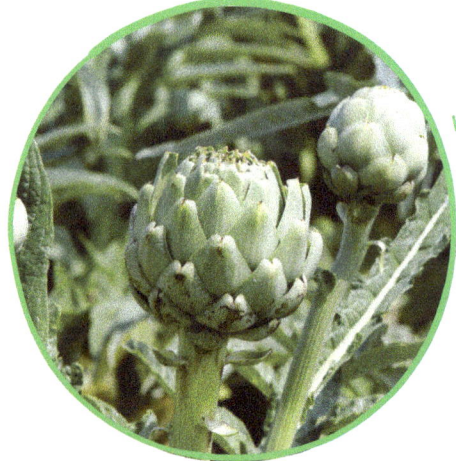

Where Does Broccoli Come From?

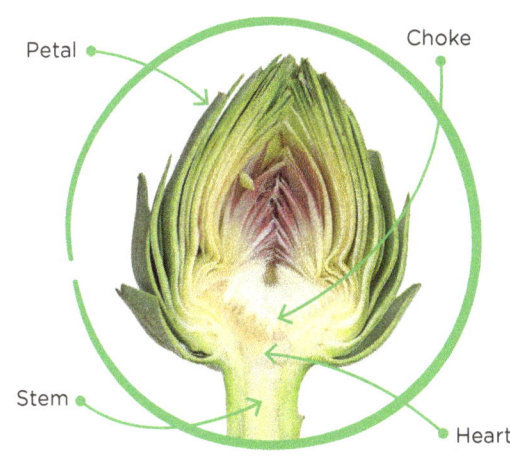

Petal · Choke · Stem · Heart

PICK
Pick dark green, crisp **flowers** with closed petals. Petals should just start to open and squeak when squeezed. Artichoke should be firm and feel heavy for their size.

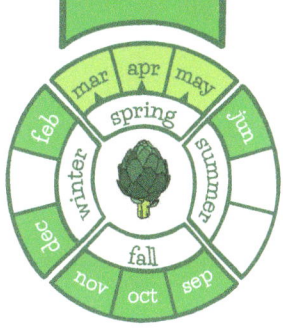

February to June; September to December; Imported year-round

Peak Season
March-May

STORE
Refrigerate raw artichoke in an open plastic bag for up to 7 days. Refrigerate cooked artichoke in an airtight container for 3-5 days.

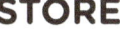

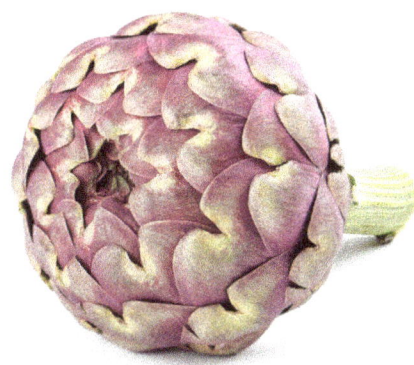

CUTTING ARTICHOKE

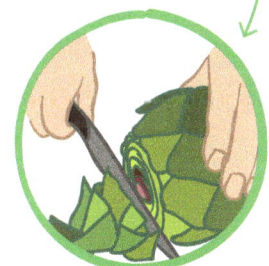

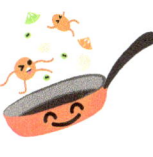

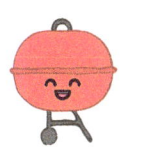

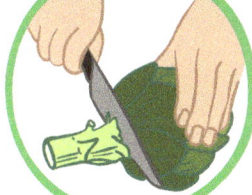

EAT
Clean the skin, slice about 1 inch off the top of the artichoke petals and slice the **stem** to be 3/4 inches long or slice off the entire stem. Spread open the petals, season, and cook.

Steamed Artichoke
Steam artichoke with the stem side up for 20-30 minutes. Artichokes are ready to eat when the petals near the center pull out easily. To eat, pull off the outer petals, dip the base of the petal in your favorite sauce such as butter, and scrape the soft **flesh** with your bottom teeth. Don't forget a bowl to throw away the petals! Once all the petals have been removed, use a spoon to scoop out the fuzzy choke and enjoy the base known as the heart!

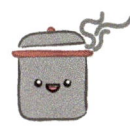

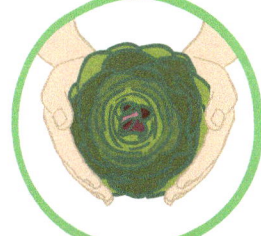

A Book of Vegetables 35

ASPARAGUS

[uh-spar-uh-guhs]

bitter, earthy, mild, sweet, tender

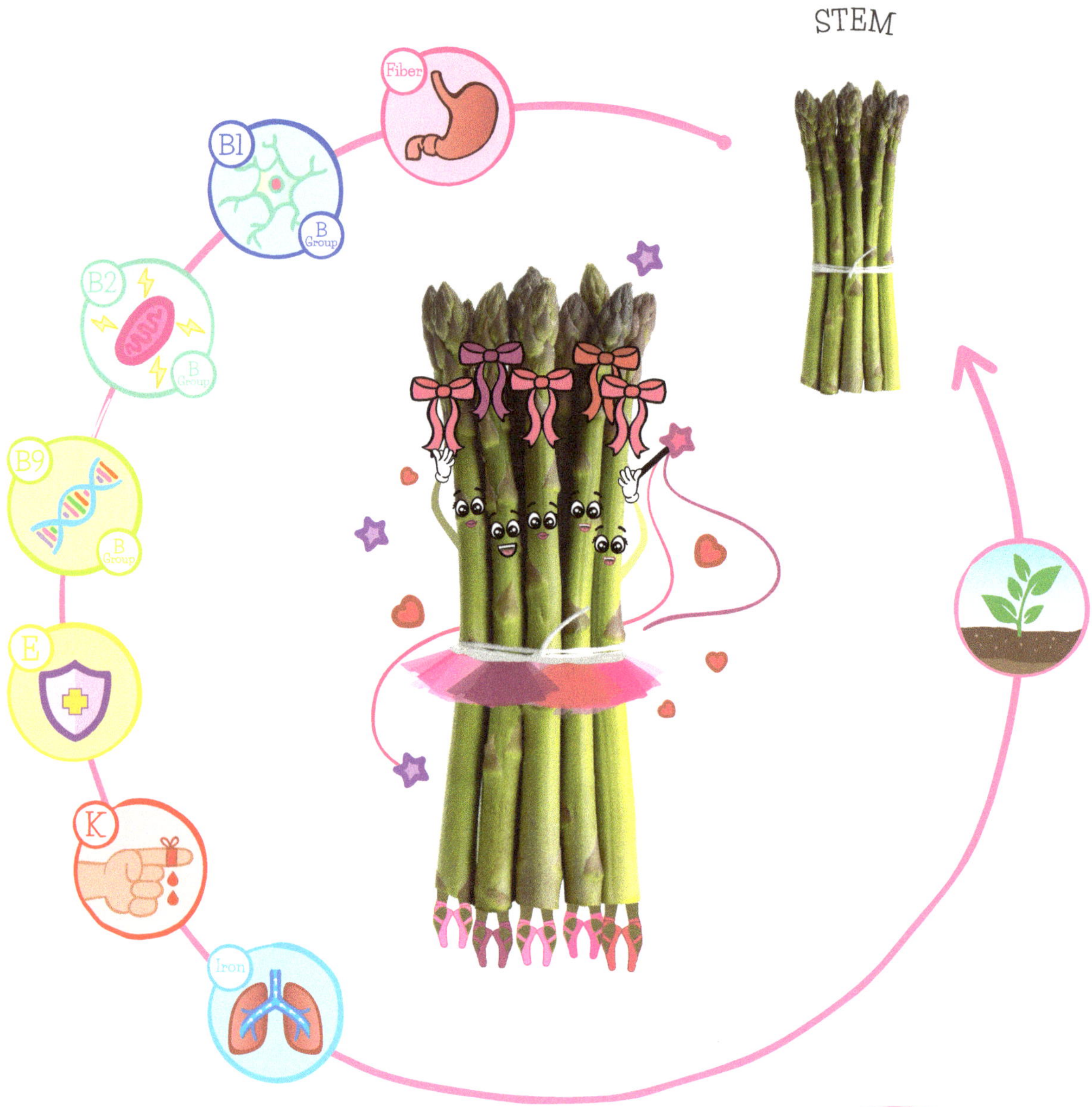

STEM

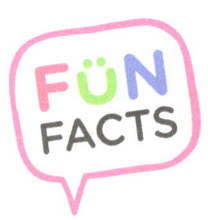
FUN FACTS

Asparagus changes the smell of your urine after you eat it because of a natural acid called **asparagusic acid**. Have you noticed a stinky smell when you pee after eating asparagus?

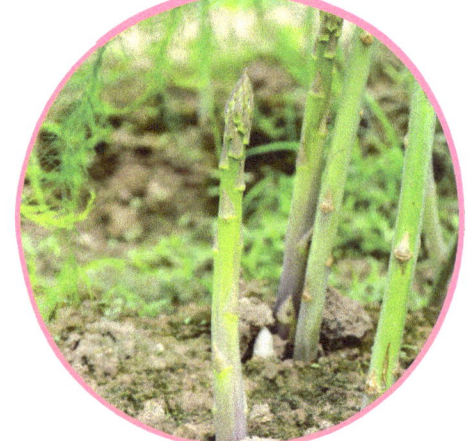

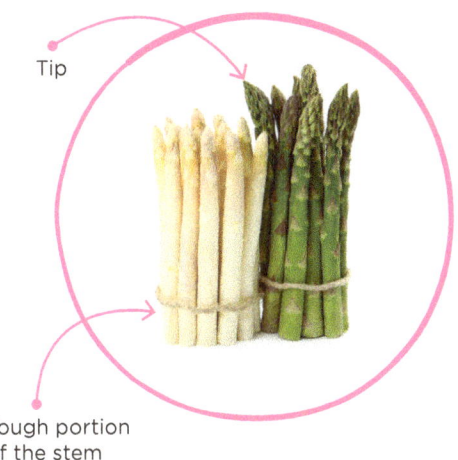

Tip

Tough portion of the stem

PICK
Pick green, purple, or white **stems** that are **uniform** in color and length. Asparagus should be smooth, firm, and have tightly closed tips. Avoid weak, rubbery, dull-colored, and dry stems or spears.

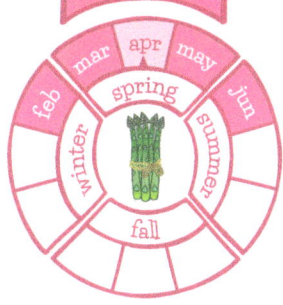

Available February to June; Imported year-round

Peak Season
April

STORE
Refrigerate raw asparagus in a jar with the stem end in 1-2 centimeters of water or wrap the stem end in a moist paper towel in an open plastic bag for up to 4 days. Refrigerate cooked asparagus in an airtight container for up to 5 days.

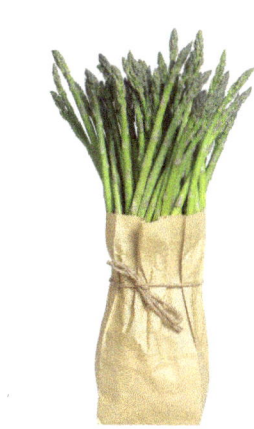

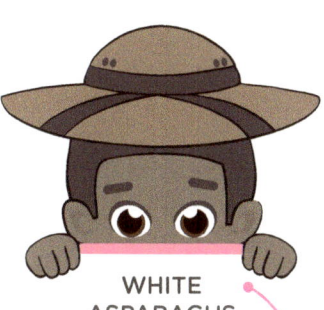

WHITE ASPARAGUS

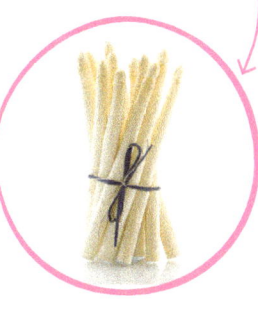

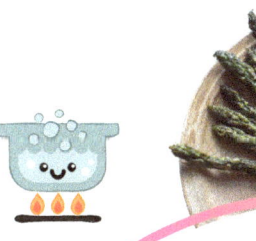

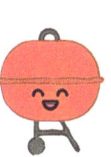

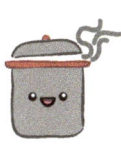

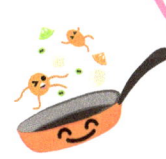

EAT
Clean the skin, slice or snap off the tough stem end, season, and cook.

Roasted Asparagus
Preheat your oven to 425 degrees F. Place asparagus on a foil-lined roasting tray, **drizzle** with olive oil and roast for about 10 minutes until asparagus are slightly tender.

White asparagus spears get their color, or absence of color, because they are grown underground. Farmers cover the spears with soil and dark plastic so the green coloring in plants known as **chlorophyll**, cannot form. White asparagus is more tender and delicate in flavor and must be peeled because the skin is thick and bitter.

A Book of Vegetables

AVOCADO

[av-o-ca-do]

buttery, creamy, floral, grassy, nutty

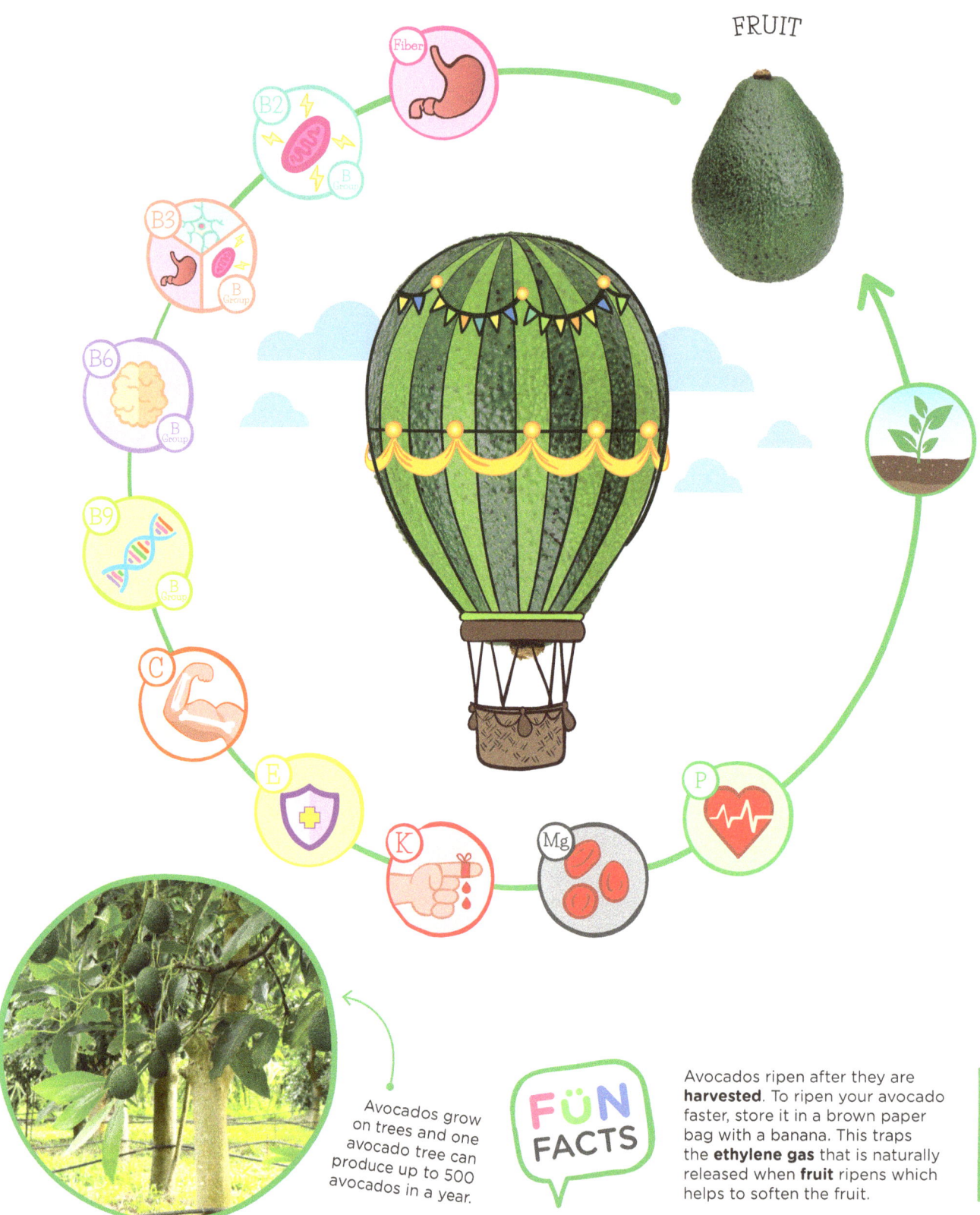

FRUIT

Avocados grow on trees and one avocado tree can produce up to 500 avocados in a year.

FUN FACTS

Avocados ripen after they are **harvested**. To ripen your avocado faster, store it in a brown paper bag with a banana. This traps the **ethylene gas** that is naturally released when **fruit** ripens which helps to soften the fruit.

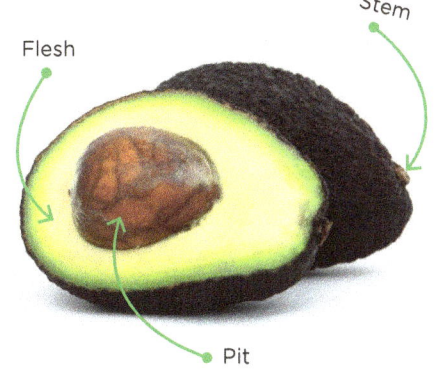
Flesh · Stem · Pit

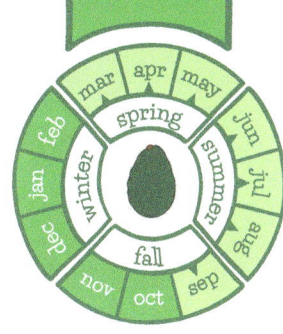

Varieties available year-round

Peak Season
March-September

PICK
Pick dark green to deep purple-black **fruit** that are soft to touch. Avoid avocados with **bruises** or mushy spots.

STORE
Keep avocado at room **temperature** on the countertop until **ripe**. Ripe avocado can be stored in the refrigerator for 2-3 days. To keep sliced avocado from browning, squeeze lemon or lime juice on slices before storing in the refrigerator.

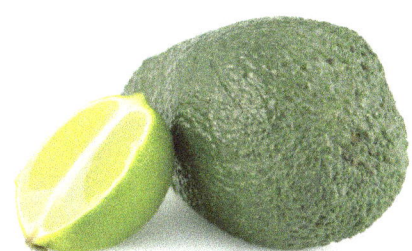

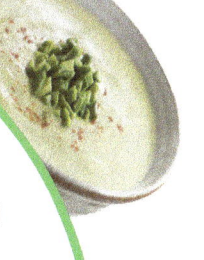

CUTTING AVOCADO

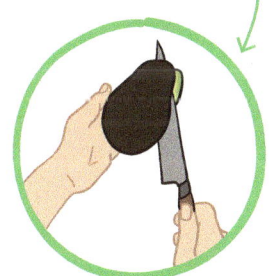
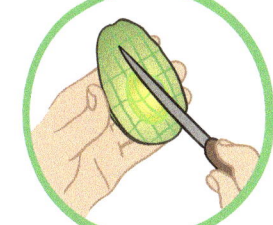
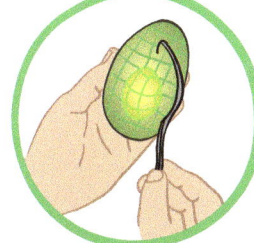

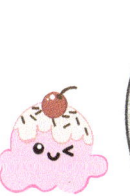
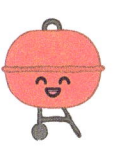

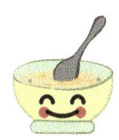

EAT
Clean the skin and slice the avocado **stem** to stem (hot dog style), tracing your knife around the pit. Twist the two sides apart, remove the pit, and slice the flesh gently without cutting through the skin. Scoop out the fruit with a spoon.

Cold Avocado Soup
Sauté 1 chopped white onion with 4 minced garlic cloves in olive oil over medium heat for about 10 minutes until they are **translucent**. Then, transfer to a blender and combine with 3 cups of water, 2 peeled and pitted avocados, 1/2 cup cilantro, and 2 tablespoons of lime juice. While blending, add 2 ounces of olive oil and season with salt and pepper. Chill in the refrigerator for at least an hour, then serve with a cilantro garnish.

A Book of Vegetables

BAMBOO SHOOT

[bam-boo shoot]

crisp, distinctive, mild, sweet, tender

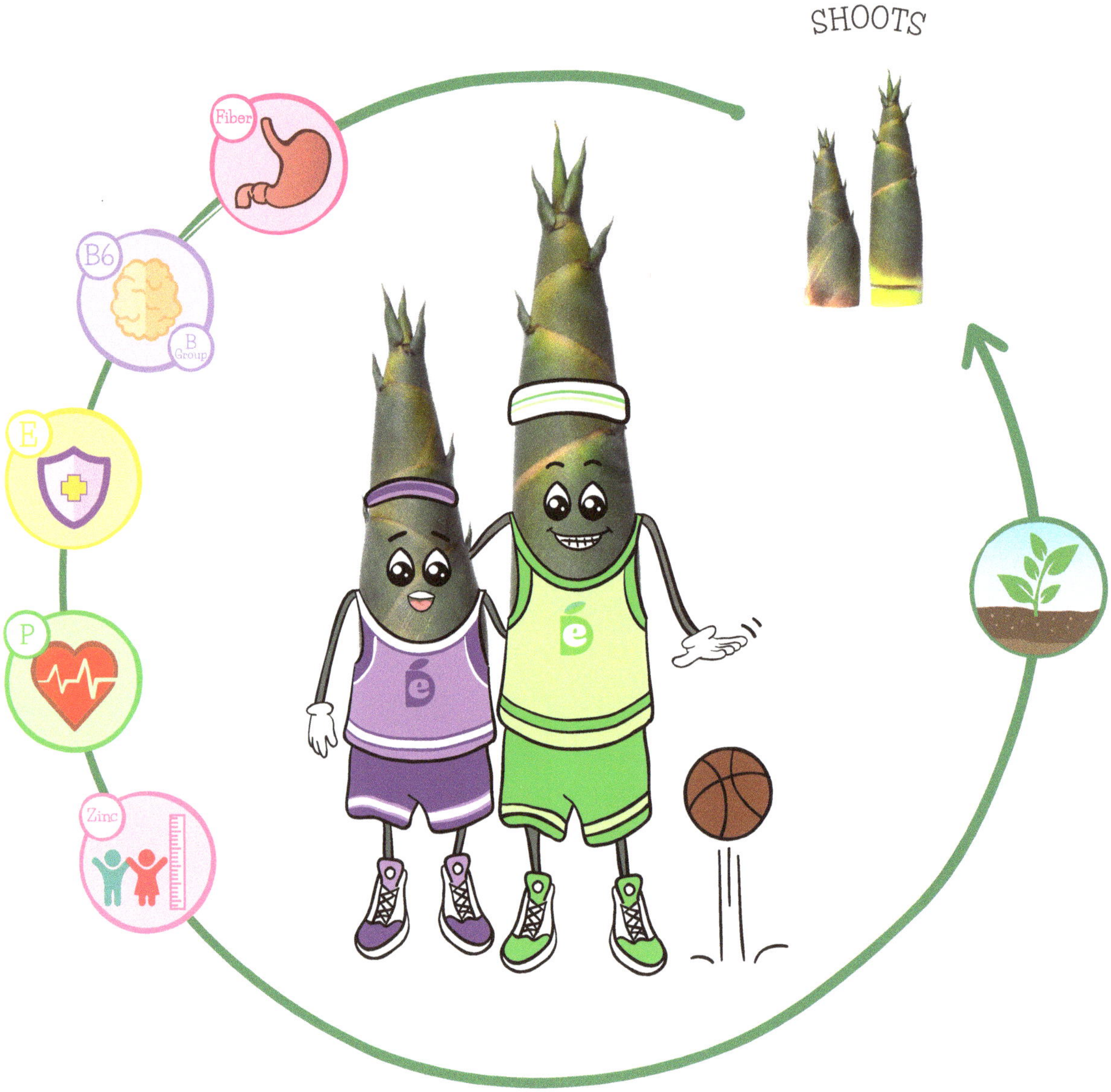

SHOOTS

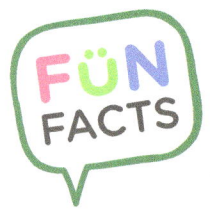

Bamboo shoots can grow up to 1 foot in 24 hours! Young, small shoots can be eaten raw, but large shoots tend to be bitter and need to be cooked.

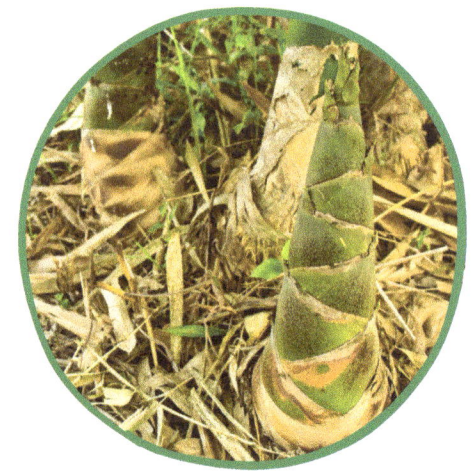

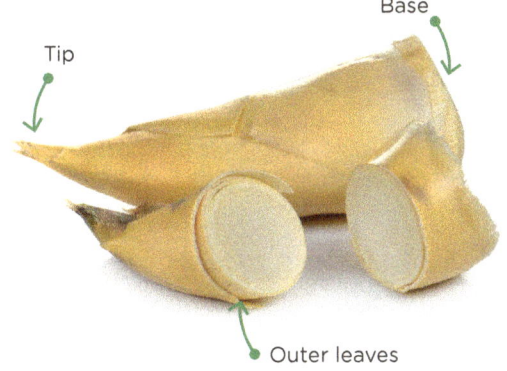

Tip · Base · Outer leaves

PICK
Pick creamy, white **shoots** that are small with a wide base that feel firm. Avoid bamboo shoots with soft, dry, or greenish color **roots**.

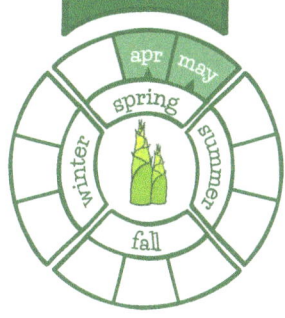

Available April to May; Imported year-round

Peak Season
April-May

STORE
Refrigerate unpeeled, raw shoots in a plastic bag for up to 7 days.

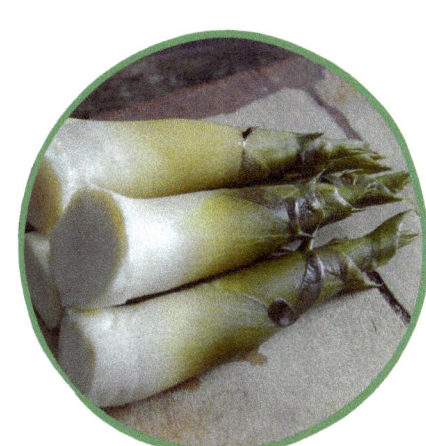

EAT
Clean the skin, slice off the tough portion at the base, slice the shoot in half lengthwise (hot dog style), and peel the tough outer leaves from the base of the shoot towards the tip. Chop or slice per recipe.

Blanched Bamboo Shoots
Blanch bamboo shoots to remove bitterness and then boil them in salted water for about 20 minutes until shoots are tender and can be easily **pierced** with a fork. If shoots are still bitter, boil them in fresh salted water for another 5-10 minutes and repeat the process until there is no more bitterness. Add to salads, stir-fry, or as a side dish with soy sauce and butter.

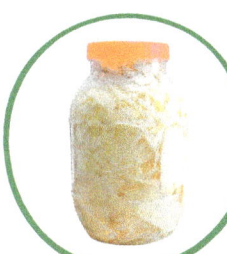

PICKLED BAMBOO SHOOTS

Bamboo shoots are typically sold canned, jarred, vacuumed sealed, or dried in the United States because the **harvest** season is very short and there is a limited need for fresh shoots.

A Book of Vegetables   41

BEET AND GREENS

[beat]

buttery, earthy, meaty, sweet, velvety

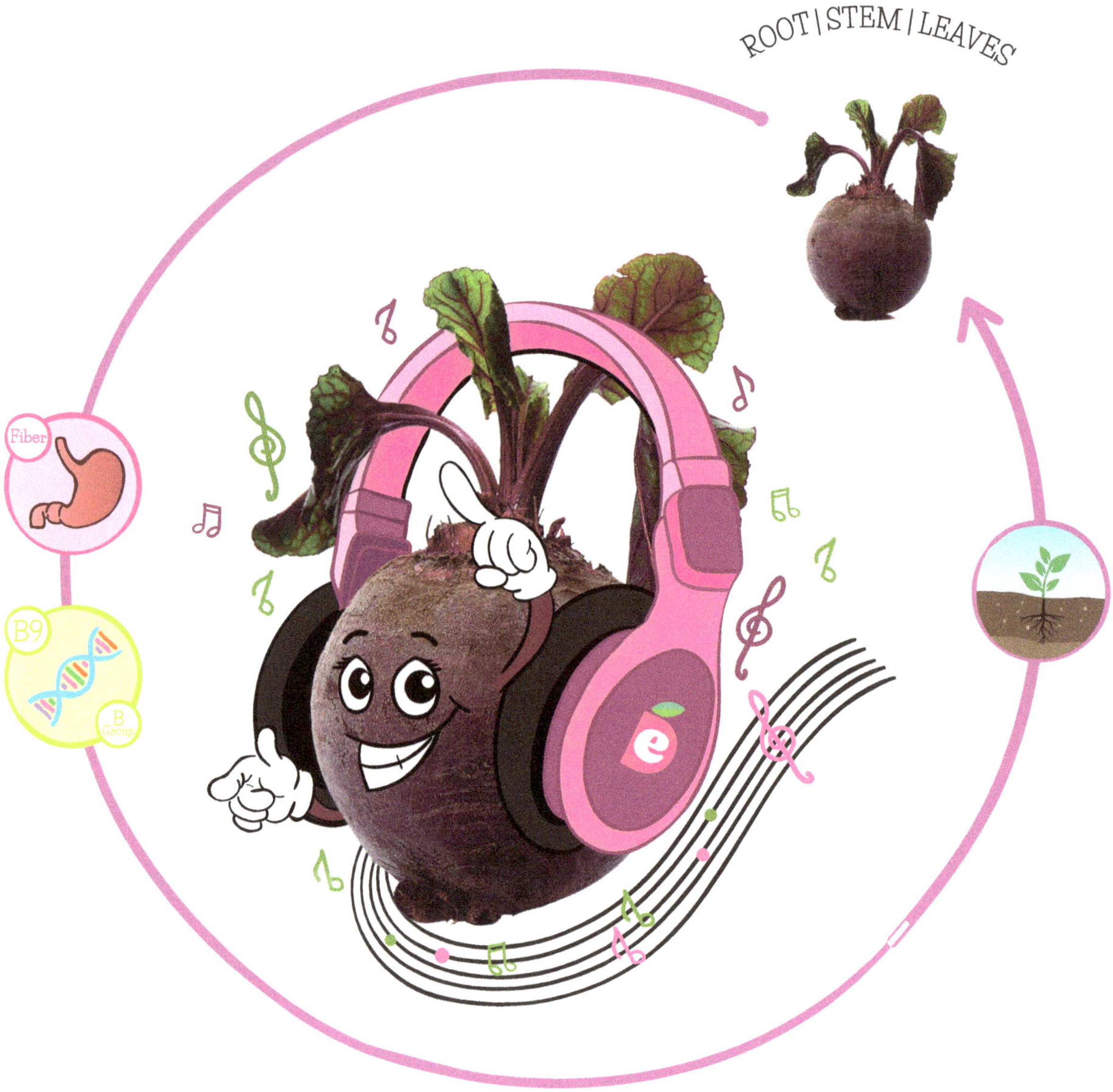

ROOT | STEM | LEAVES

FUN FACTS

Beets are known for their powerful red **pigment** or color which **stains** everything, including your hands! If your hands get stained, try scrubbing them with salt.

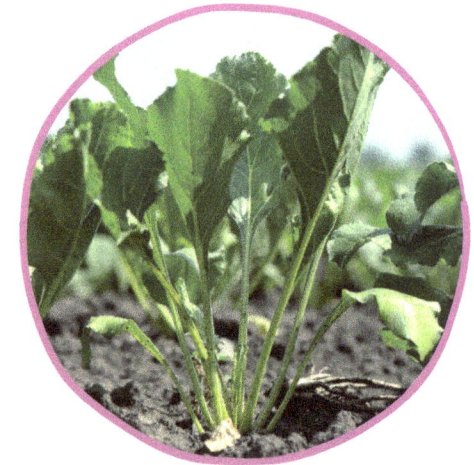

42 | Where Does Broccoli Come From?

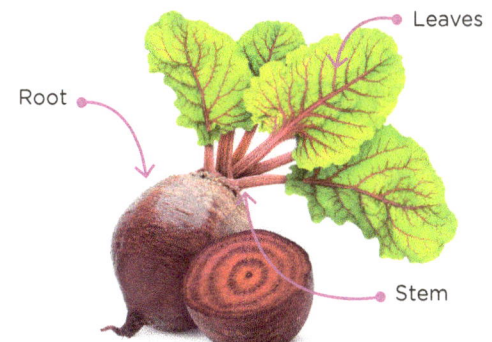

Root · Leaves · Stem

PICK
Pick small to medium **roots** with firm, smooth skin that feel heavy for their size. Avoid beets with cuts and mushy spots. Attached greens should be bright green and crisp. Colors and shapes are different depending on **variety**.

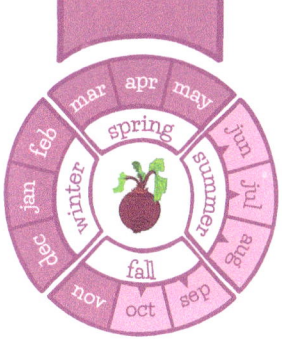

Varieties available year-round

Peak Season
June-October

STORE
Refrigerate raw beet in a moist paper towel in an open plastic bag for up to 2 weeks and cooked beet in an air tight container for 3-5 days. Raw beet greens should be refrigerated separately in an airtight container for 2-3 days.

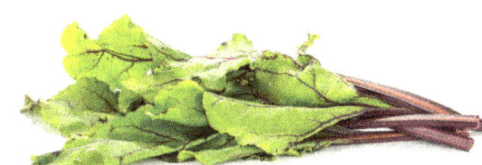

BEET VARIETIES

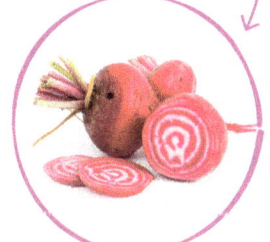

Chioggia Beet

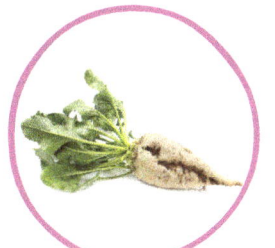

Sugar Beet

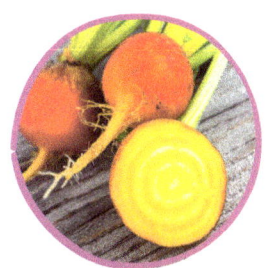

Golden Beet

EAT
Clean the skin with a vegetable brush and slice the greens off about 1 inch from the root.

Roasted Beets
Preheat your oven to 400 degrees F. Place beets on a foil-lined roasting tray, **drizzle** with olive oil, and roast for about 1 hour until roots are tender and can be easily **pierced** with a fork. Allow beets to cool, then peel off the tough outer skin, and chop or slice per recipe! Greens can be eaten raw or stir-fried!

A Book of Vegetables 43

BROCCOLI

[broc-co-lee]

bitter, bland, crisp, mild, mustardy

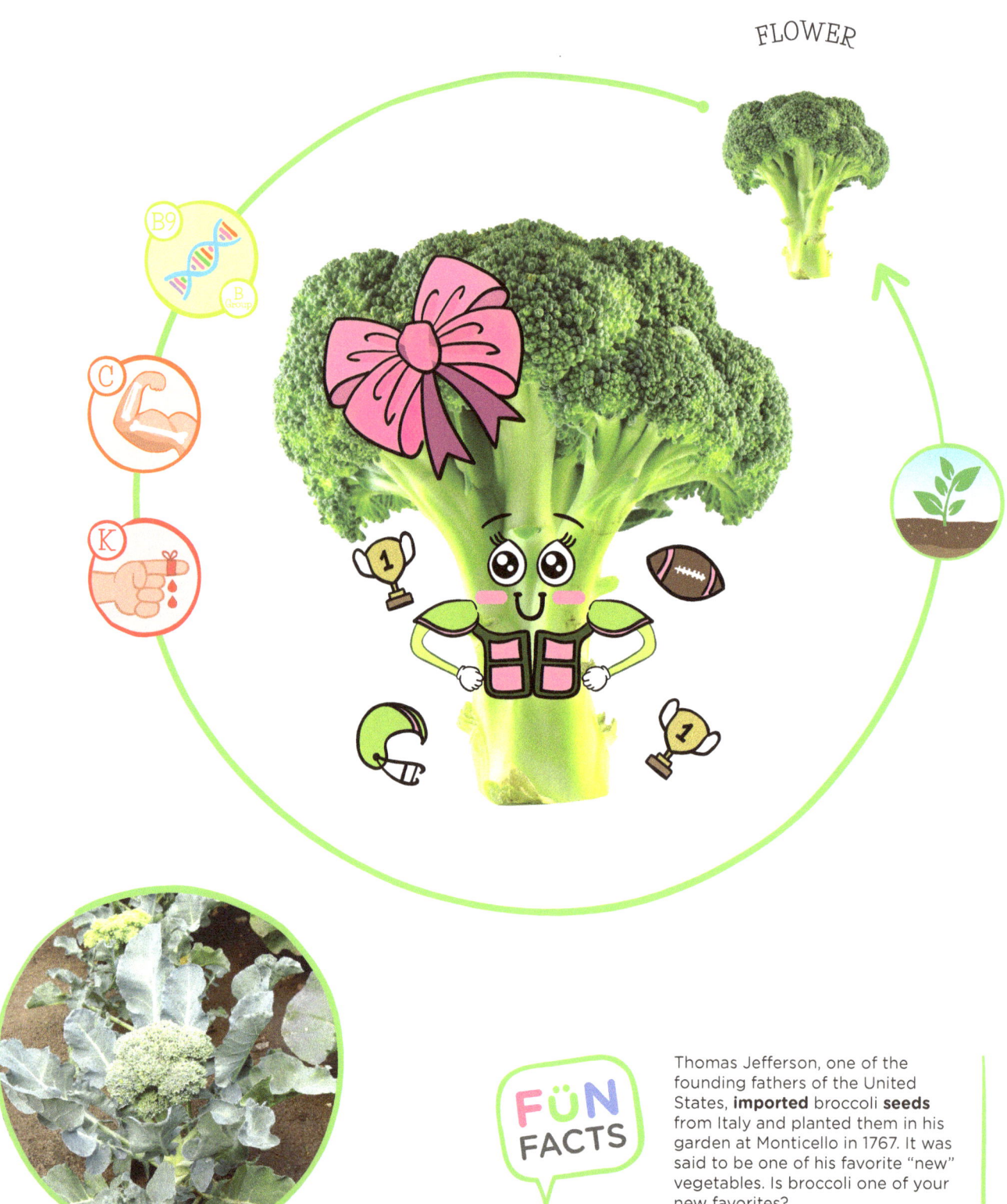

FLOWER

Fun Facts

Thomas Jefferson, one of the founding fathers of the United States, **imported** broccoli **seeds** from Italy and planted them in his garden at Monticello in 1767. It was said to be one of his favorite "new" vegetables. Is broccoli one of your new favorites?

Where Does Broccoli Come From?

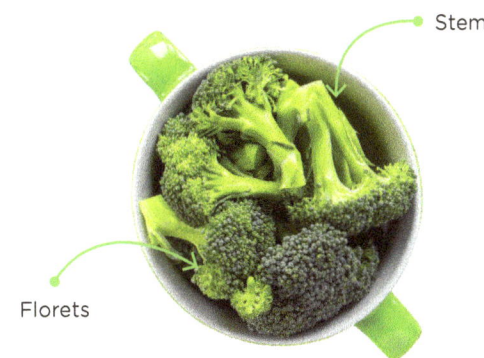

Stem

Florets

PICK
Pick dark green to bluish-green **florets** with firm, **compact buds**, and firm **stems** that feel heavy for their size. Avoid broccoli with open buds, yellowing in color, or soft **wilted** stems.

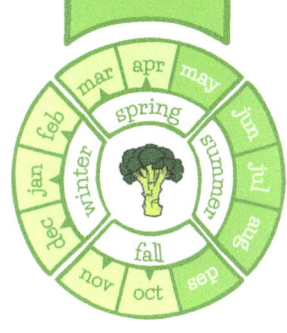

Varieties available year-round

Peak Season
October-April

STORE
Refrigerate unwashed, raw broccoli in an open plastic bag for up to 5 days. Refrigerate cooked broccoli in an airtight container for 3-5 days.

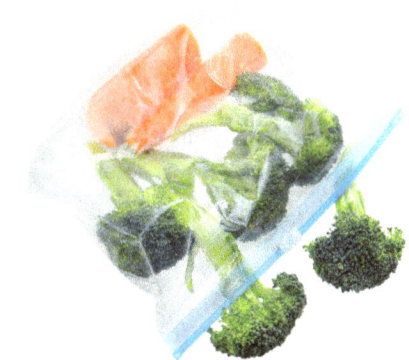

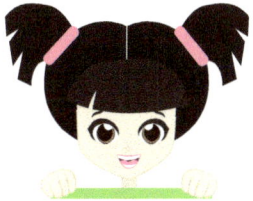

BROCCOLI TIDBITS

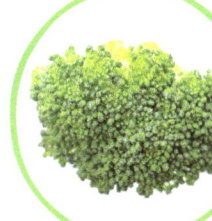

EAT
Clean the skin, cut the florets off the stem, and chop florets and stems into **uniform** sized pieces.

Steamed Broccoli
Steam florets and stems for 5-7 minutes. Broccoli is ready to eat when the pieces are tender.

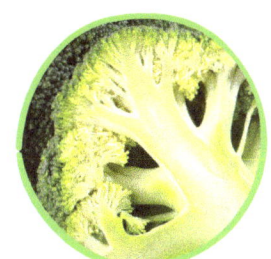

The part of the broccoli you eat are actually baby **flowers** that haven't opened yet!

A Book of Vegetables 45

CABBAGE

[cab-bage]

crunchy, earthy, peppery, sweet, tender

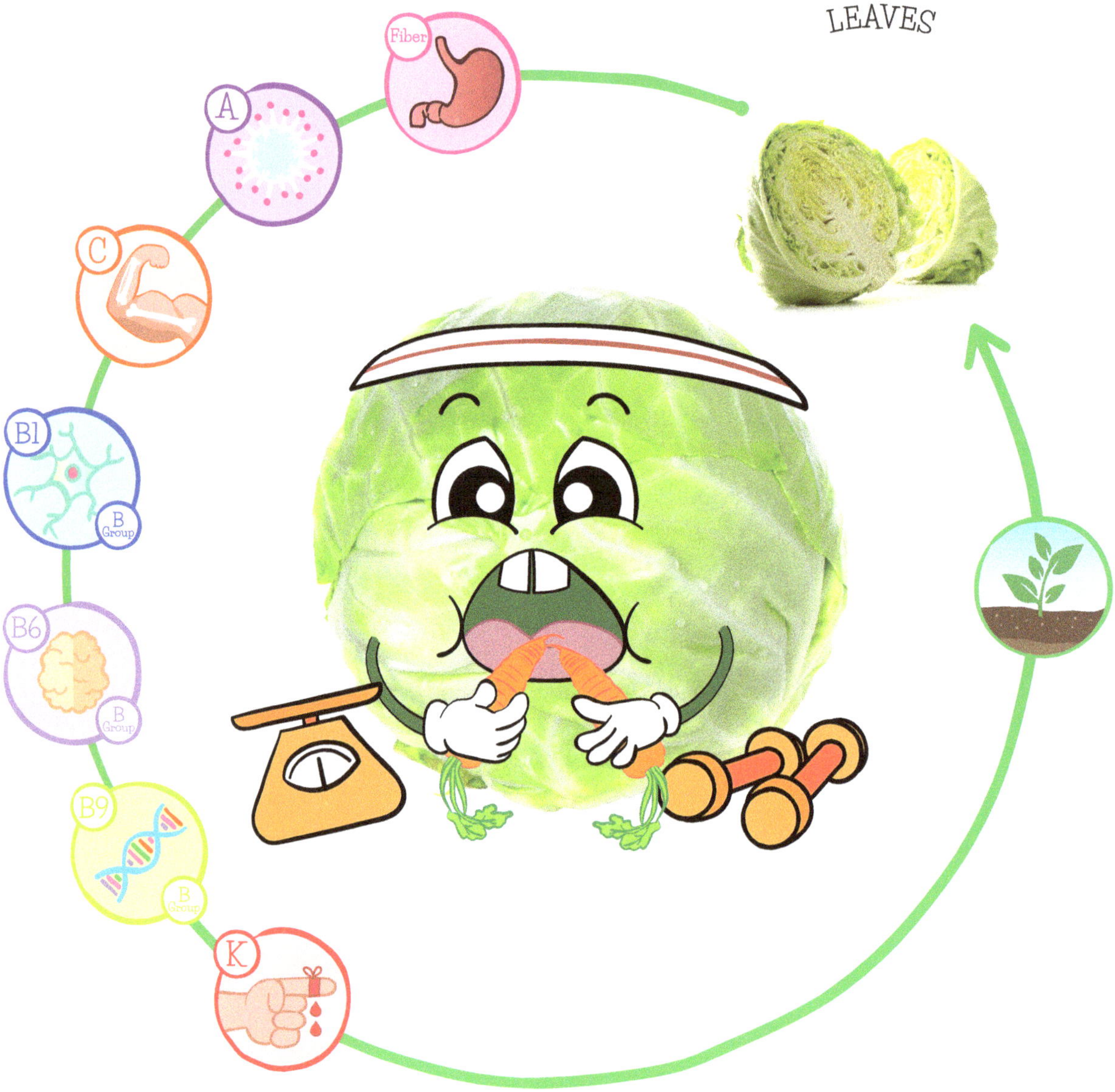

LEAVES

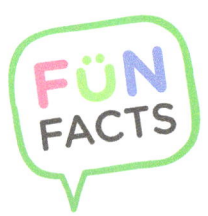

One of the world's oldest vegetables. Cabbage grows well in cold **climates** and has been **harvested** for more than 4,000 years!

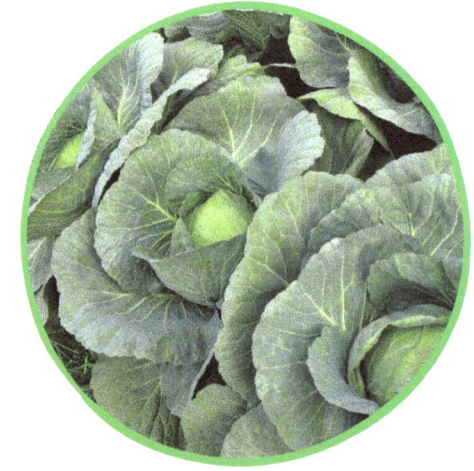

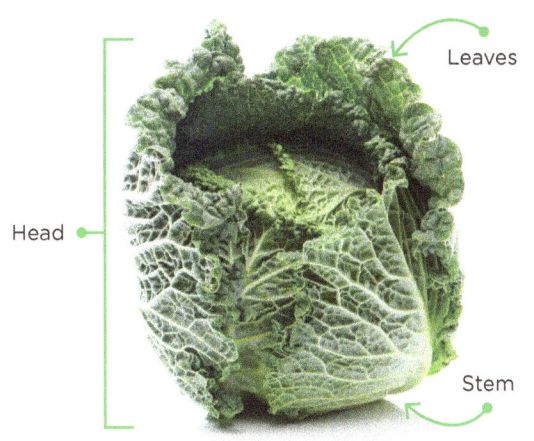
Leaves
Head
Stem

PICK
Pick cabbage with **compact** heads and tender **leaves** that feel heavy for their size. Avoid cabbage with insects and damaged leaves. Colors are different depending on **variety**.

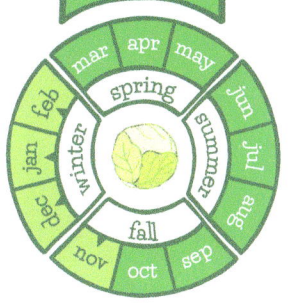

Varieties available year-round

Peak Season
November-February

STORE
Refrigerate unwashed, raw cabbage in an open plastic bag for up to 10 days. Refrigerate cooked cabbage in an airtight container for up to 7 days.

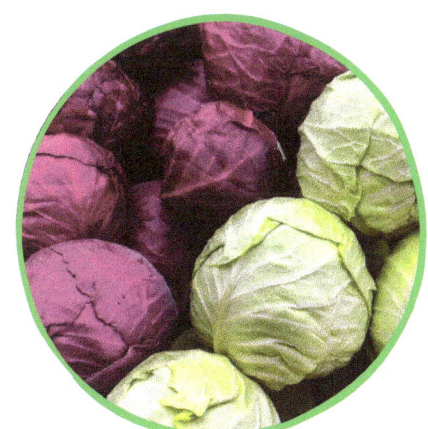

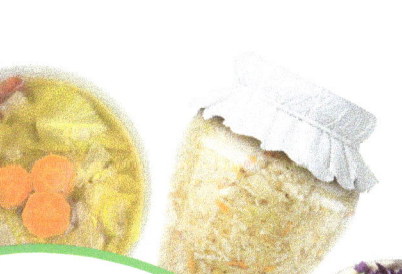

EAT
Remove the tough outer leaves, clean the skin, slice off the **stem**, and chop or slice per recipe.

Sautéed Cabbage
Place shredded cabbage into an oiled pan and cook over medium-low heat for 6-8 minutes until lightly **wilted**.

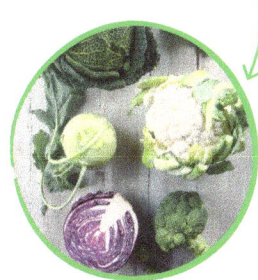

CABBAGE FAMILY

Broccoli, cauliflower, kale, and kohlrabi are in the cabbage family.

A Book of Vegetables 47

CABBAGE VARIETIES

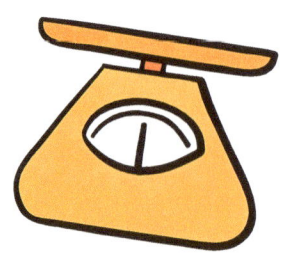

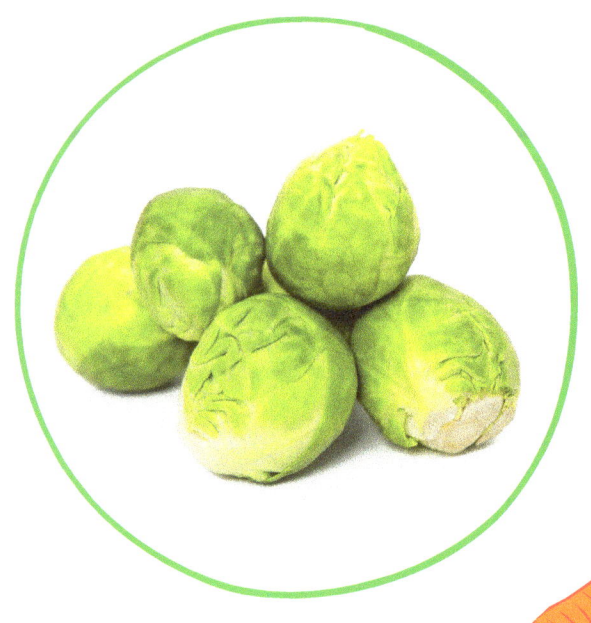

BRUSSELS SPROUT
[BRUS-SELS SPROUT]

Brussels **sprouts** grow on a thick stemmed **stalk** with many rows of miniature cabbage-like heads. Roasting Brussels sprouts brings out their sweet, nutty flavor.

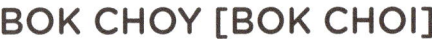

BOK CHOY [BOK CHOI]

A type of Chinese cabbage, bok choy do not form heads. They grow spoon-shaped **leaves** with a crunchy **texture** and have a sweet, mild, and mustardy flavor.

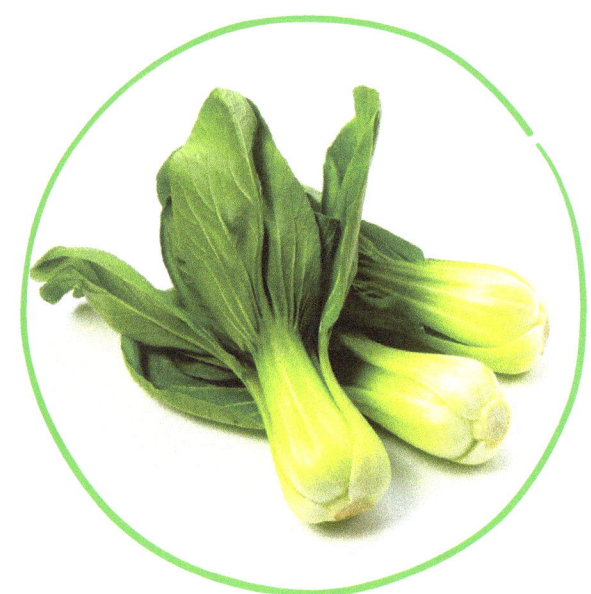

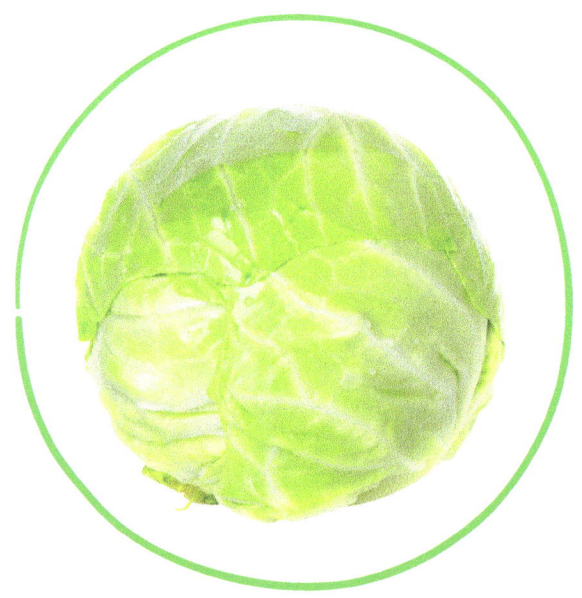

GREEN CABBAGE
[GREEN CAB-BAGE]

The Guinness Book World Record for the heaviest cabbage weighed 138.25 pounds and was presented at the Alaska State Fair in 2012.

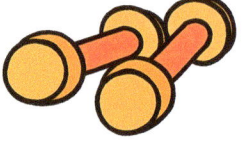

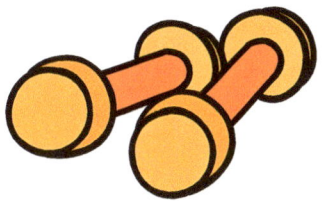

RED CABBAGE [RED CAB-BAGE]

Smaller and more dense than green cabbage, red cabbage is often pickled or cooked with vinegar to preserve its vibrant color and peppery flavor.

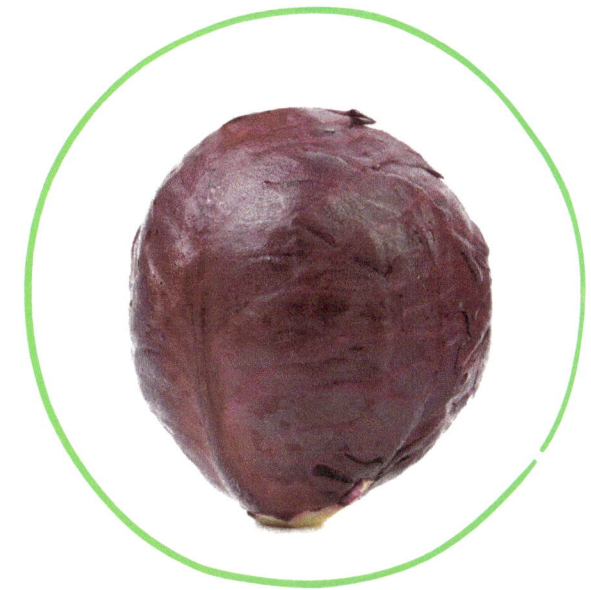

NAPA [NAP-UH]

Napa cabbage is **cylindrical** in shape with crisp, crinkled, light green leaves. Napa cabbage is commonly used to make kimchi, a traditional spicy fermented Korean dish.

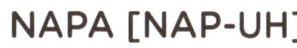

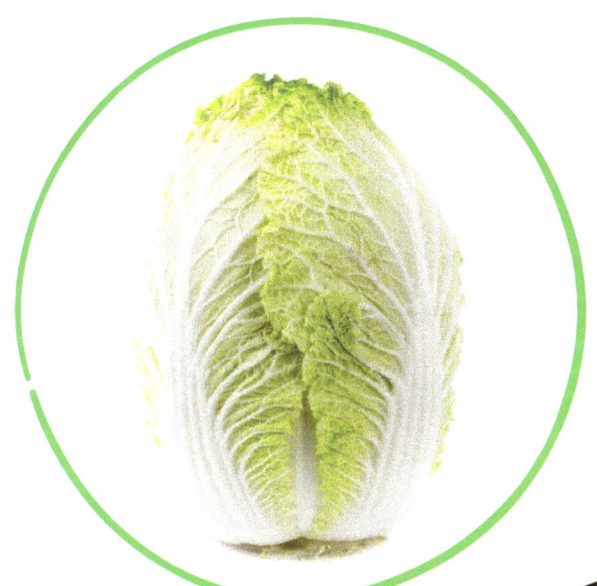

SAVOY [SA-VOY]

Considered the most beautiful and **versatile** of all the cabbages, the tender, sweet, curly leaves of Savoy can be **prepared** many ways and are great in place of tortillas for sandwich wraps.

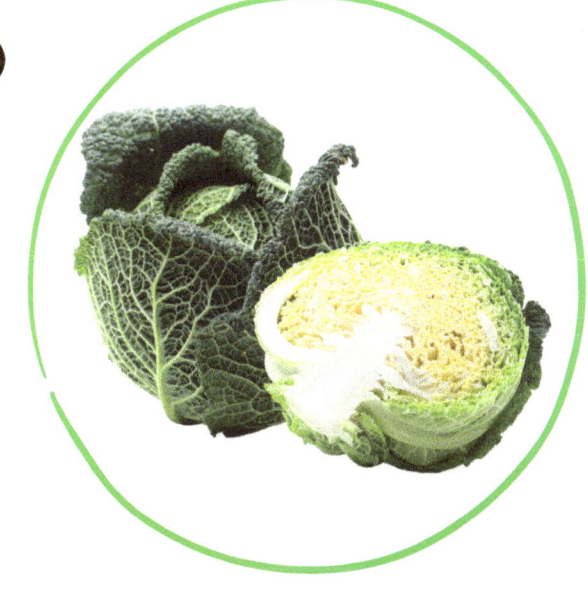

CARROT AND GREENS

[car-rot]

bitter, crisp, crunchy, fruity, sweet

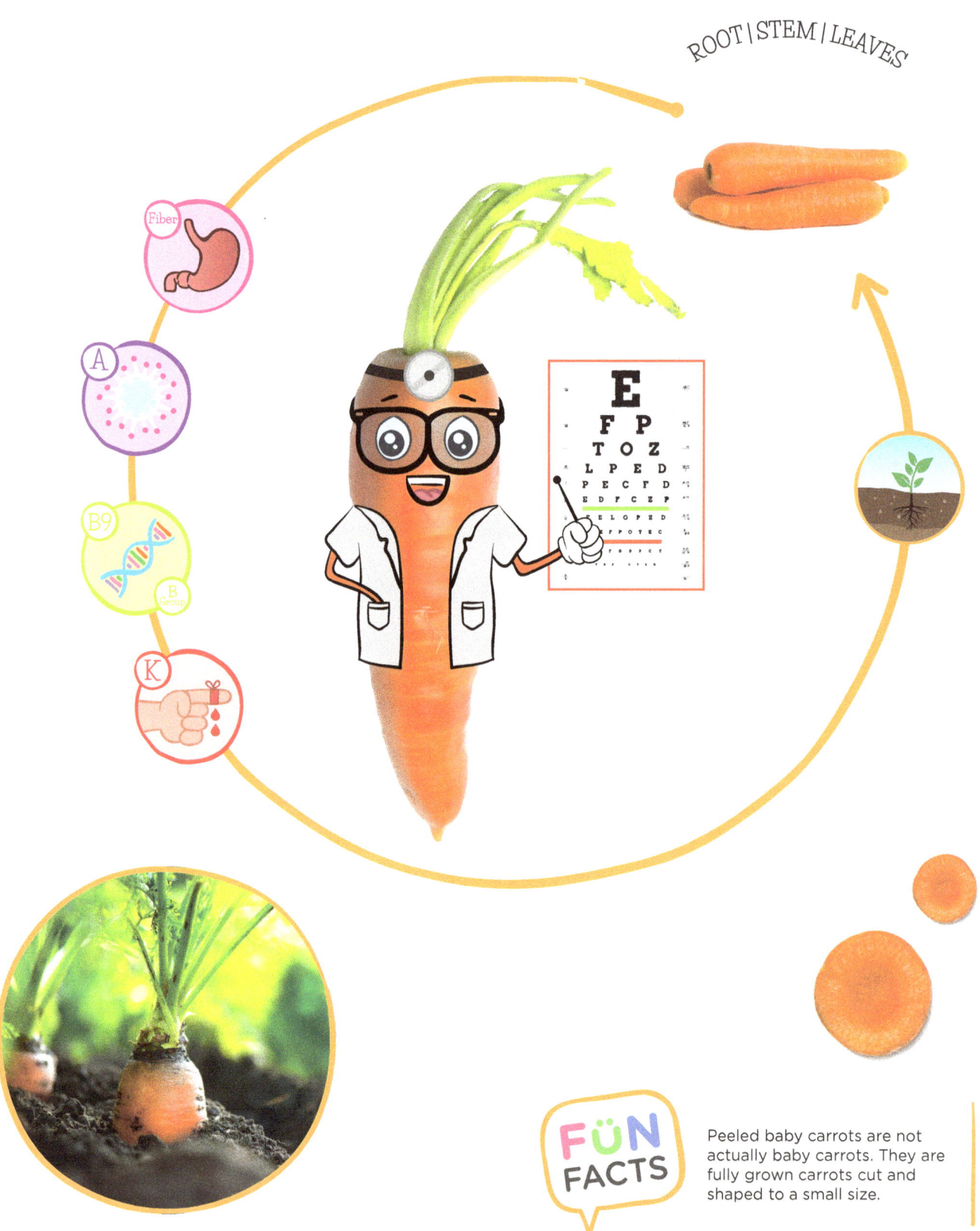

ROOT | STEM | LEAVES

Fun Facts: Peeled baby carrots are not actually baby carrots. They are fully grown carrots cut and shaped to a small size.

Where Does Broccoli Come From?

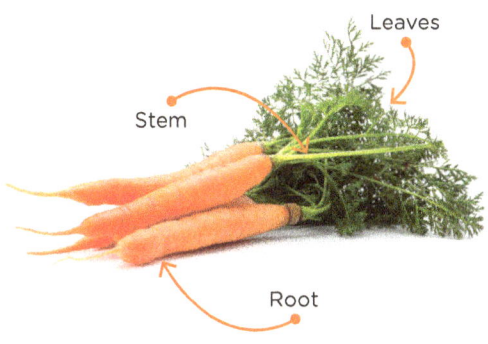
Leaves
Stem
Root

PICK
Pick firm, smooth, moist, well-shaped **roots**. Avoid dry, rubbery carrots. Attached greens should be bright green and crisp. Colors are different depending on **variety**.

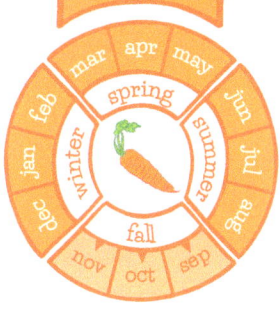

Varieties available year-round

Peak Season
September-November

STORE
Refrigerate raw, unpeeled carrot in a moist paper towel in a closed plastic bag or container for up to 4 weeks, chopped carrots in a closed container for 2-3 weeks, and cooked carrots in an airtight container for 3-5 days. Raw carrot greens should be refrigerated separately in an airtight container for 2-3 days.

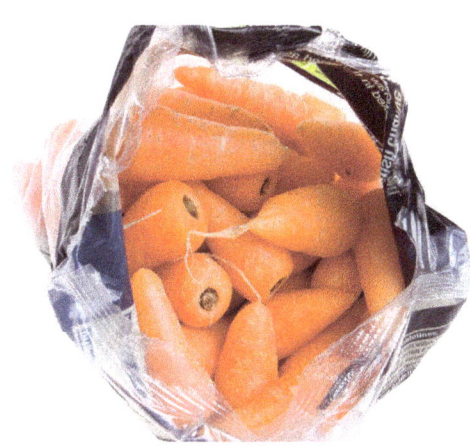

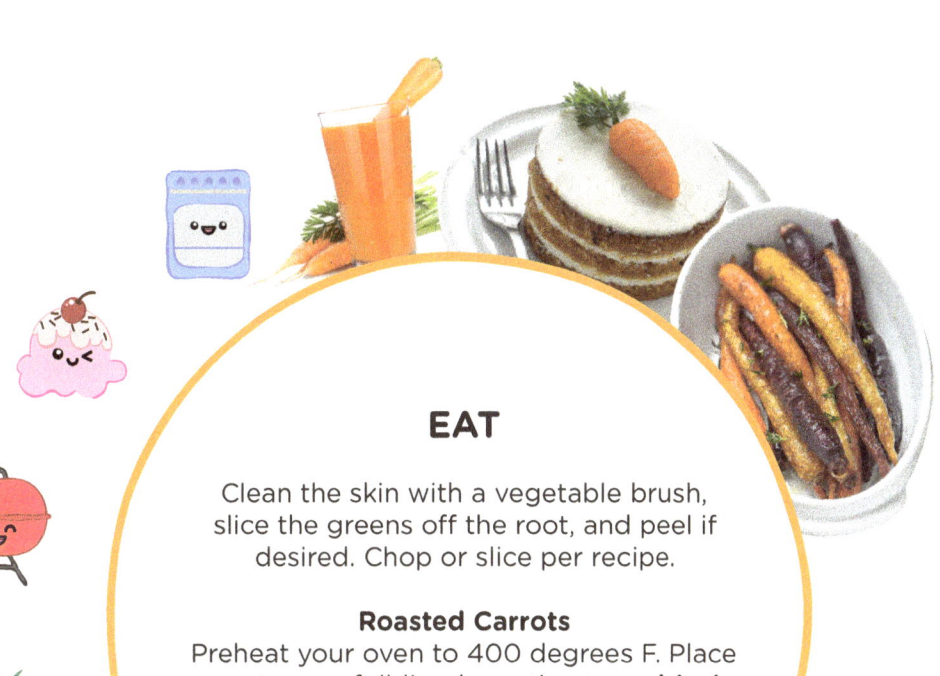

EAT
Clean the skin with a vegetable brush, slice the greens off the root, and peel if desired. Chop or slice per recipe.

Roasted Carrots
Preheat your oven to 400 degrees F. Place carrots on a foil-lined roasting tray, **drizzle** with olive oil, and roast for about 20 minutes (depending on size) until roots are tender and can be easily **pierced** with a fork.

CARROT TIDBITS

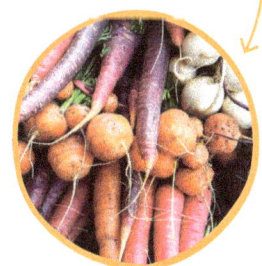

Carrots come in many different colors and shapes.

 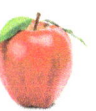

Do not store carrots near apples because the **ethylene gas** released from the **fruit** during ripening will make carrots taste bitter.

A Book of Vegetables   51

CASSAVA
YUCA

[cas-sa-va] | [yu-ca]

buttery, chewy, glutinous, starchy, sweet

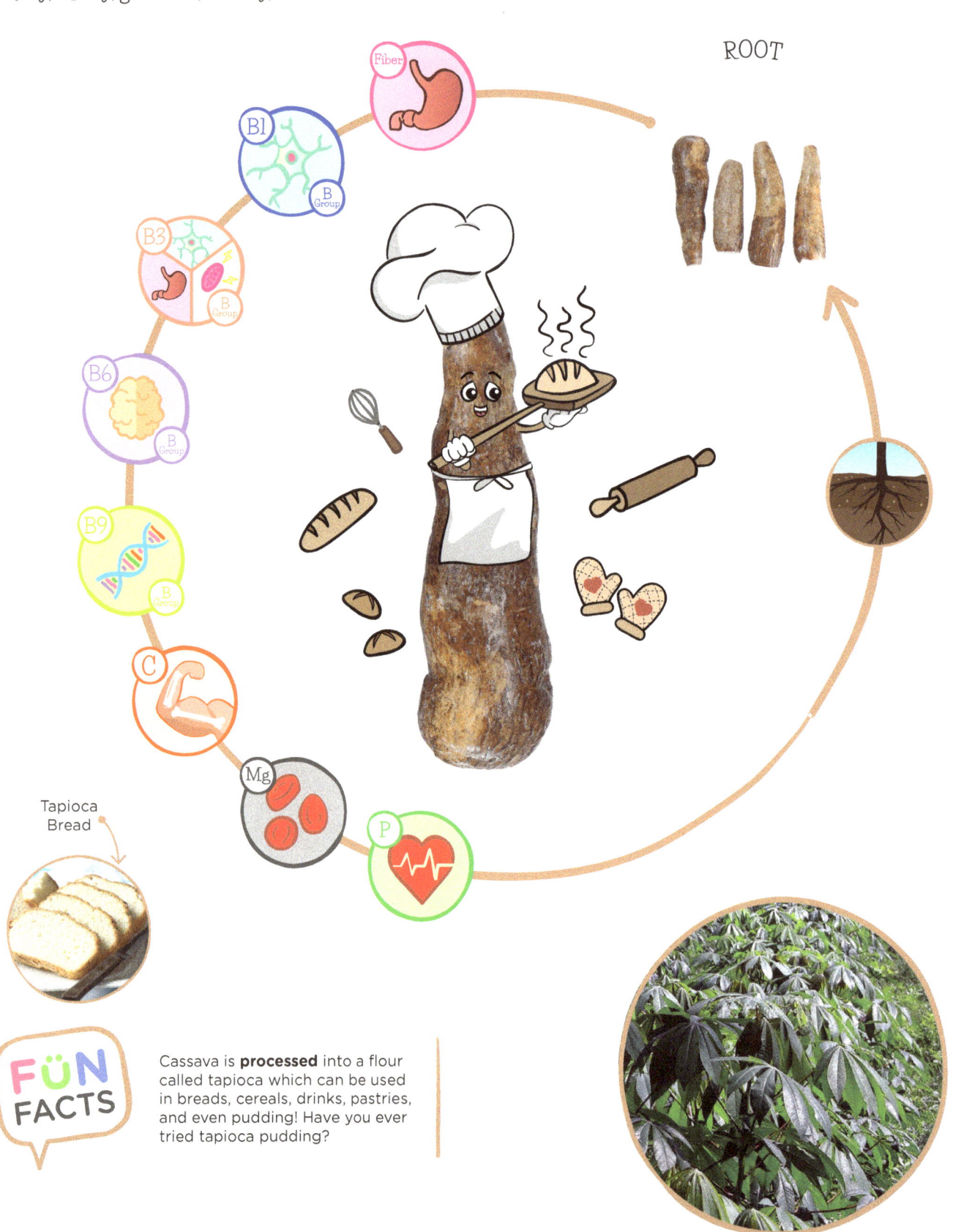

ROOT

Tapioca Bread

FUN FACTS

Cassava is **processed** into a flour called tapioca which can be used in breads, cereals, drinks, pastries, and even pudding! Have you ever tried tapioca pudding?

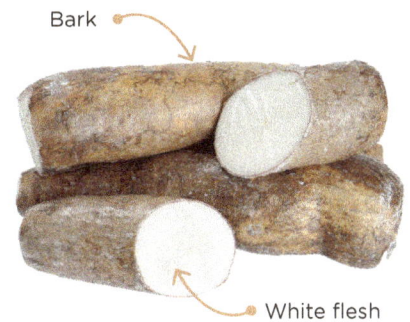
Bark
White flesh

PICK

Pick brown, bark-covered **roots** with white to yellow **flesh**. Avoid cassava with cuts, cracks, slime, **mold**, dark areas in the flesh, or smell rotten.

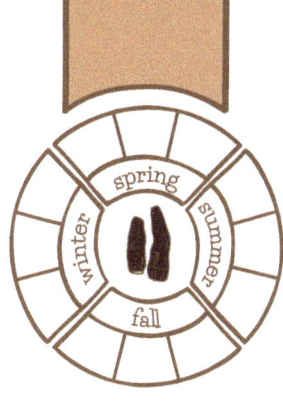

Available imported year-round

STORE

Refrigerate raw cassava in an airtight plastic bag or plastic wrap for up to 2 days. Cassava **spoils** very quickly!

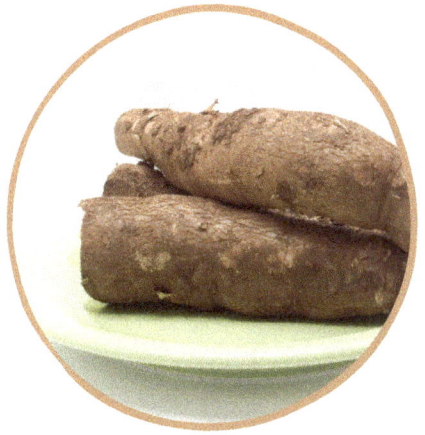

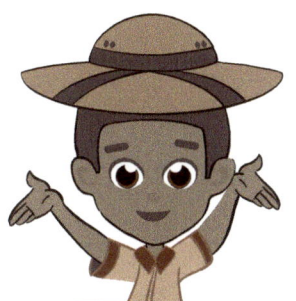

CASSAVA PLANT

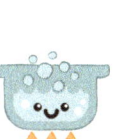

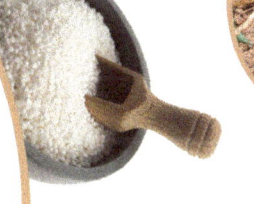

EAT

Clean the skin then peel and chop into **uniform** sized pieces.

Boiled Cassava
Boil cassava in salted water for about 20 minutes or until roots are tender and can be easily **pierced** with a fork. Try them boiled or mash like you would potatoes.

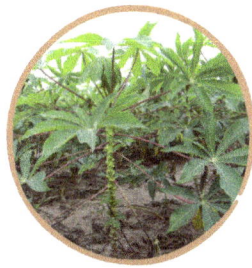

Cassava (Roots)

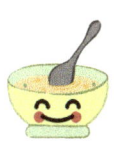

Cassava Plant

A Book of Vegetables 53

CAULIFLOWER

[cau-li-flow-er]

bitter, crunchy, mild, nutty, sweet

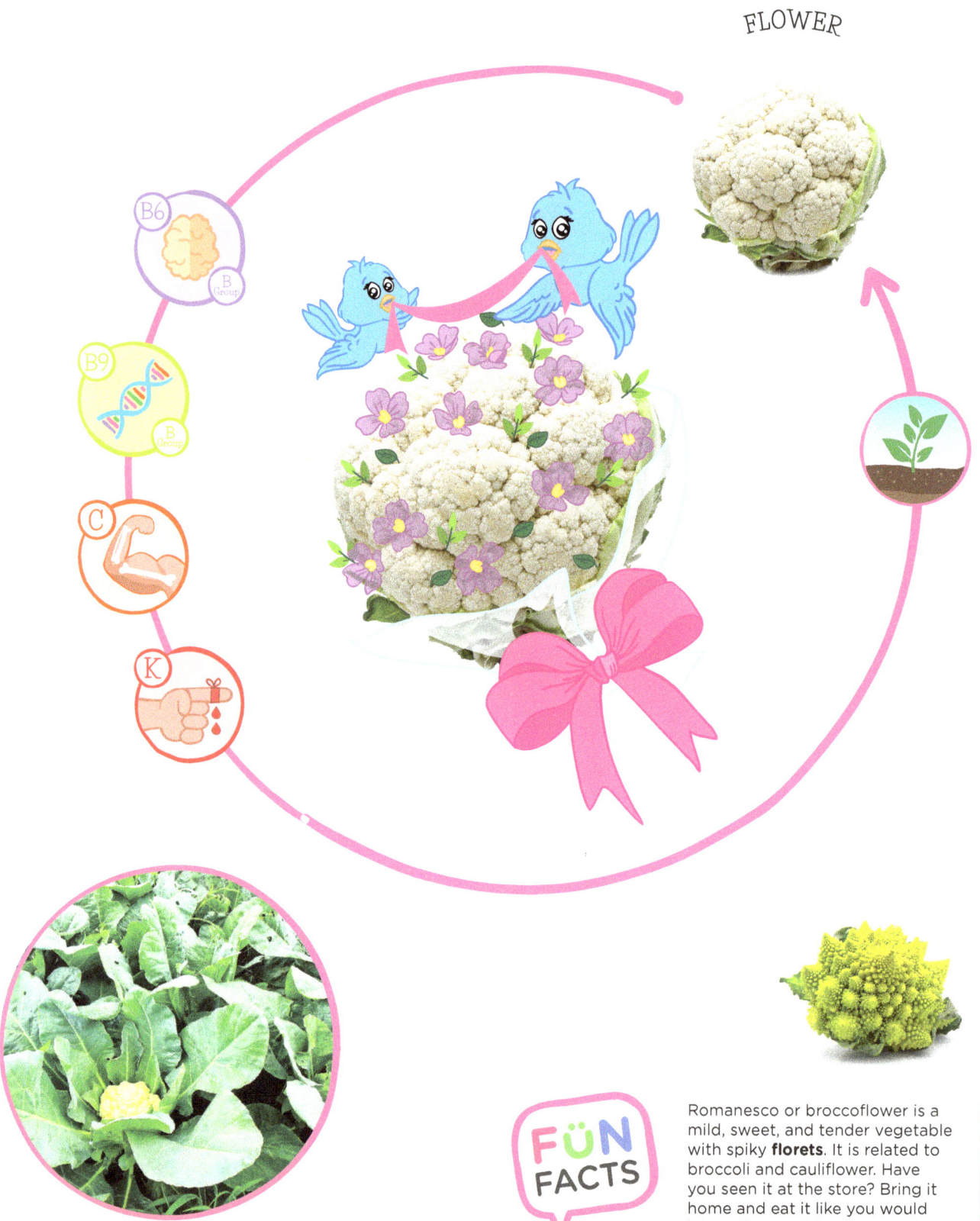

FLOWER

Fun Facts: Romanesco or broccoflower is a mild, sweet, and tender vegetable with spiky **florets**. It is related to broccoli and cauliflower. Have you seen it at the store? Bring it home and eat it like you would broccoli or cauliflower.

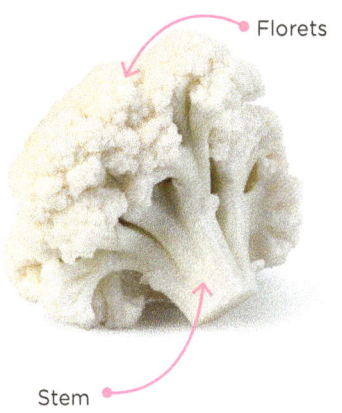
Florets
Stem

PICK
Pick creamy or snowy white, clean, florets with firm, **compact buds**, and firm **stems** that feel heavy for their size. Avoid cauliflower that have buds with a rice-like or grainy appearance.

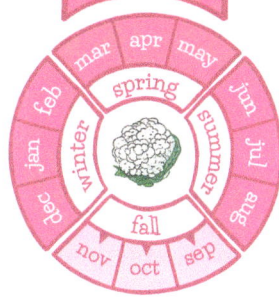

Varieties available year-round

Peak Season
September-November

STORE
Refrigerate unwashed, raw cauliflower in a closed plastic bag for up to 7 days. Refrigerate cooked cauliflower in an airtight container for 3-5 days.

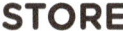
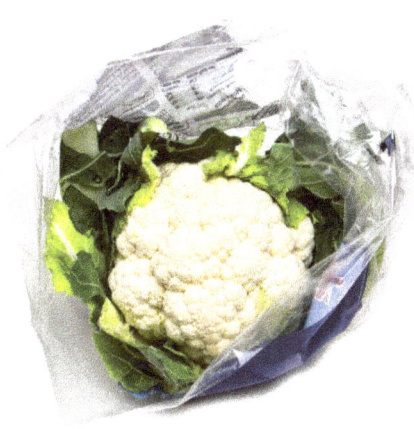

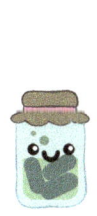
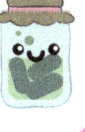

CAULIFLOWER TIDBITS

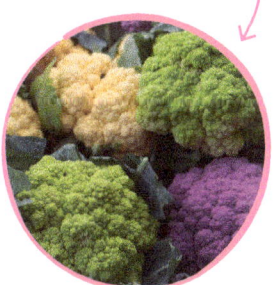

There are several colors of cauliflower: orange, purple, green, and brown.

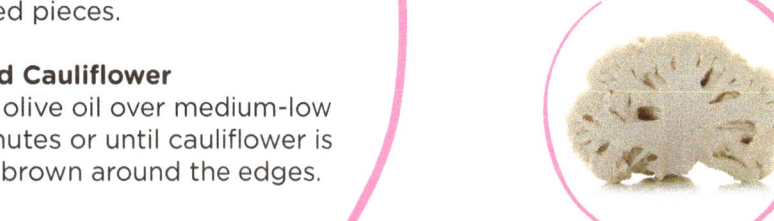

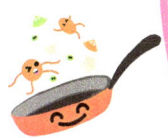

EAT
Clean the skin, cut the florets off the stem, and chop florets and stems into **uniform** sized pieces.

Sautéed Cauliflower
Sauté cauliflower in olive oil over medium-low heat for about 8 minutes or until cauliflower is tender and golden brown around the edges.

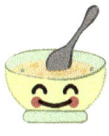
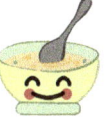

Flower heads are sometimes called curds.

A Book of Vegetables

CELERIAC
CELERY ROOT

[sell-air-e-ak] | [sell-ery root]

celery-like, crunchy, earthy, nutty, starchy

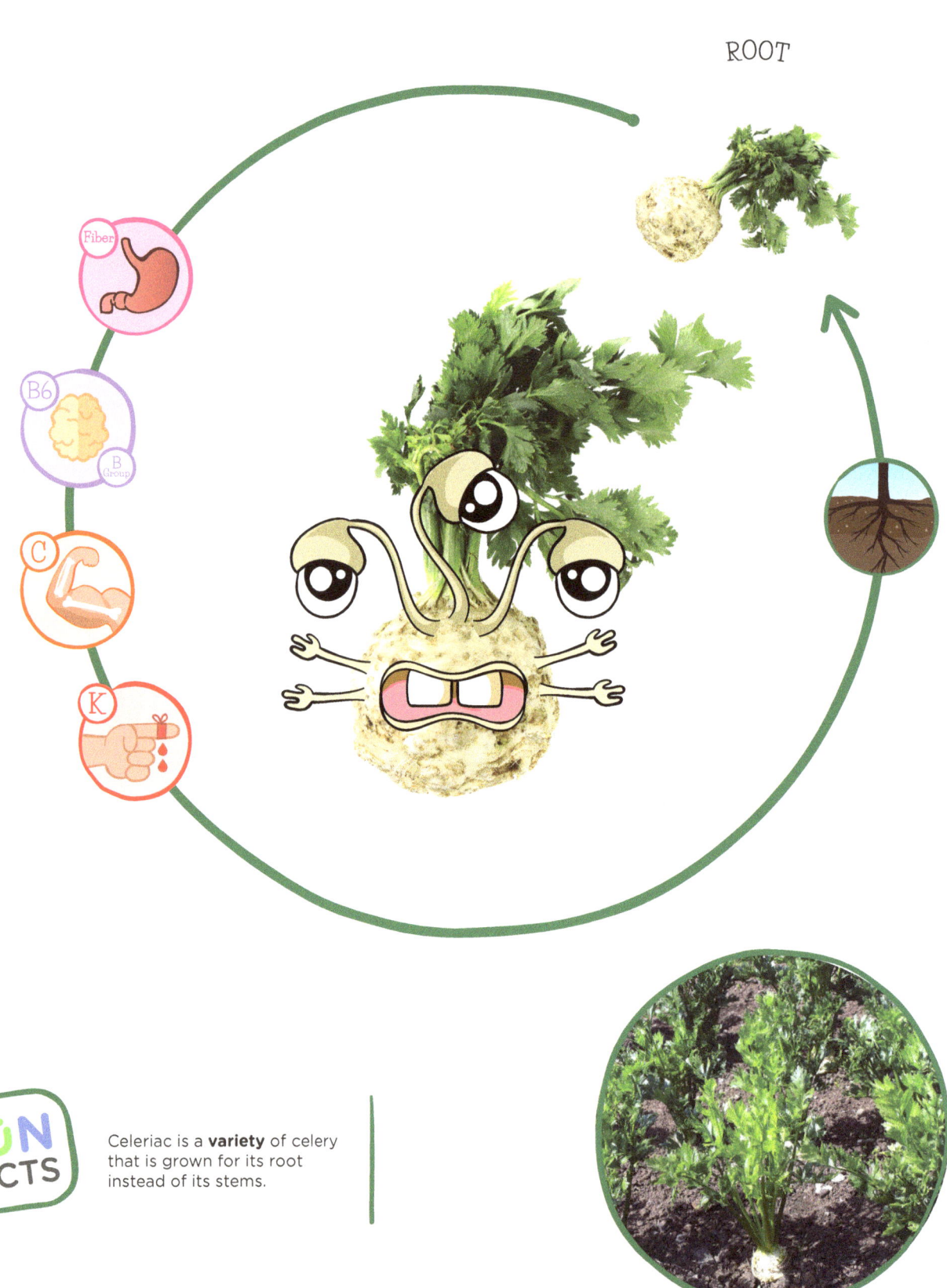

ROOT

FUN FACTS: Celeriac is a **variety** of celery that is grown for its root instead of its stems.

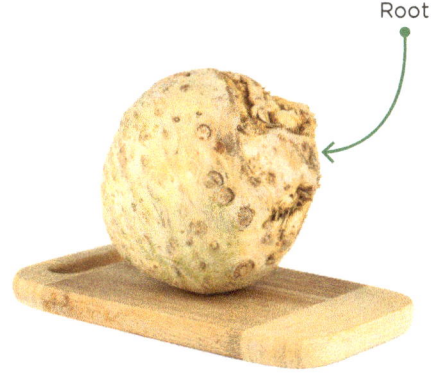
Root

PICK
Pick small, firm **roots** that feel heavy for their size. Celeriac should have minimal deep ridges. Avoid celeriac that have cuts and **bruises**. Attached greens should be bright green and crisp.

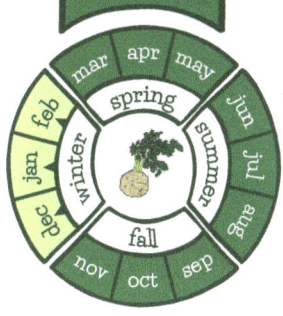

Varieties available year-round

Peak Season
December-February

STORE
Refrigerate raw celeriac in a moist paper towel in a closed plastic bag for up to 14 days. Refrigerate cooked celeriac in an airtight container for 3-4 days.

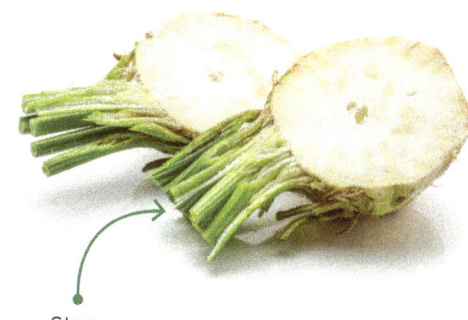
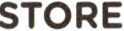
Stem

CELERIAC TIDBITS

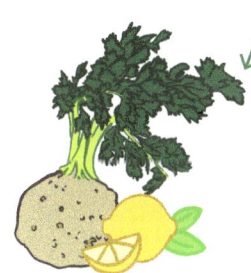

Celeriac discolors quickly. After chopping or slicing per recipe, place celeriac in a bowl of water with lemon juice or vinegar to prevent browning.

EAT
Clean the skin and slice off the **stem** end and root end, peel, and then chop or slice per recipe.

Mashed Celeriac
Chop celeriac into small chunks, simmer in salted water for about 20 minutes or until the celeriac can be easily **pierced** with a fork. Drain water, add butter, and mash or whip with an electric mixer until smooth and creamy, then season with salt and pepper.

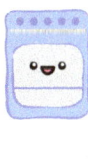
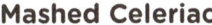
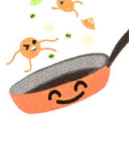

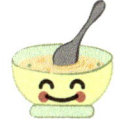
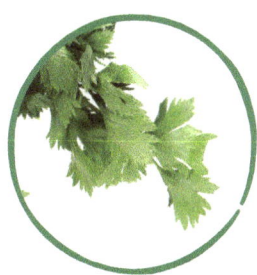

The stem and the **leaves** are not eaten as they are bitter and stringy.

A Book of Vegetables

CELERY

[sell-ery]

aromatic, bright, crispy, refreshing, tangy

STEM

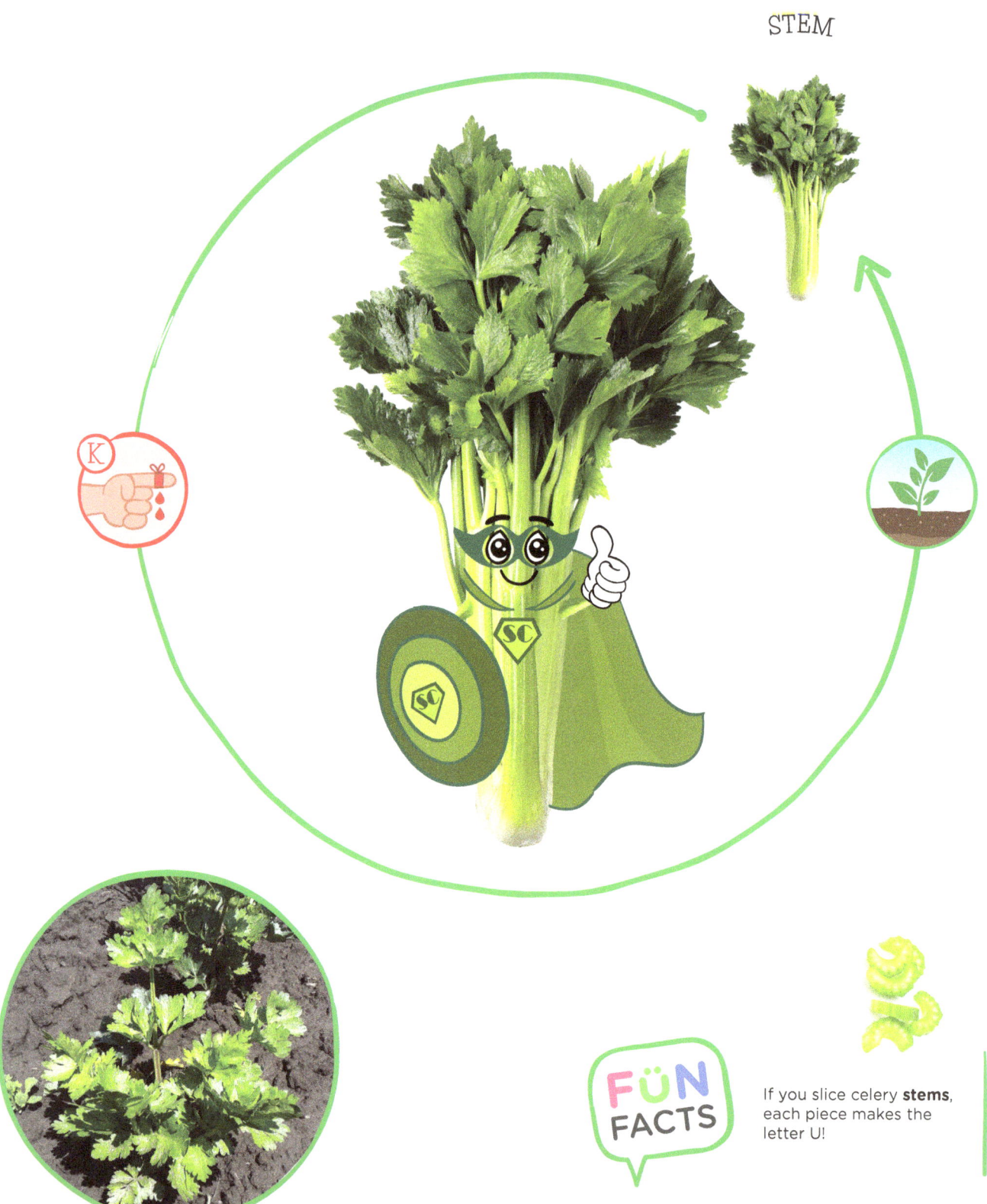

FUN FACTS

If you slice celery **stems**, each piece makes the letter U!

58 | Where Does Broccoli Come From?

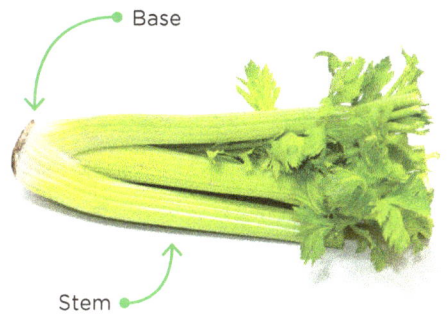

PICK
Pick green, clean, tightly formed bunches that are firm and crisp when snapped. Avoid celery that are cracked, brown, or have **wilted leaves**.

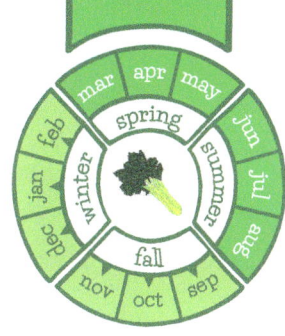

Varieties available year-round

Peak Season
September-February

STORE
Refrigerate raw celery in a closed plastic bag or aluminum foil for up to 14 days. Refrigerate cooked celery in an airtight container for 3-4 days.

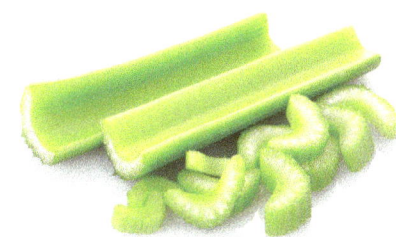

Celery **seeds** are often used as a spice or flavoring for recipes.

Celery sticks are also called ribs and can be eaten raw.

EAT
Separate stems from the base, clean the skin, and chop or slice per recipe.

Raw Celery
Try them raw, filled with peanut butter, and topped with raisins for a fun treat called Ants on a Log.

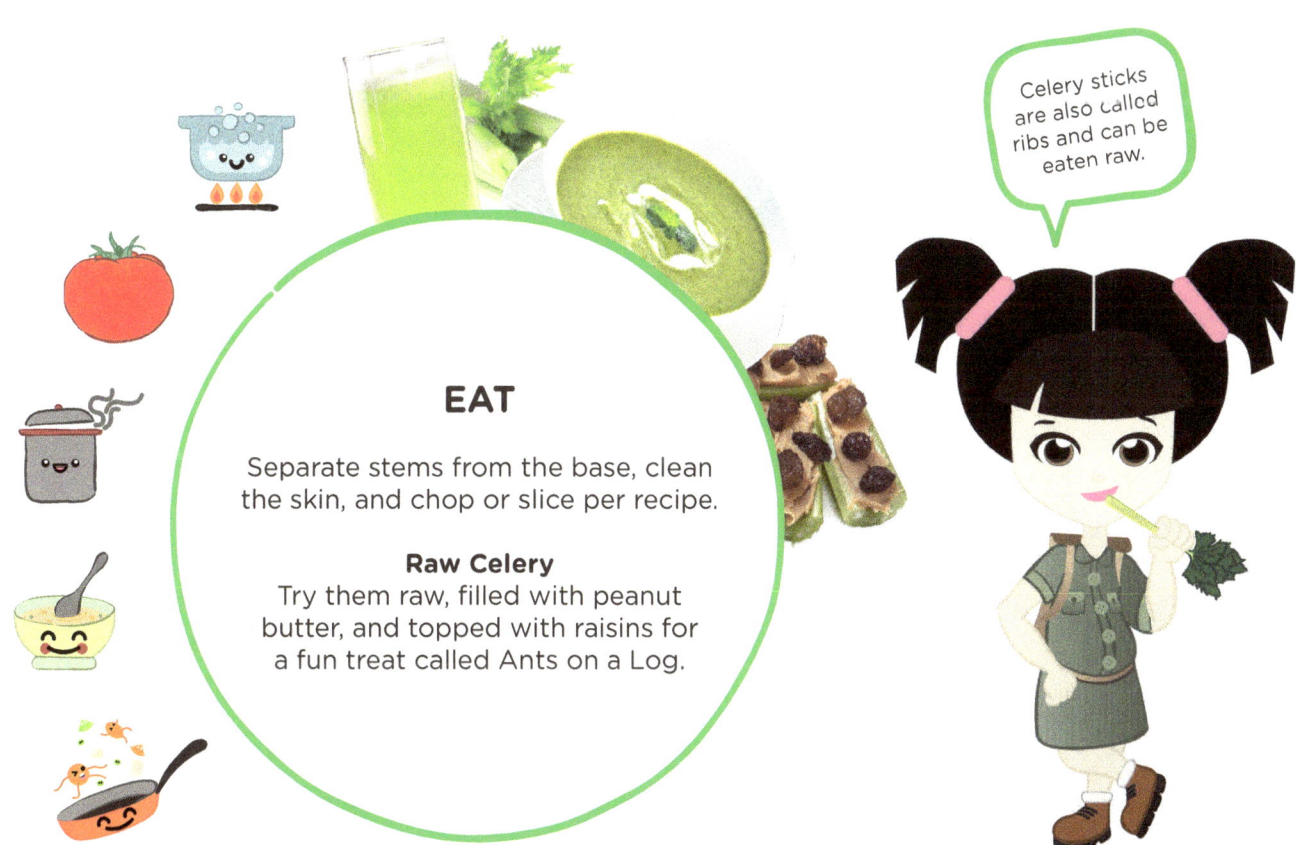

A Book of Vegetables

COLLARD GREENS

[col-lard greens]

acidic, bitter, fibrous, hearty, mild

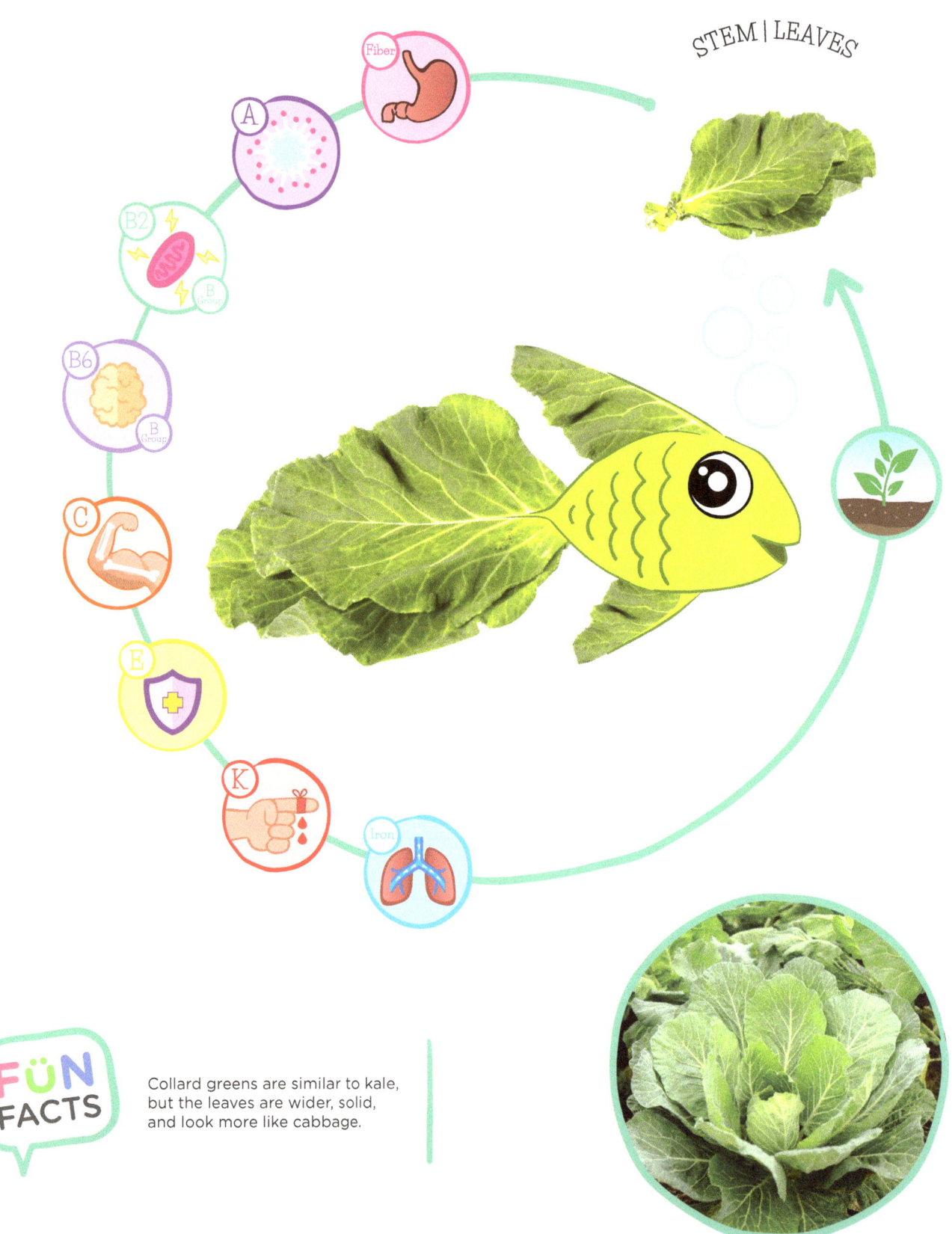

STEM | LEAVES

FUN FACTS: Collard greens are similar to kale, but the leaves are wider, solid, and look more like cabbage.

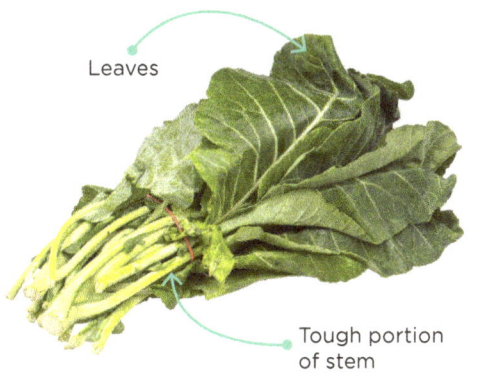
Leaves
Tough portion of stem

PICK
Pick green, crisp, firm **leaves**. Avoid collard greens that are **wilting**, yellowing, and have browning leaves.

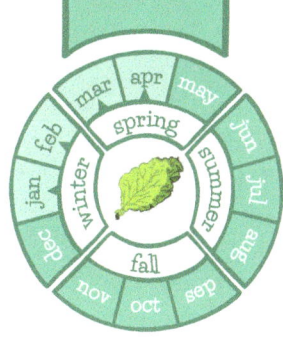

Varieties available year-round

Peak Season
January–April

STORE
Refrigerate unwashed, raw collard greens in a closed plastic bag up to 5 days. Refrigerate cooked collard greens in an airtight container for 3-4 days.

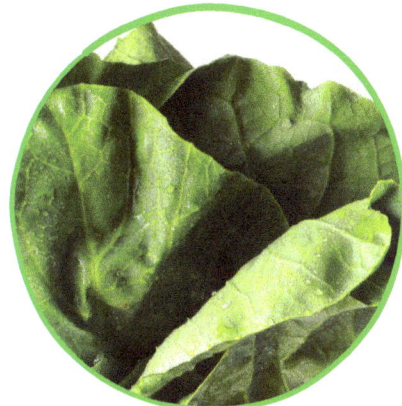

CUTTING COLLARD GREENS

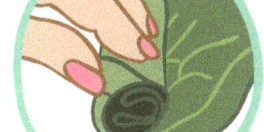
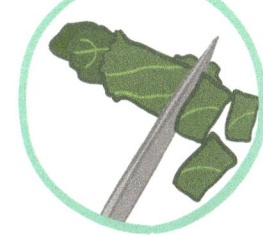

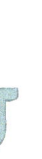

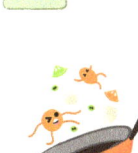

EAT
Clean the leaves several times to remove all dirt and sand. For large, mature leaves, fold each leaf in half lengthwise (hot dog style) and slice off the tough portion of the **stem**. For young, tender leaves, stems do not need to be removed. Stack several leaves on top of each other, roll into a large bunch, and cut leaves into thick slices or chop per recipe.

Soup, Stews, and Stir-Fried Collard Greens
Add collard greens to soups and stews. Collard greens may also be stir-fried in olive oil over medium heat for 3-4 minutes until they are bright green.

A Book of Vegetables 61

CORN
MAIZE

[core-n] | [mayz]

creamy, juicy, sugary, sweet, tender

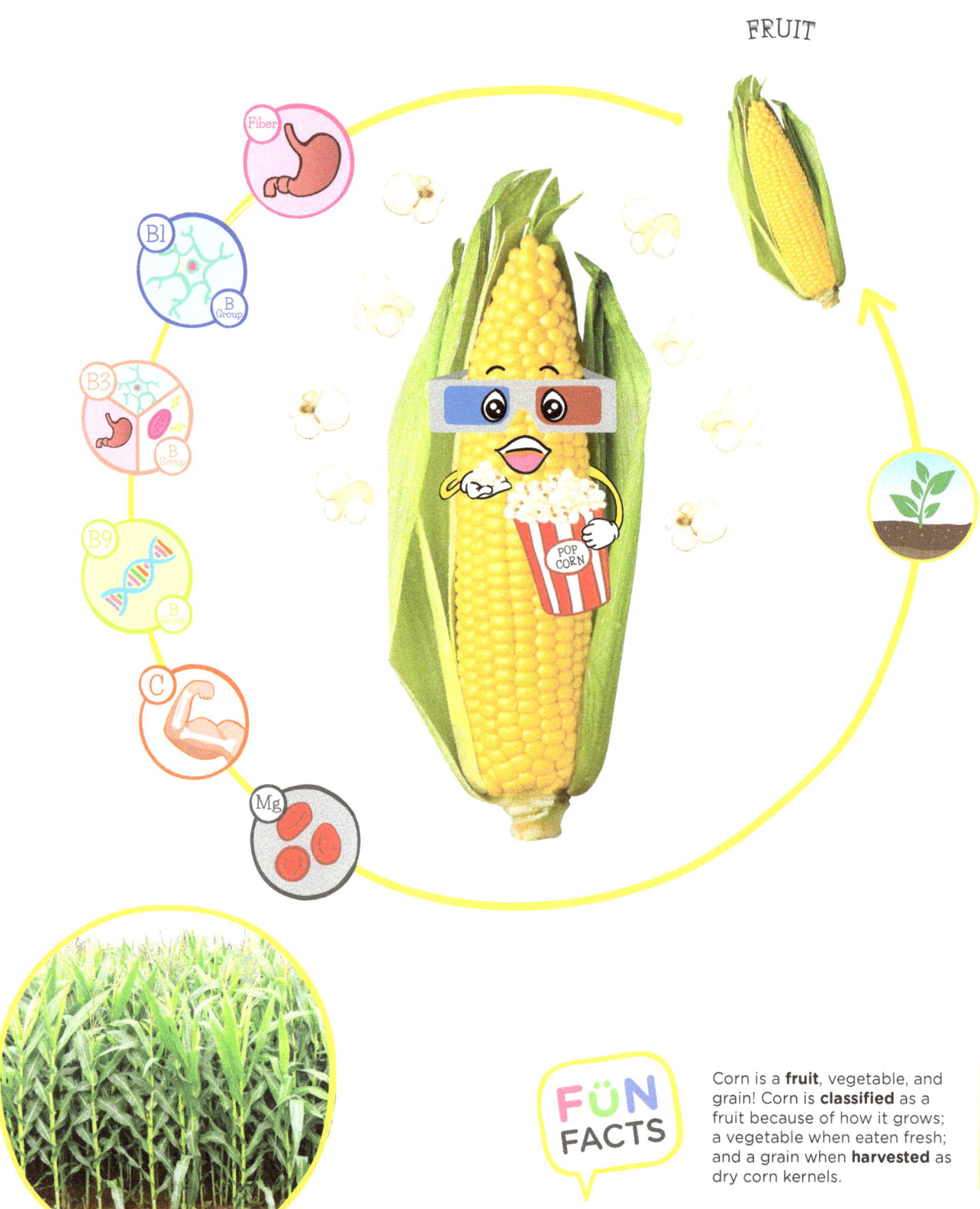

FRUIT

FUN FACTS

Corn is a **fruit**, vegetable, and grain! Corn is **classified** as a fruit because of how it grows; a vegetable when eaten fresh; and a grain when **harvested** as dry corn kernels.

| Where Does Broccoli Come From?

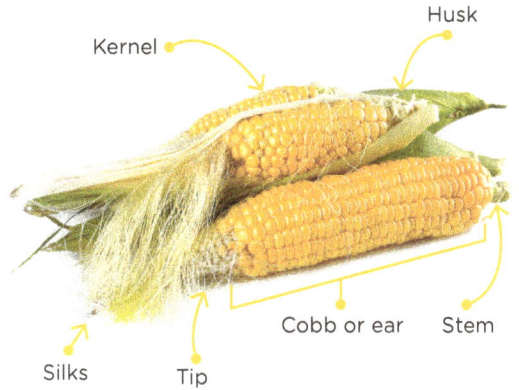

Kernel, Husk, Silks, Tip, Cobb or ear, Stem

PICK
Pick green, crisp, outer **husks** that are tightly wrapped around the cob, with sticky brown silks, that feel heavy for their size. Feel the corn kernels through the husk to ensure they feel **plump** and firm. Avoid corn cobbs with holes or missing kernels, dry silks, and husks with small brown holes near the top.

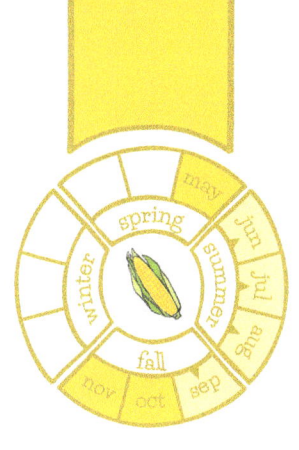

Available May to November

Peak Season
June-September

SHUCKING CORN

To shuck corn, peel off the outer husk from the tip and peel the inner **leaves** back until you see the first row of kernels. Hold the **stem** of the ear with one hand and pull the silks and leaves downward toward the stem with your other hand. Repeat until all leaves and silks are removed.

STORE
Refrigerate corn with the husk on in an open container for up to 3 days. If husks have been removed, wrap corn in plastic or aluminum foil. Refrigerate cooked corn in an airtight container for 3-5 days.

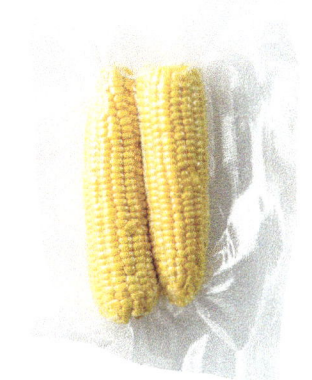

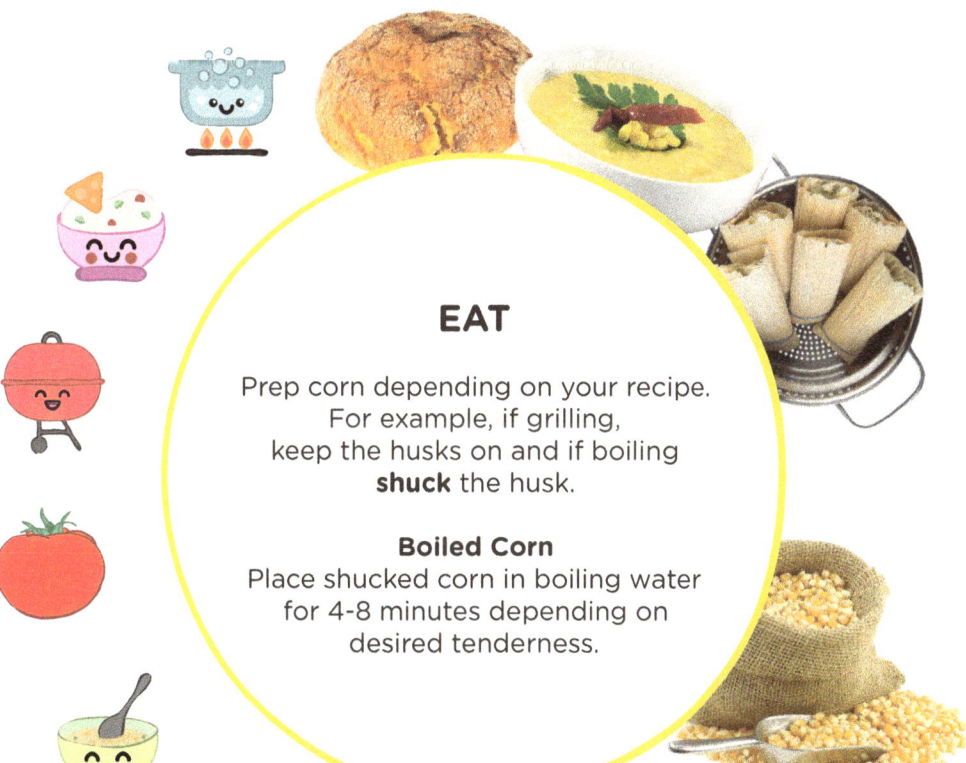

EAT
Prep corn depending on your recipe. For example, if grilling, keep the husks on and if boiling **shuck** the husk.

Boiled Corn
Place shucked corn in boiling water for 4-8 minutes depending on desired tenderness.

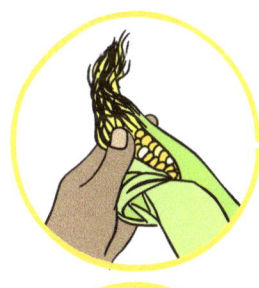
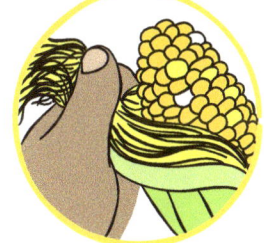
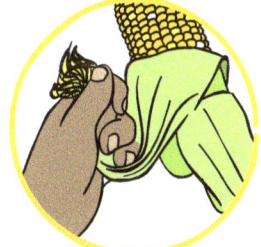

A Book of Vegetables

CUCUMBER

[cu-cum-ber]

bitter, crisp, mild, refreshing, tender

FRUIT

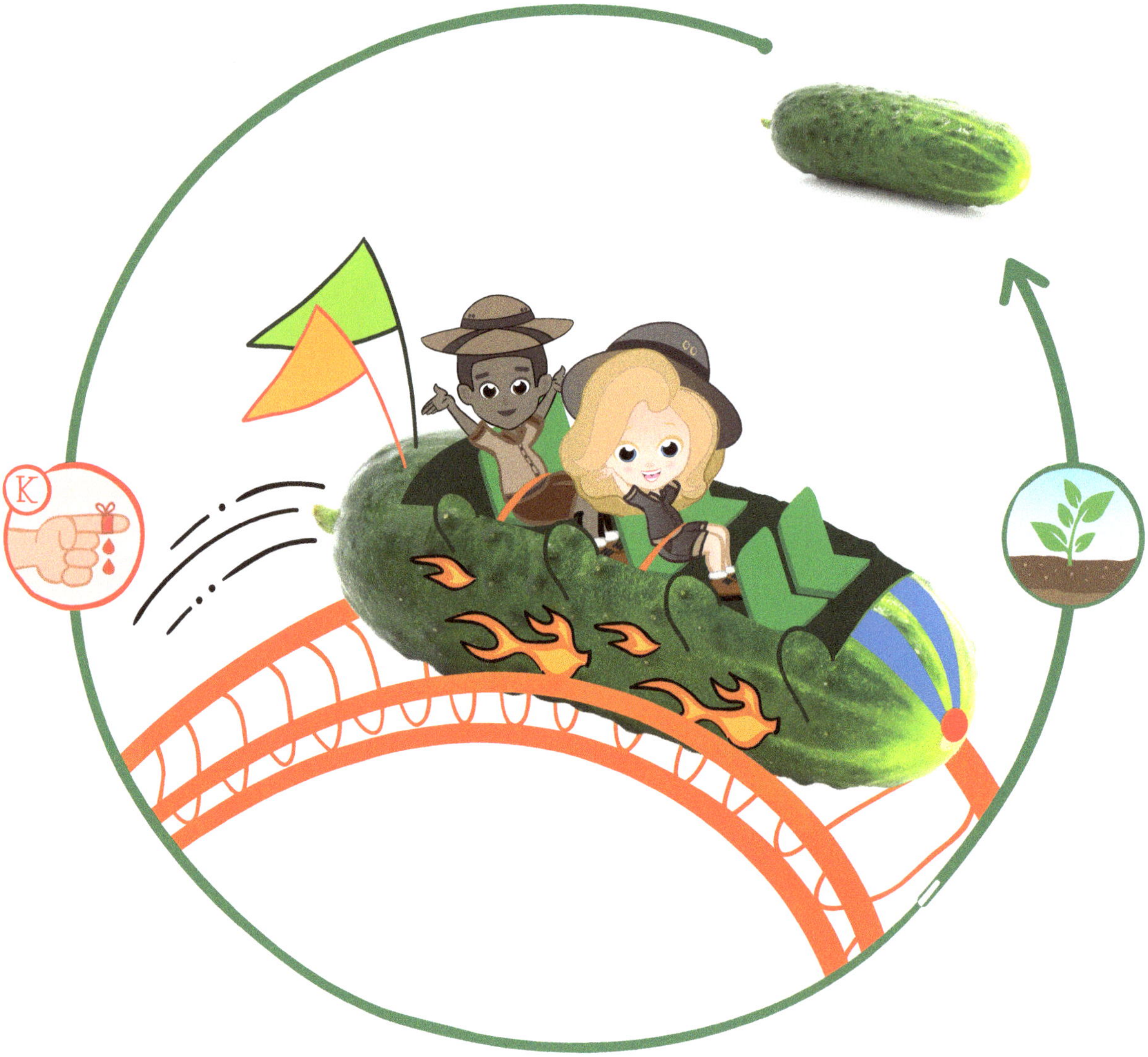

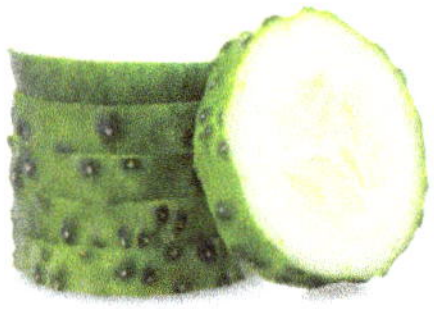

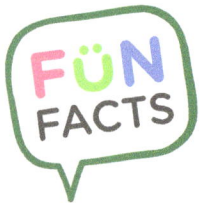

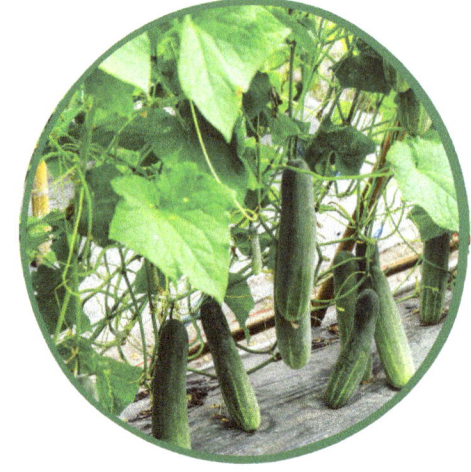

FUN FACTS

Have you ever heard the saying "cool as a cucumber?" The inside **flesh** of a cucumber growing in a field on a hot summer day is 20 degrees cooler than the outside air **temperature**!

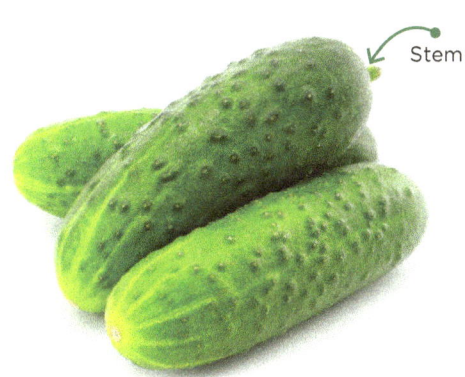
Stem

PICK
Pick dark green, evenly colored, firm **fruit**. Avoid cucumbers with soft spots and cuts.

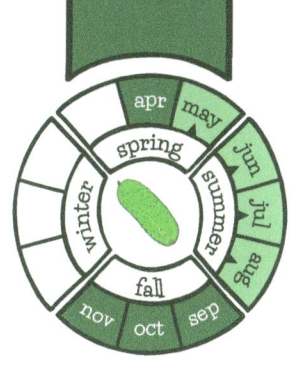

Available April to November; Imported year-round

Peak Season
May-August

STORE
Refrigerate unwashed, raw cucumber in a closed plastic bag for up to 7 days. Refrigerate sliced or chopped cucumber in an airtight container for 1-2 days.

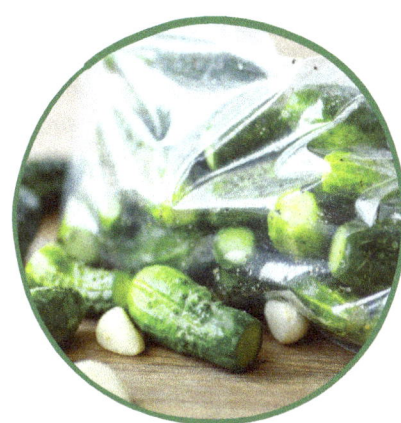

CUCUMBER TIDBITS

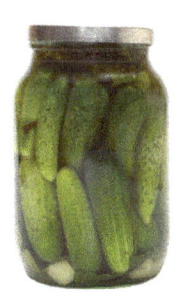

Cucumbers soaked in vinegar or **brine** with spices are known as pickles. Do you like pickles?

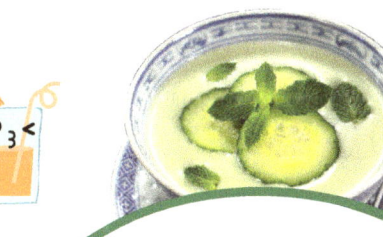

EAT
Clean the skin and chop or slice per recipe. Peeling may be necessary for **varieties** with tough skin.

Raw Cucumber
Slice and dip cucumbers in your favorite dressing, add them to salads, or top with spreadable cheese for a snack.

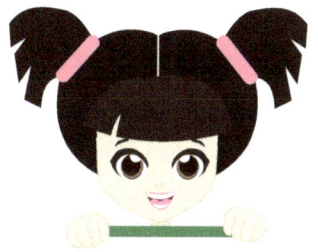

Cucumber is in the gourd family along with pumpkins and melons.

A Book of Vegetables 65

DAIKON AND GREENS

[dye-kon]

crisp, juicy, mild, sweet, tangy

ROOT | STEM | LEAVES

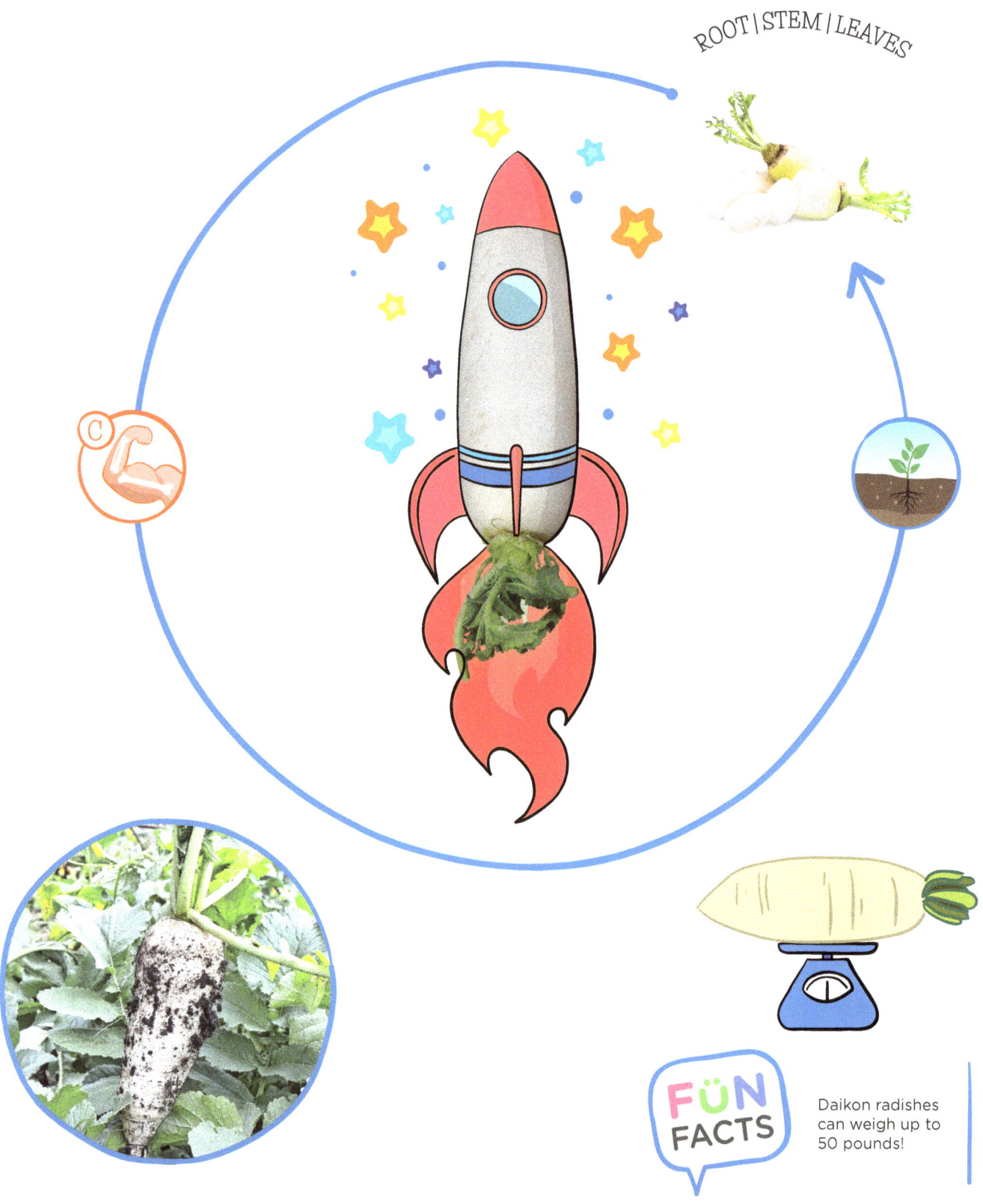

FUN FACTS Daikon radishes can weigh up to 50 pounds!

66 | Where Does Broccoli Come From?

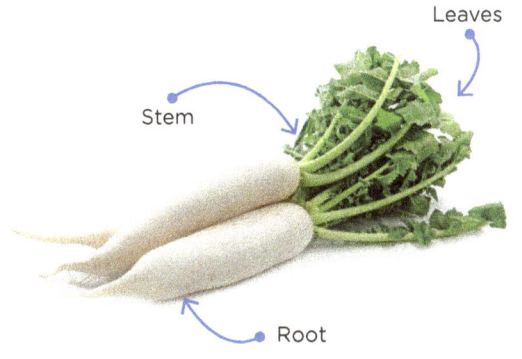

Leaves
Stem
Root

PICK
Pick white, firm, well-shaped **roots**, with smooth skin. Avoid daikon with deep ridges and cuts. Attached greens should be bright green and crisp.

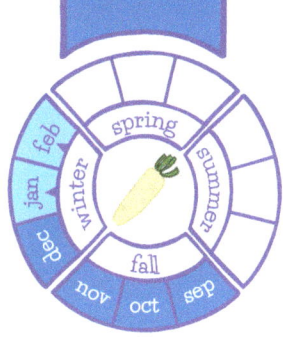

Available September to February; Imported year-round

Peak Season
January-February

STORE
Refrigerate unpeeled raw daikon in an open plastic bag for up to 14 days. Refrigerate raw, sliced daikon in an airtight container for 2-3 days and cooked daikon in an airtight container for 3-5 days. Daikon greens should be refrigerated separately in an airtight container for 2-3 days.

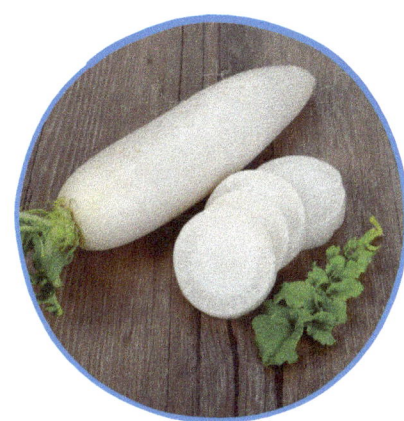

DAIKON TIDBITS

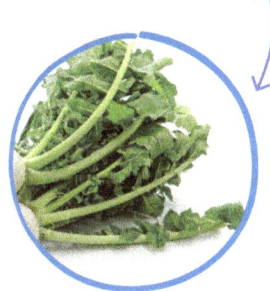

Daikon greens can be used the same way as beet and carrot greens. They can be sautéed, added to soups, or eaten as salad greens.

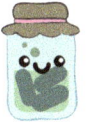
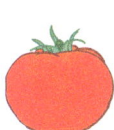
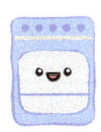

EAT
Clean the skin with a vegetable brush, slice the greens off the **root**, peel and chop or slice per recipe.

Pickled Daikon
Thinly chop 1/2 pound of daikon and 1/2 pound of carrots into small strips, mix together and then place in a clean jar. Combine 4 cups of warm water, 3 tablespoons of sugar, 3 tablespoons of salt, and 4 ounces of rice vinegar and mix until salt and sugar are **dissolved**. Pour vinegar mixture over daikon and carrots until they are completely coated in liquid. Cover jar and place in the refrigerator for 3 days and enjoy.

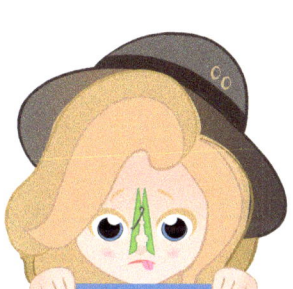

Chopped daikon may make your fridge smell like rotten eggs!

A Book of Vegetables 67

EGGPLANT
AUBERGINE

[egg-plant] | [aw-ber-jean]

bitter, complex, meaty, rich, tender

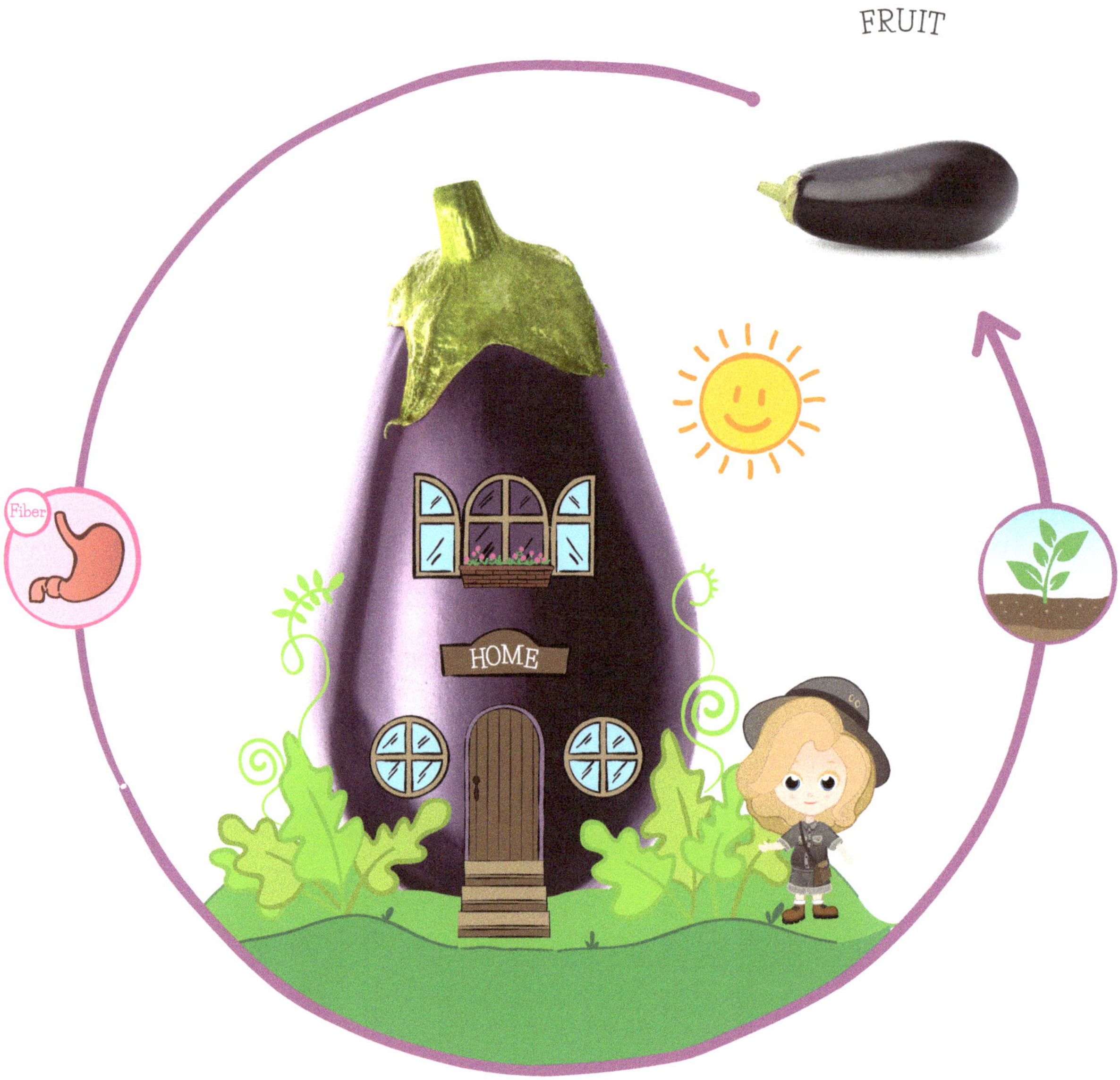

FRUIT

FUN FACTS

The soft airy flesh of the eggplant acts like a sponge with oil. It soaks up every drop! To decrease the sponge effect while cooking, "sweat" the eggplant. To sweat an eggplant sprinkle slices with salt and allow them to sit on the counter for 30-60 minutes for the salt to pull moisture from the flesh. Be sure to rinse off the salt before using them.

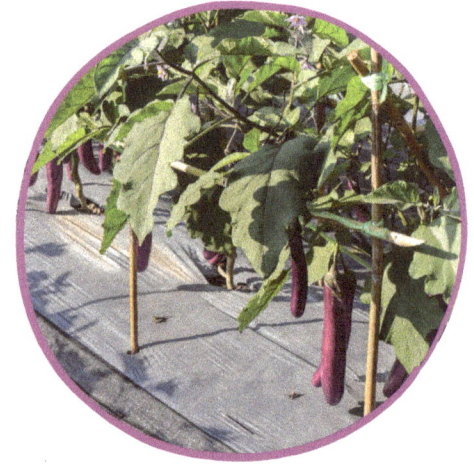

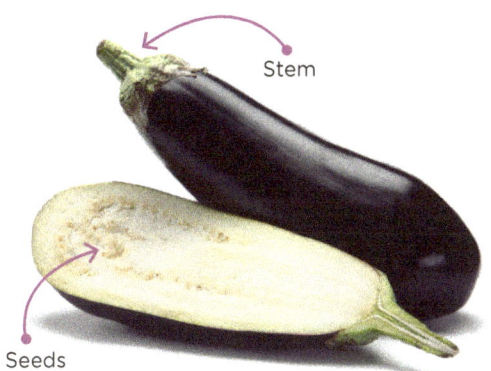

PICK
Pick glossy, smooth **fruit** that are firm to touch and heavy for their size. Avoid eggplant with dark or soft spots. **Flesh** should be creamy white with no brown **seeds**. Flesh with brown seeds may have a bitter taste.

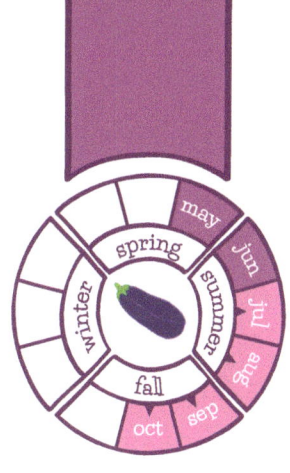

Available May to October; Imported year-round

Peak Season
July-October

STORE
Refrigerate unwashed, raw eggplant in an open plastic bag for up to 7 days. Refrigerate cooked eggplant in an airtight container for 3-5 days.

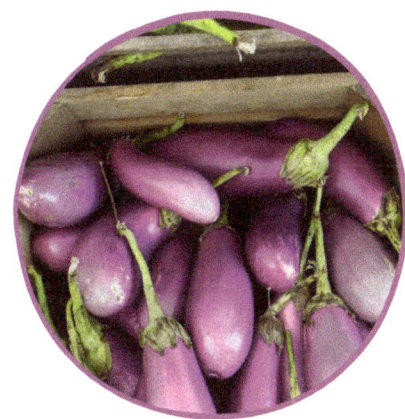

Eggplant is a great meat substitute in recipes and do not need to be peeled.

EGGPLANT TIDBITS

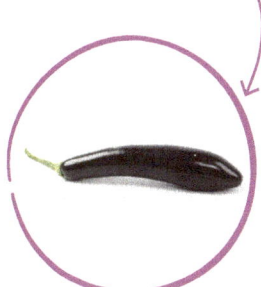

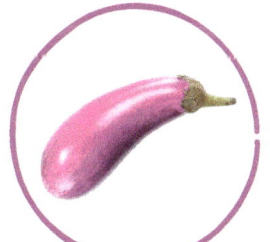

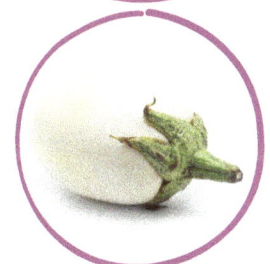

Eggplant colors vary from deep purple or almost black, to light purple with creamy stripes, to all white. Eggplants also vary in shape from round, to pear-shaped, to long and **cylindrical**.

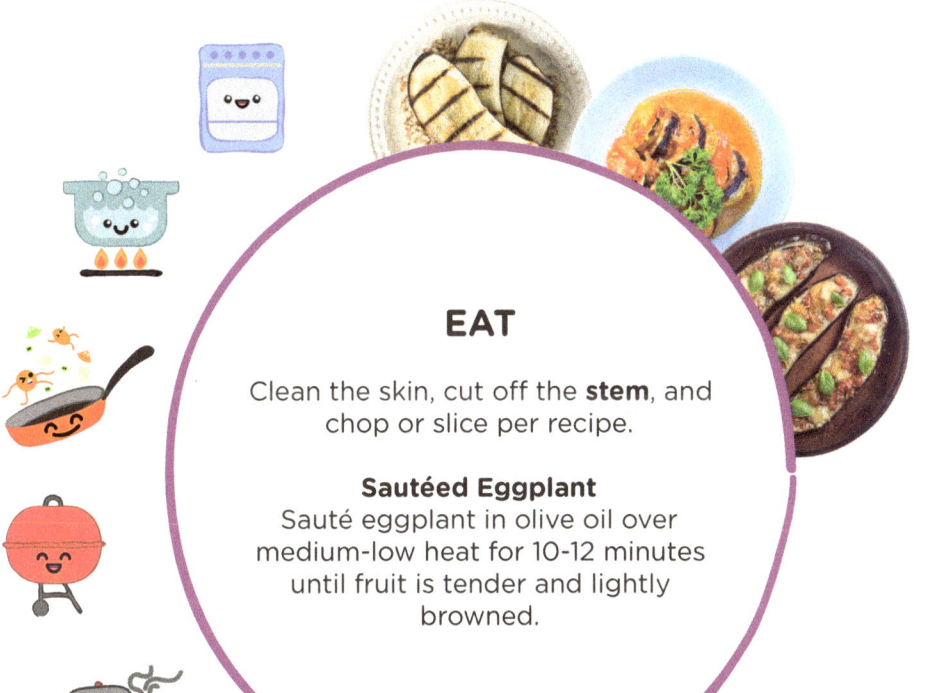

EAT
Clean the skin, cut off the **stem**, and chop or slice per recipe.

Sautéed Eggplant
Sauté eggplant in olive oil over medium-low heat for 10-12 minutes until fruit is tender and lightly browned.

A Book of Vegetables

FENNEL

[fen-nel]

anise, aromatic, bright, crunchy, sweet

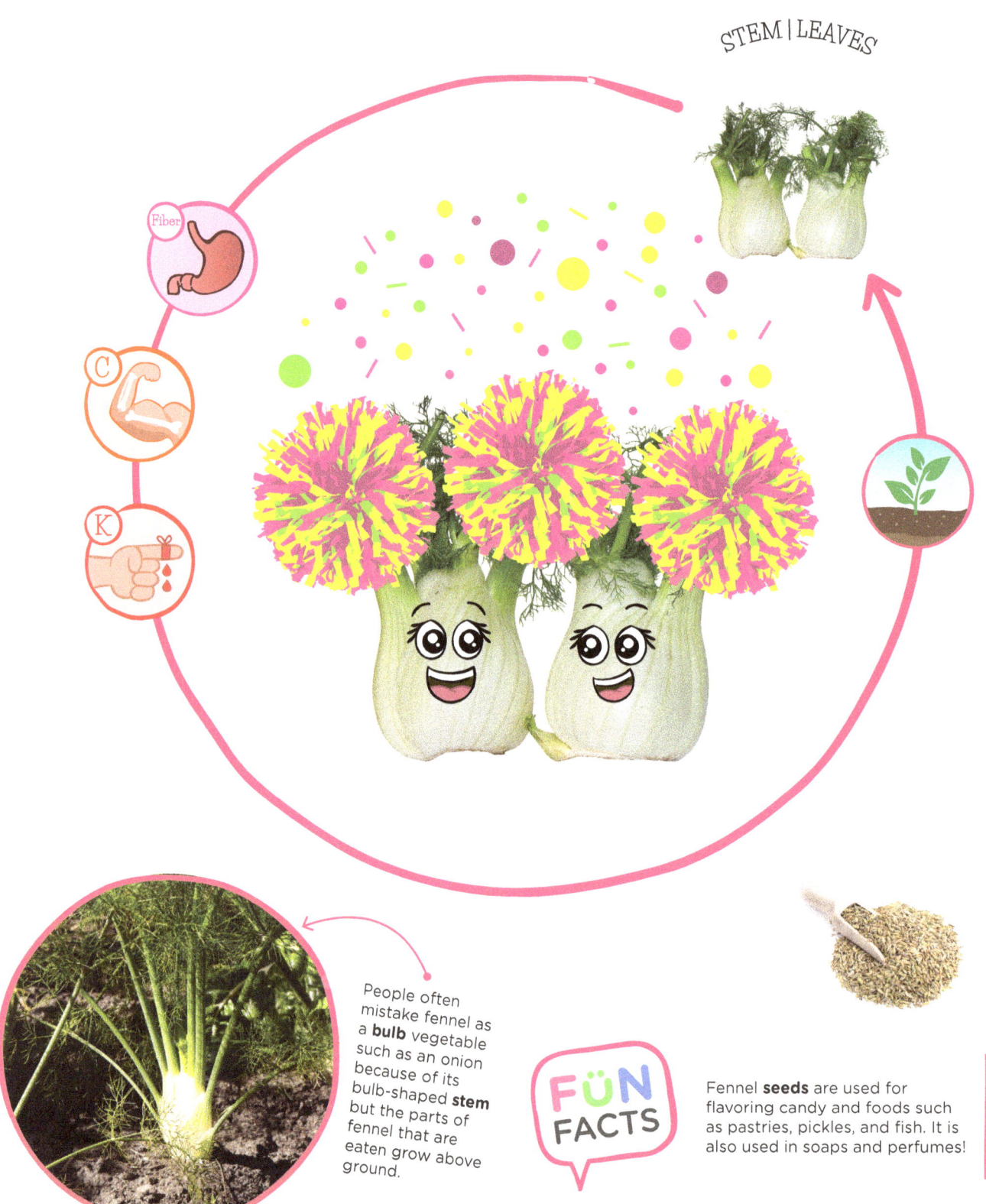

STEM | LEAVES

People often mistake fennel as a **bulb** vegetable such as an onion because of its bulb-shaped **stem** but the parts of fennel that are eaten grow above ground.

FUN FACTS

Fennel **seeds** are used for flavoring candy and foods such as pastries, pickles, and fish. It is also used in soaps and perfumes!

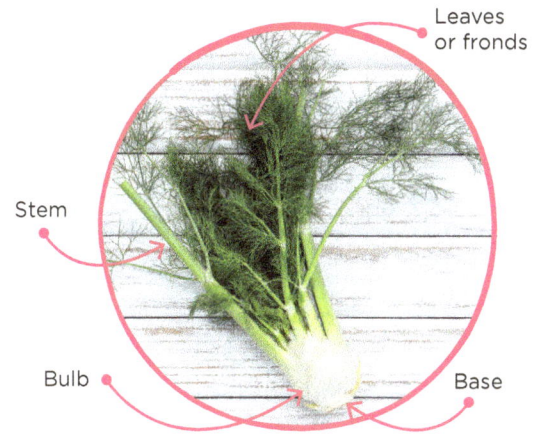

- Leaves or fronds
- Stem
- Bulb
- Base

PICK
Pick white, small, firm, **plump**, clean bulbs that feel heavy for their size. Fennel stems and **leaves** should be crisp and look clean. Avoid fennel with any browning or signs of cracking.

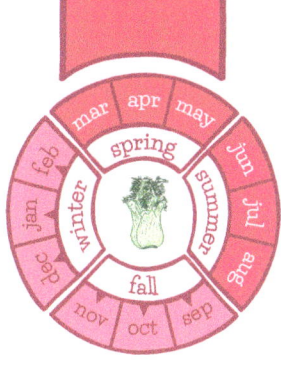

Varieties available year-round

Peak Season
September-February

STORE
Refrigerate unwashed, raw fennel in a closed plastic bag for up to 10 days. Refrigerate cooked fennel in an airtight container for 3-5 days.

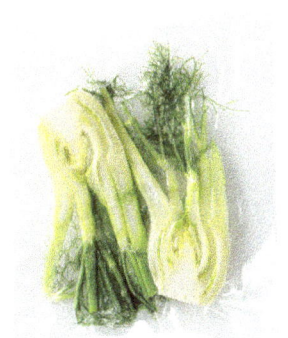

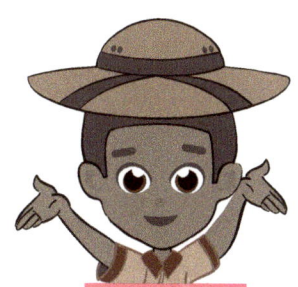

FENNEL TIDBITS

Do you like licorice? Fennel is known for having a licorice-like flavor!

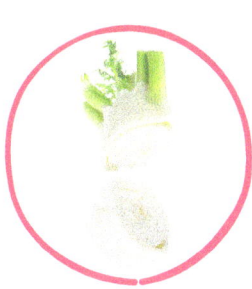

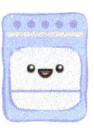
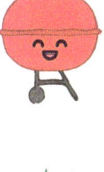
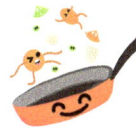

EAT
Clean the skin, cut off the base, and slice or chop bulb per recipe. Save the **fronds** to garnish your dish!

Raw Fennel Slaw
Thinly chop 1 large fennel bulb into small strips. Make a **vinaigrette** by combining 1 small chopped shallot, 2 ounces of olive oil, 2 tablespoons of lemon juice, 1 tablespoon of chopped fresh mint, 1 1/2 teaspoons of sugar, 1/2 teaspoon Dijon mustard, and 1/2 teaspoon salt in a blender and mix until smooth. Combine fennel and vinaigrette then **marinate** in the refrigerator for at least an hour.

There are two types of **edible** fennel. One is **classified** as a bulb-like vegetable and the other is treated as an **herb**. The bulb-like vegetable has stems that can be eaten raw like celery and the bulb can be **prepared** like onions. The herb's fronds and seeds are used as a seasoning in many dishes from soups to sausages.

A Book of Vegetables

FIDDLEHEAD FERN

[fid-dle-head furn]

bitter, crunchy, earthy, grassy, nutty

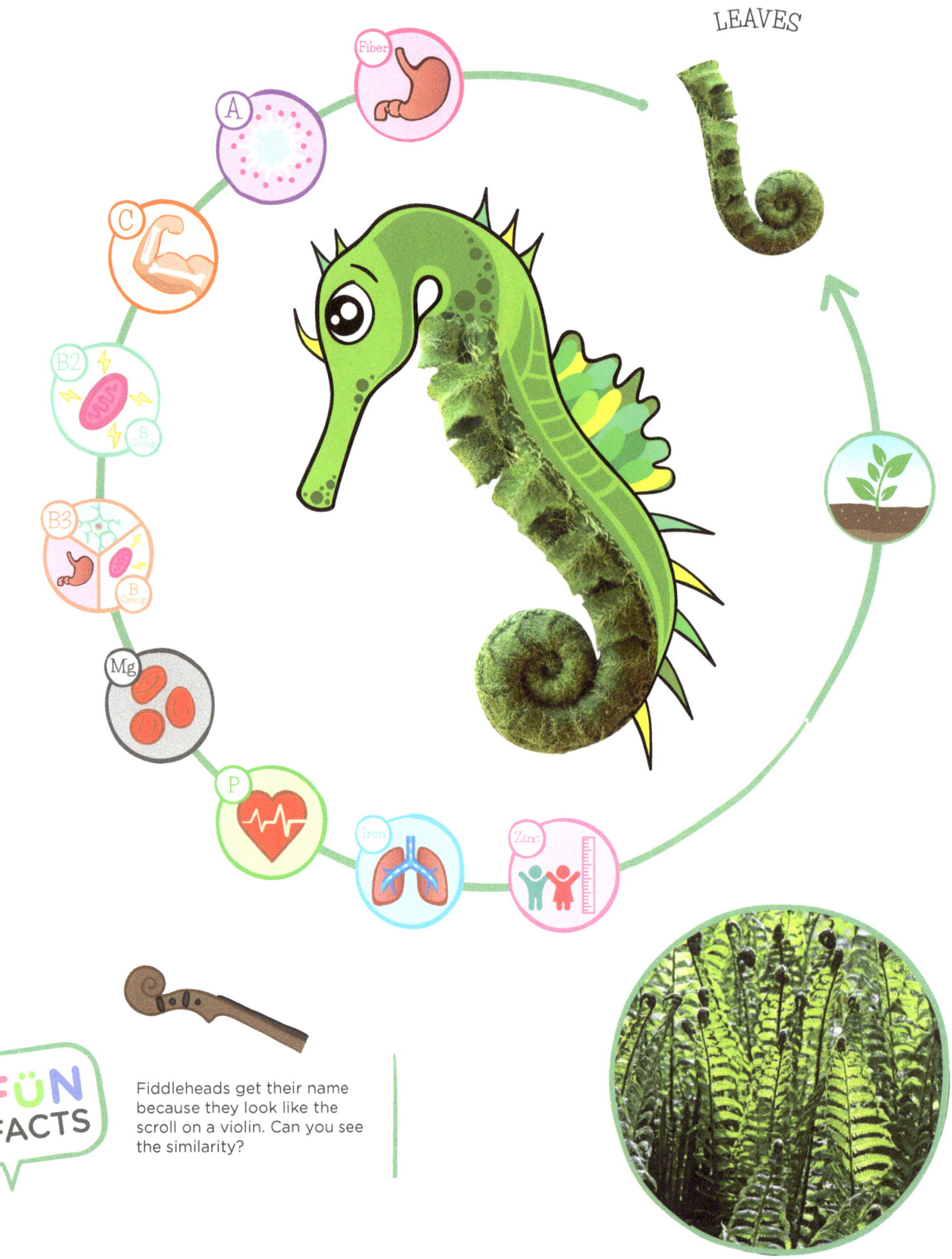

LEAVES

FUN FACTS

Fiddleheads get their name because they look like the scroll on a violin. Can you see the similarity?

72 | Where Does Broccoli Come From?

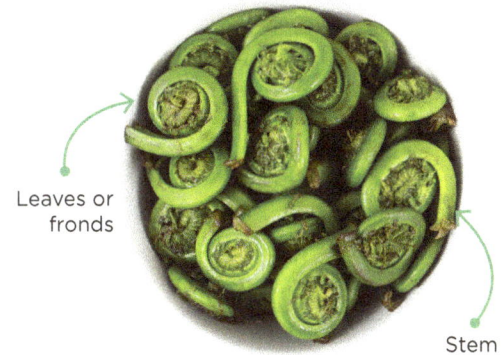
Leaves or fronds
Stem

PICK
Pick bright green, small, tightly curled **fronds**. Avoid fiddleheads with browning, yellowing, or soft spots.

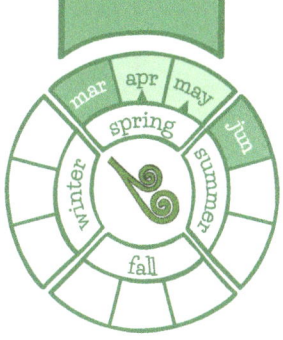
Available March to June

Peak Season
April-May

STORE
Refrigerate unwashed, raw fiddleheads in a closed plastic bag for up to 2 days. Refrigerate cooked fiddleheads in an airtight container for 3-5 days.

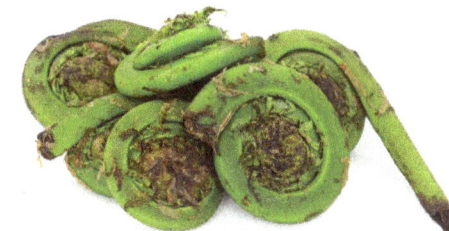

Fiddleheads are grown close to the ground and should be cooked thoroughly before eating to prevent **food borne illnesses**.

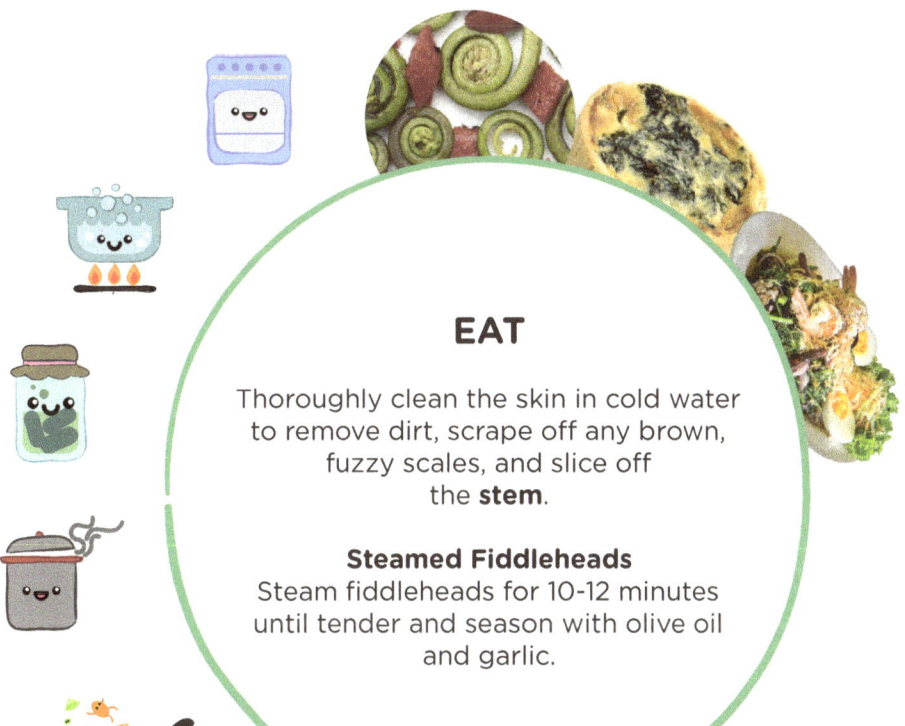

EAT
Thoroughly clean the skin in cold water to remove dirt, scrape off any brown, fuzzy scales, and slice off the **stem**.

Steamed Fiddleheads
Steam fiddleheads for 10-12 minutes until tender and season with olive oil and garlic.

FIDDLEHEADS TIDBITS

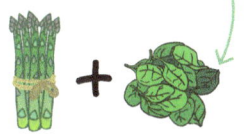

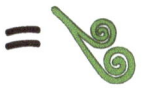

The flavor of fiddleheads is often compared to a cross between asparagus and baby spinach.

Not all fiddlehead ferns are edible. If you **forage**, be sure to talk to a local plant expert to ensure they are safe to eat.

A Book of Vegetables

HEARTS OF PALM
PALMITO

[harts of pal-mm] | [palm-e-to]

crisp, delicate, nutty, sweet, tender

SHOOTS

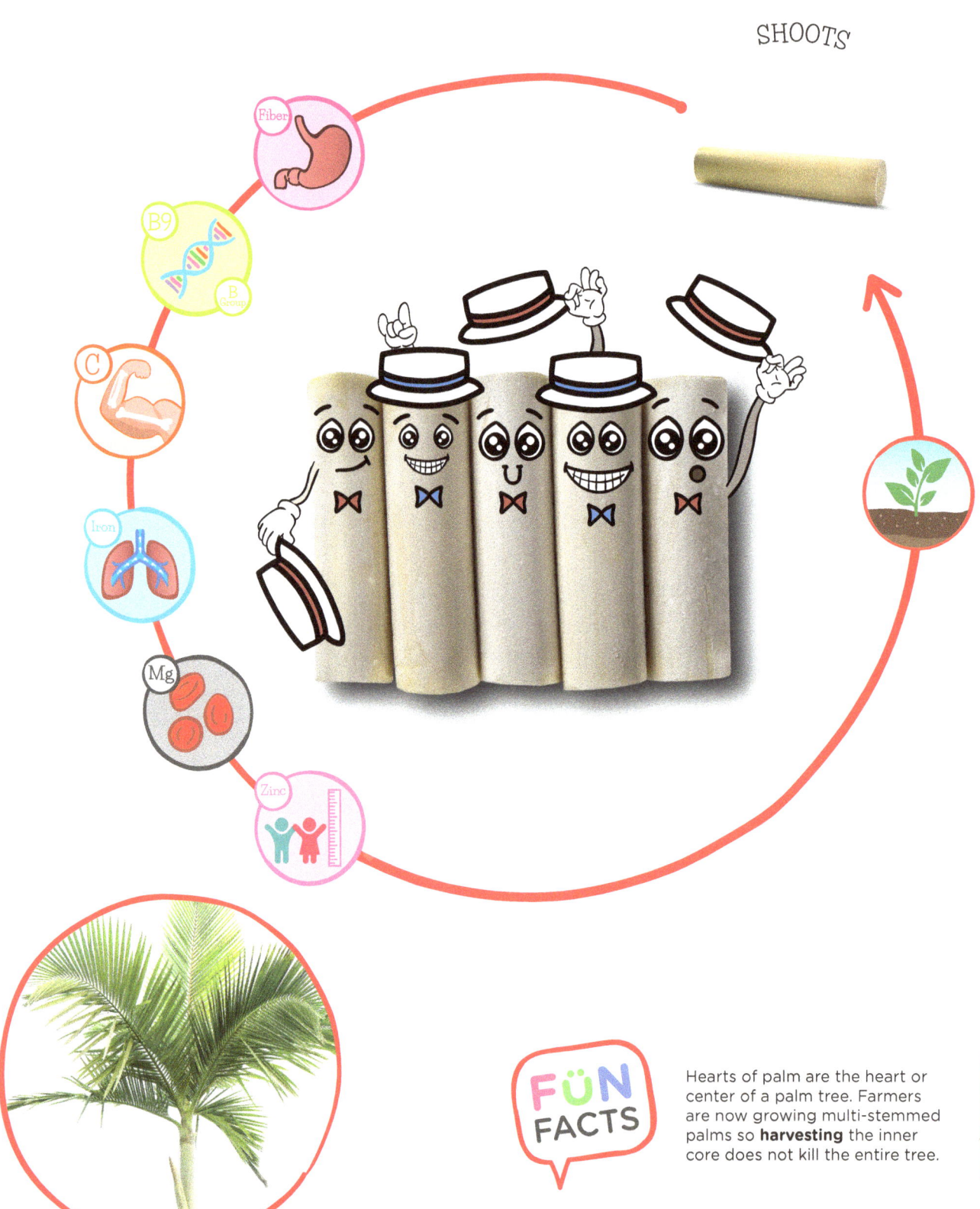

FUN FACTS: Hearts of palm are the heart or center of a palm tree. Farmers are now growing multi-stemmed palms so **harvesting** the inner core does not kill the entire tree.

74 | Where Does Broccoli Come From?

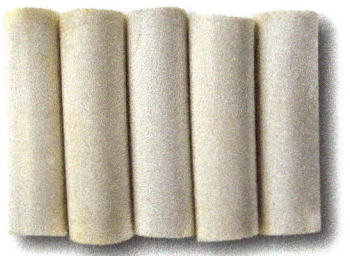

PICK
Hearts of palm are typically only sold canned or jarred outside of the countries where they grow because they **spoil** very quickly. For fresh hearts of palm, pick firm, intact **shoots** with a smooth surface. Avoid hearts of palm with soft spots and browning.

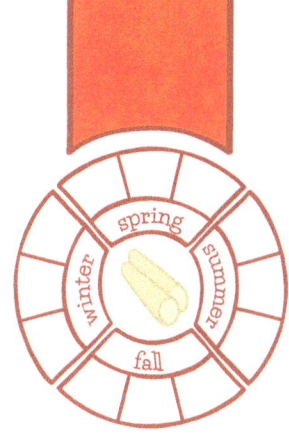

Available imported year-round

STORE
Refrigerate fresh hearts of palm in an airtight container for up to 14 days and opened canned or jarred hearts of palm for 3-4 days.

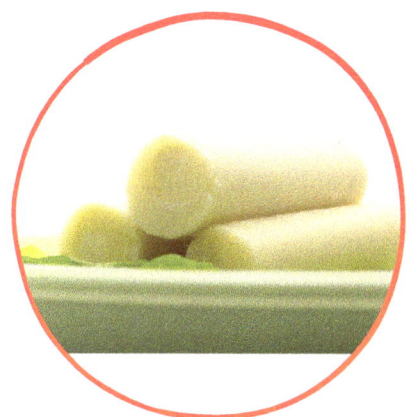

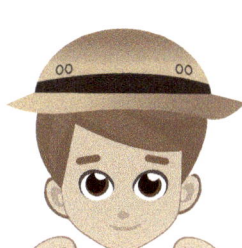

HEARTS OF PALM TIDBITS

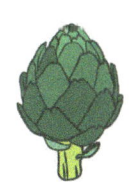

The flavor of hearts of palm is often compared to the earthy, nutty flavor of artichoke.

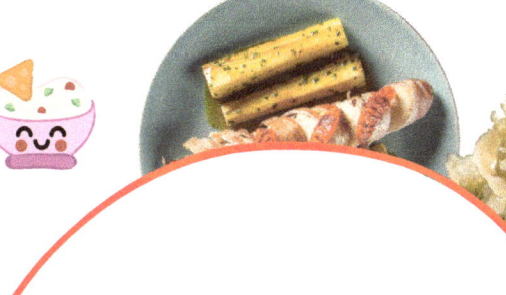

EAT
Clean the skin of fresh hearts of palm or drain canned or jarred shoots. Chop or slice per recipe.

Raw Hearts of Palm
Add hearts of palm to your favorite salad or try adding slices to a stir-fry.

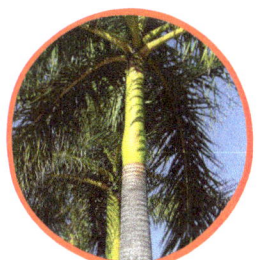

Varieties come from many different palm trees including the coconut palm and the acai palm.

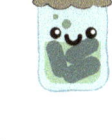
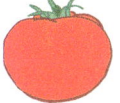
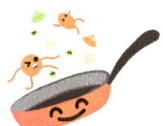
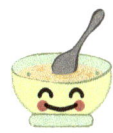
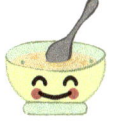

A Book of Vegetables

JERUSALEM ARTICHOKE
SUNCHOKE

[Je-ru-sa-lem ar-ti-choke] | [sun-choke]

crunchy, delicate, nutty, starchy, sweet

TUBER

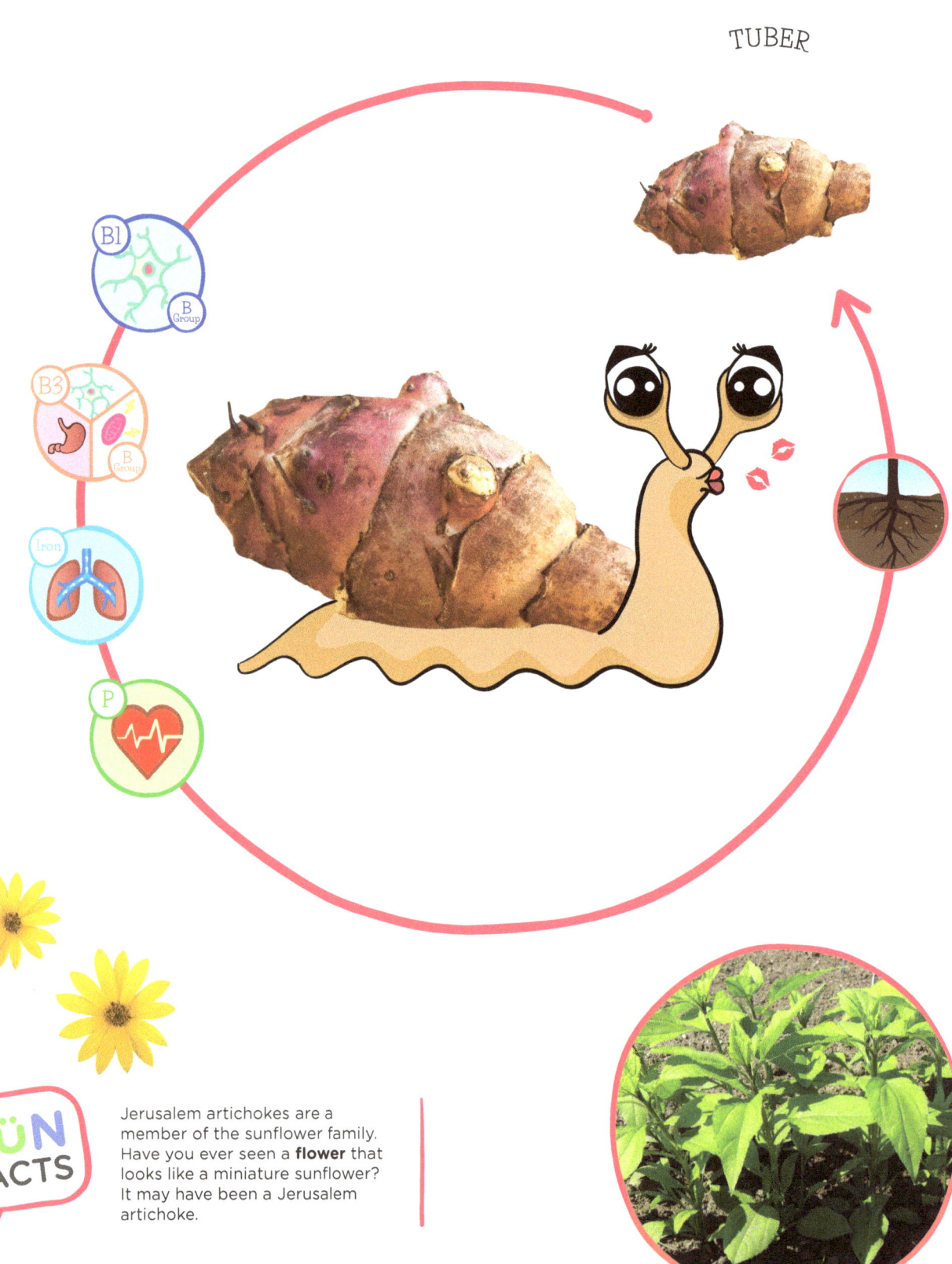

FUN FACTS

Jerusalem artichokes are a member of the sunflower family. Have you ever seen a **flower** that looks like a miniature sunflower? It may have been a Jerusalem artichoke.

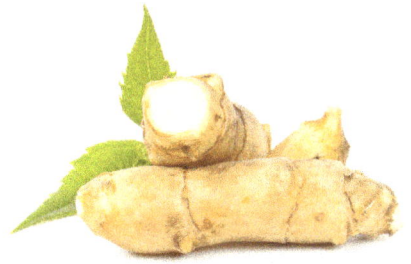

PICK
Pick tan, brown, or rose-colored **tubers** with skin that have few knobby bumps. Avoid Jerusalem artichokes with wrinkled skin, soft spots, and **sprouts**.

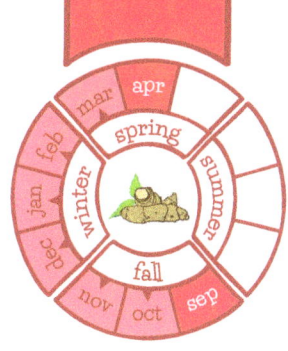

Available September to April; Imported year-round

Peak Season
October-March

STORE
Refrigerate raw Jerusalem artichoke in a dry paper towel in an open plastic bag for up to 14 days. Refrigerate cooked Jerusalem artichoke in an airtight container for 3-5 days.

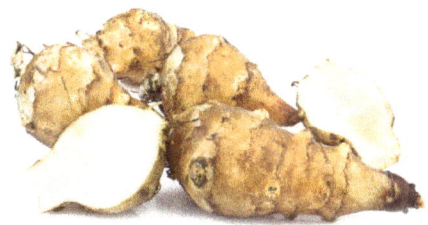

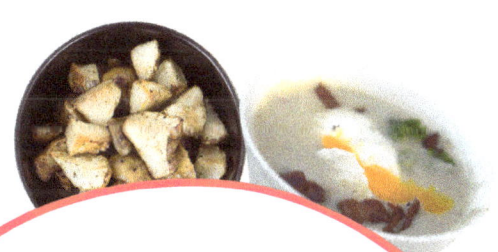

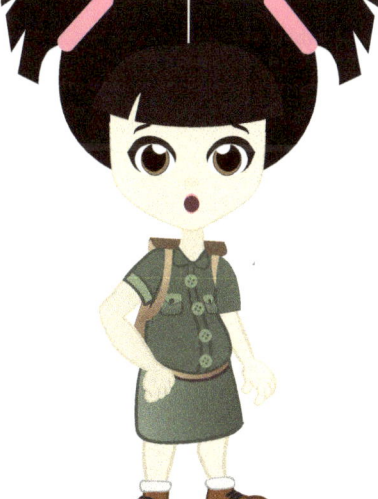

Jerusalem artichoke is a natural source of **inulin**, a type of fiber that cannot be digested by the body and may make you toot!

EAT
Clean the skin with a vegetable brush, peel if desired, and chop or slice per recipe.

Grilled Jerusalem Artichokes
Slice Jerusalem artichokes into 1/2 inch chunks, toss with olive oil, and season with salt and pepper. Then place directly on a well-**greased** hot grill for 6-8 minutes. Turn chunks occasionally until tender and can be easily **pierced** with a fork.

A Book of Vegetables 77

JICAMA
YAM BEAN

[hee-kah-ma] | [yeah-m been]

crisp, juicy, mild, nutty, sweet

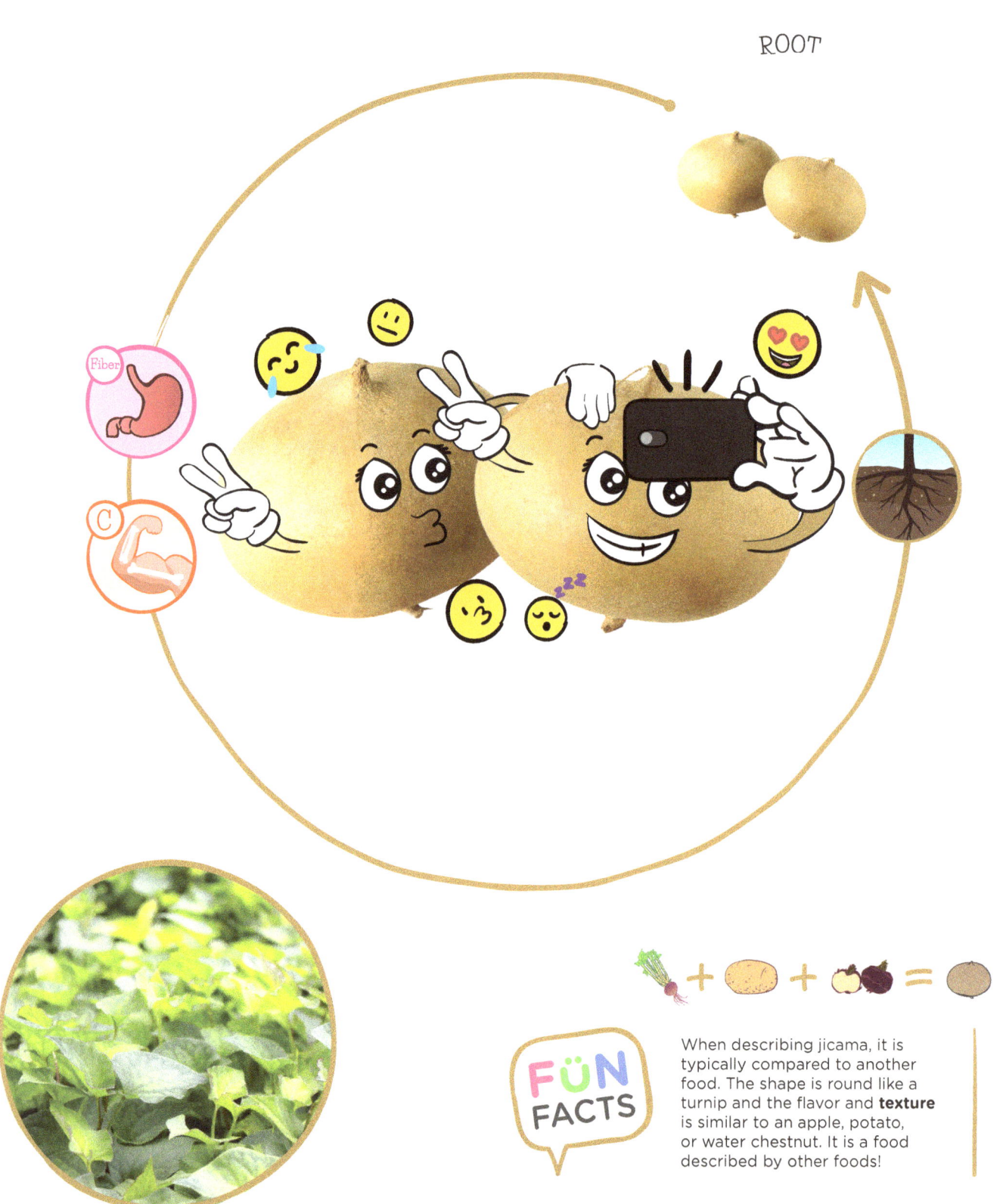

ROOT

When describing jicama, it is typically compared to another food. The shape is round like a turnip and the flavor and **texture** is similar to an apple, potato, or water chestnut. It is a food described by other foods!

78 | Where Does Broccoli Come From?

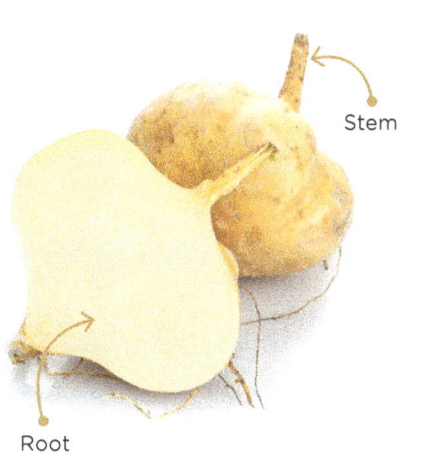

Stem

Root

PICK
Pick firm, smooth, small to medium-sized **roots** that feel heavy for their size. Avoid jicama with soft spots.

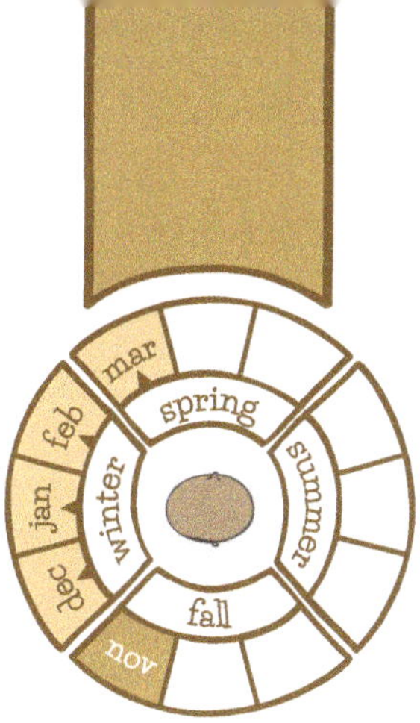

STORE
Refrigerate raw, loose, jicama without plastic for up to 14 days. Refrigerate cooked jicama in an airtight container for 3-5 days.

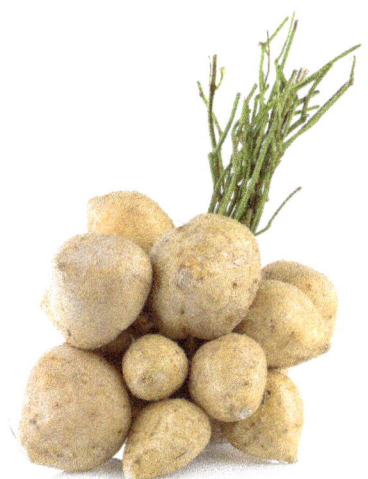

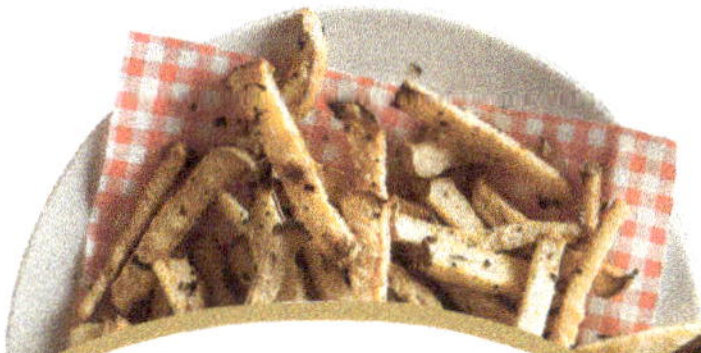

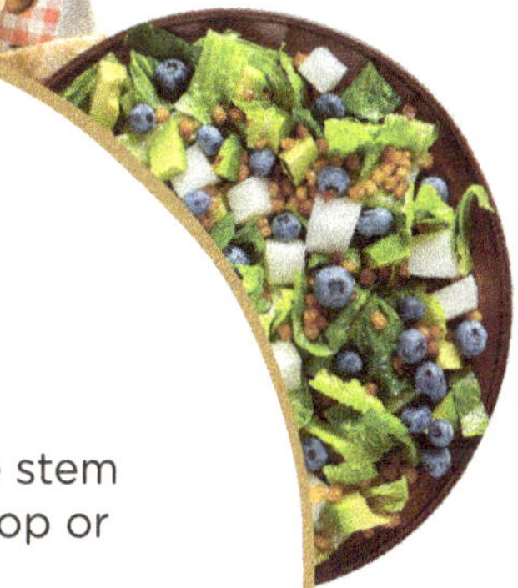

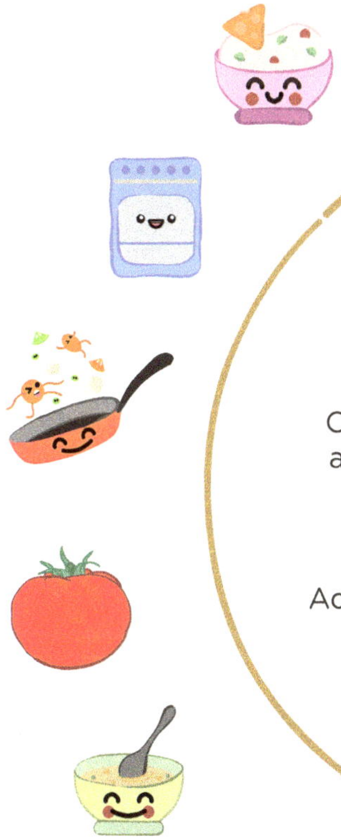

Available November to March; Imported year-round

Peak Season
December-March

EAT
Clean the skin, slice off the stem and root end, peel, and chop or slice per recipe.

Stir-fried Jicama
Add jicama to your favorite stir-fry recipe for a juicy crunch.

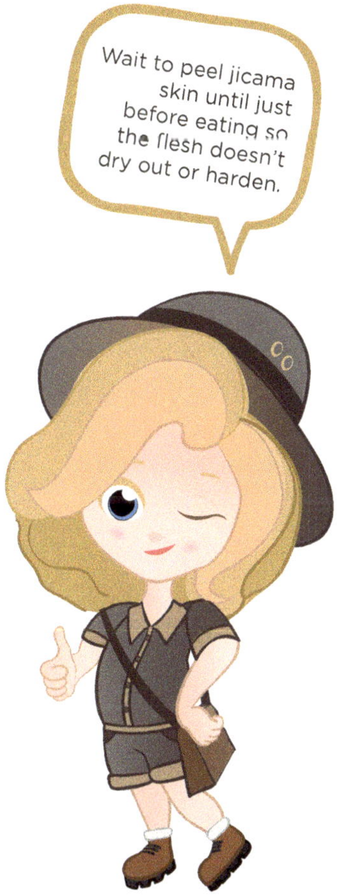

Wait to peel jicama skin until just before eating so the flesh doesn't dry out or harden.

A Book of Vegetables

KALE

[kay-el]

bitter, earthy, mild, tender, tough

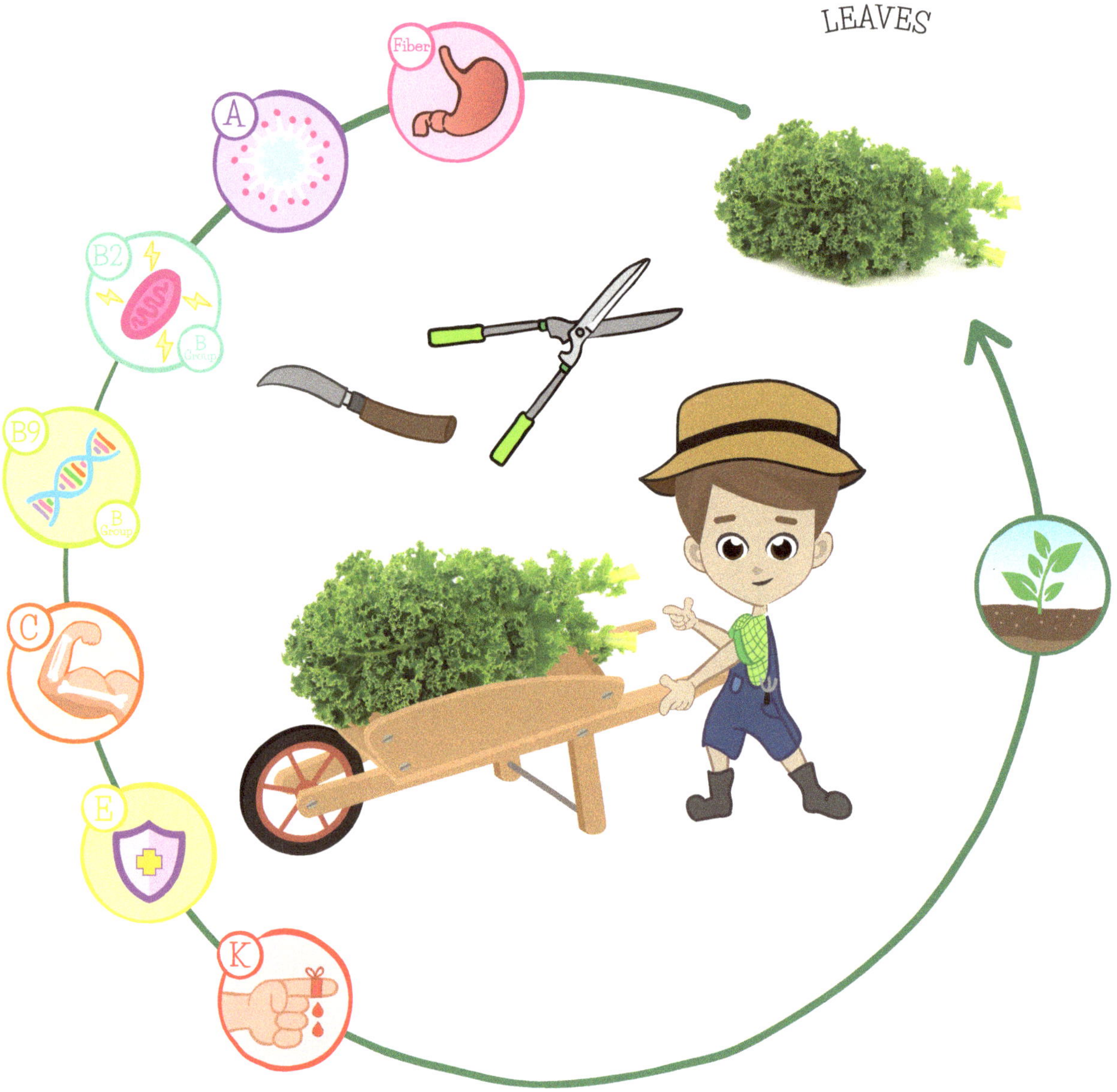

LEAVES

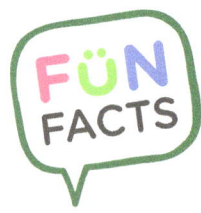

Kale comes in all different shapes, sizes, and colors. Kale can be red like red curly kale, ruffled and vibrant like purple kale, or have blue green leaves like dinosaur kale. Whichever kale you choose, a serving of kale may have more **calcium** than a glass of milk!

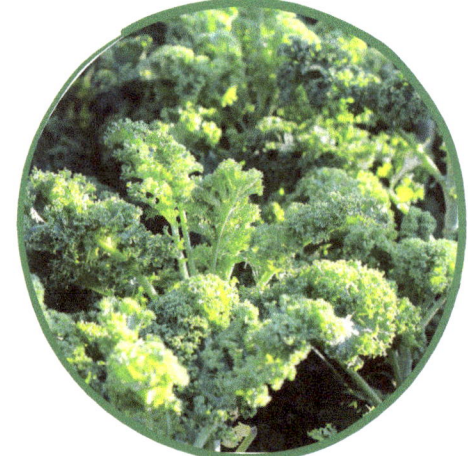

80 | Where Does Broccoli Come From?

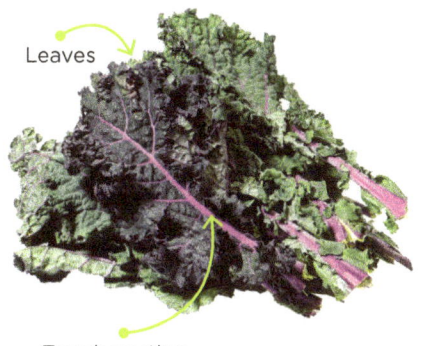

Leaves

Tough portion of the stem

PICK
Pick deep, vibrantly colored **leaves** that feel crisp to touch. Avoid dull, limp, kale with brown or yellow leaves.

STORE
Refrigerate unwashed, raw kale in an open plastic bag for up to 7 days. Refrigerate cooked kale in an airtight container for 3-5 days.

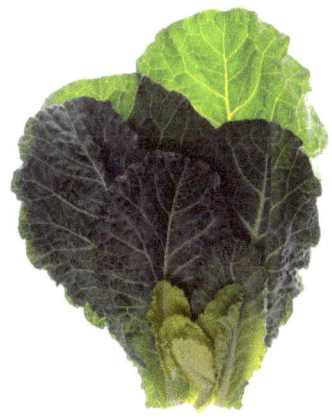

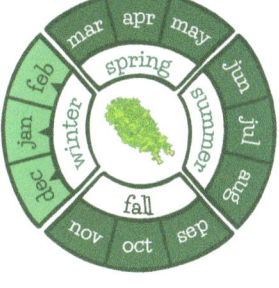

Varieties available year-round

Peak Season
December-February

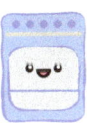

Check out page 61 (Collard Greens) for tips on how to remove the tough portion of the **stem**.

KALE TIDBITS

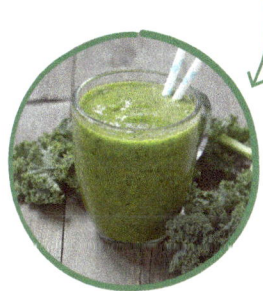

Kale stems are **edible**! Decrease food waste and save the tough stems for juicing, pesto, sautéing, or vegetable **stock**.

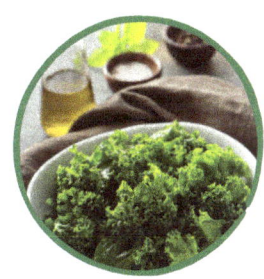

If you are planning to eat raw kale, massage tough leaves with olive oil, lemon juice, and salt, then allow it to **marinate** for about 30 minutes to soften the leaves.

EAT
Clean the leaves several times to remove all dirt and sand. For large, mature leaves, fold each leaf in half lengthwise (hot dog style) and slice off the tough portion of the stem or **spine**. Stack several of the leaves on top of each other, roll into a large bunch, and cut leaves into thick slices or chop per recipe. For baby kale, **prepare** it the same way as spinach.

Baked Kale Chips
Preheat your oven to 350 degrees F. Chop kale leaves into chip-sized pieces, toss with olive oil, and season with salt. Spread kale in a single layer on a parchment paper-lined roasting tray and bake for 10-15 minutes until the edges are crisp and brown.

A Book of Vegetables

KOHLRABI AND GREENS

[cole-ra-be]

crisp, mild, peppery, sweet, tangy

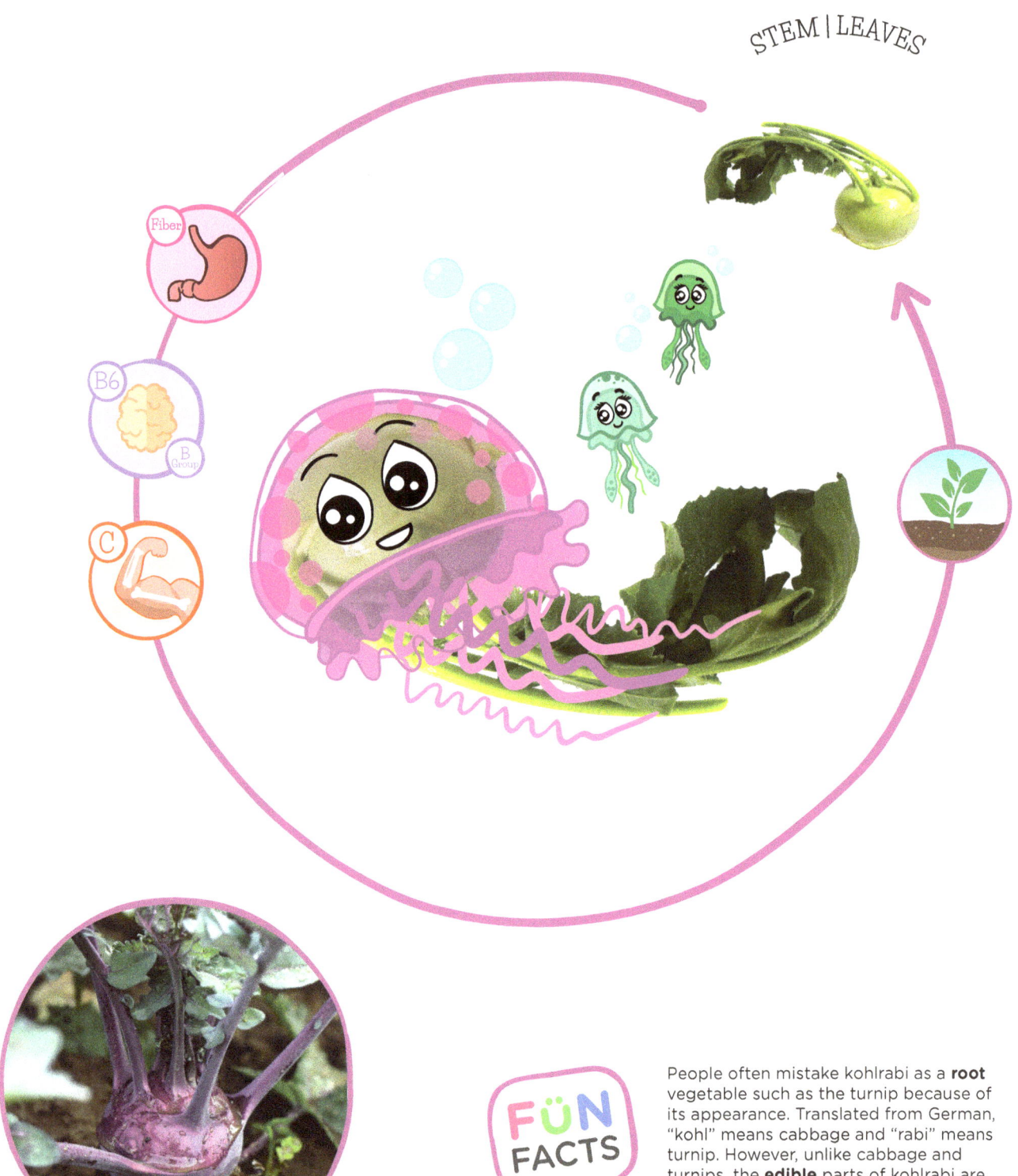

STEM | LEAVES

FUN FACTS

People often mistake kohlrabi as a **root** vegetable such as the turnip because of its appearance. Translated from German, "kohl" means cabbage and "rabi" means turnip. However, unlike cabbage and turnips, the **edible** parts of kohlrabi are the swollen stem and leaves that grow above ground.

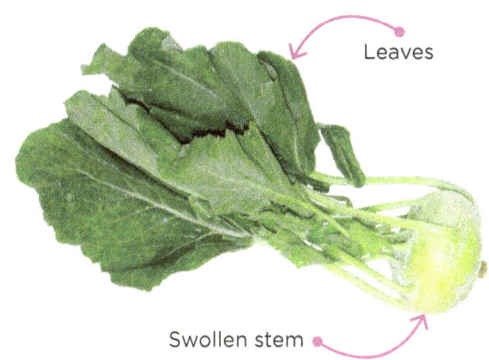
Leaves
Swollen stem

PICK
Pick small, firm **stems** with crisp, green **leaves**. Avoid kohlrabi with soft spots.

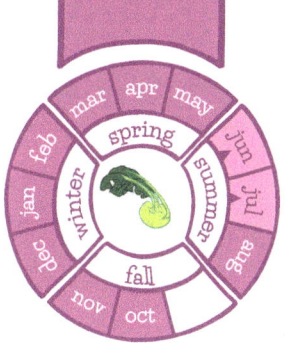

Available October to August; Imported year-round

Peak Season
June-July

STORE
Refrigerate raw kohlrabi in an open plastic bag for up to 5 days. Refrigerate cooked kohlrabi in an airtight container for 3-5 days. Kohlrabi greens should be refrigerated separately in an airtight container for 2-3 days.

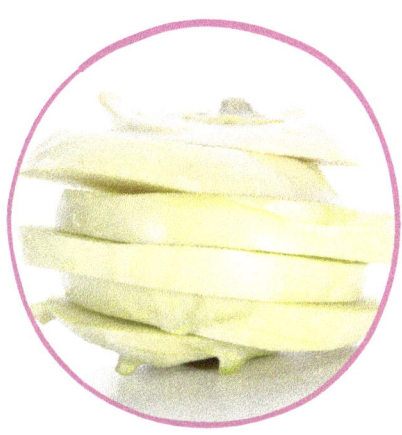

KOHLRABI COLORS

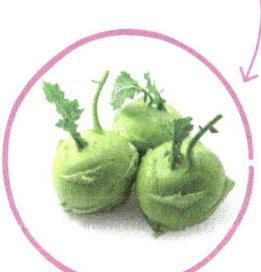

Save the stems and leaves of kohlrabi to use in place of collard greens or kale in recipes.

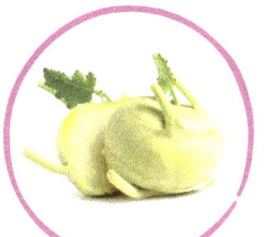

EAT
Clean the skin, slice off the leaves if they are still attached, peel skin if desired, and chop or slice per recipe.

Roasted Kohlrabi
Preheat your oven to 450 degrees F. Chop kohlrabi into wedges, toss with olive oil, and season with garlic salt and pepper. Spread in a single layer on a foil-lined roasting tray, roast for 15-20 minutes, turning occasionally, until evenly browned.

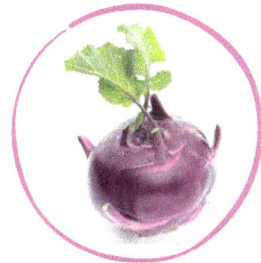

Colors vary depending on **variety**. Kohlrabi can be green, white, or purple.

A Book of Vegetables 83

LETTUCE AND SALAD GREENS

[lett-us]

crisp, mild, peppery, sweet, watery

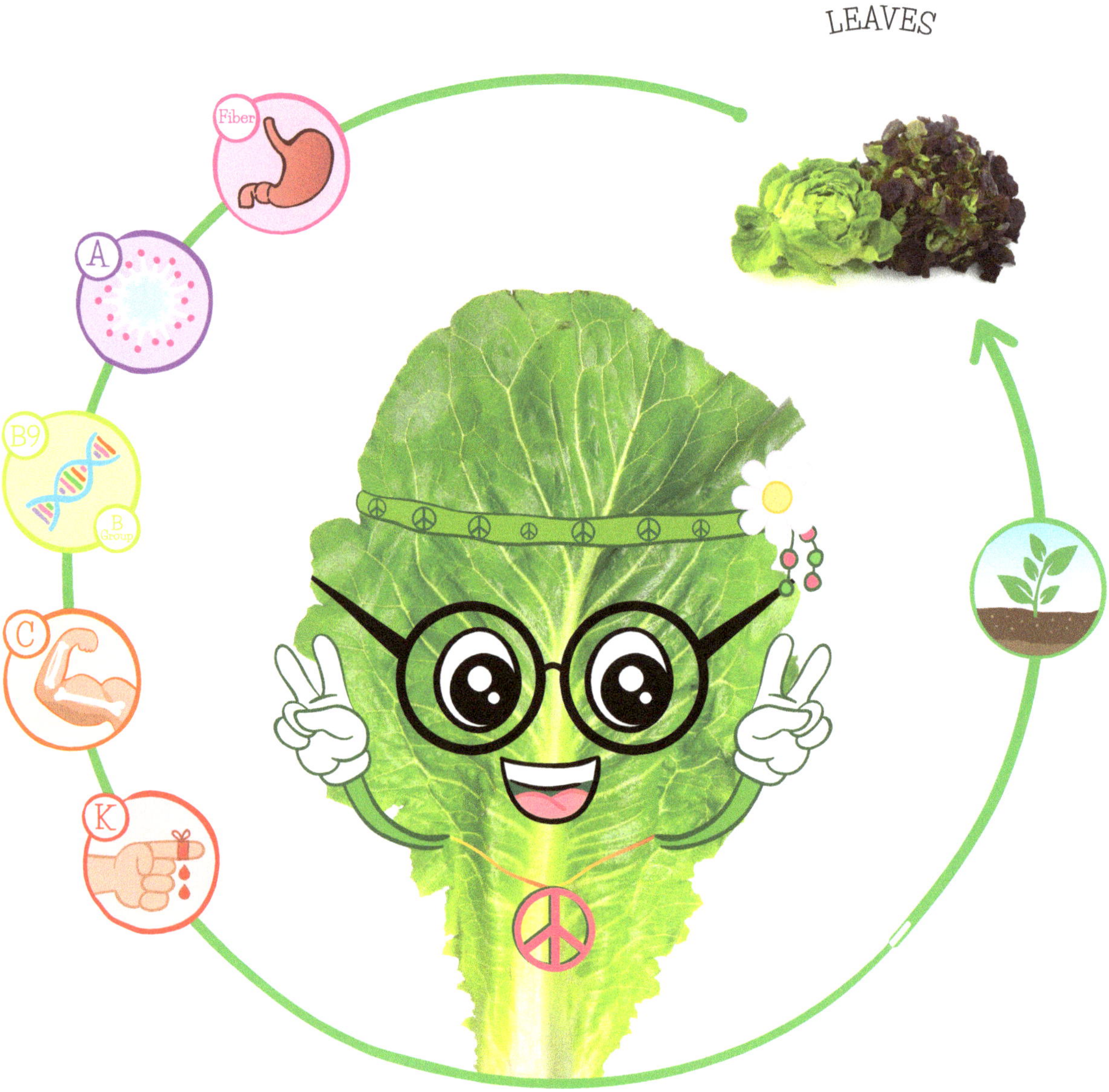

LEAVES

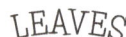

Heads

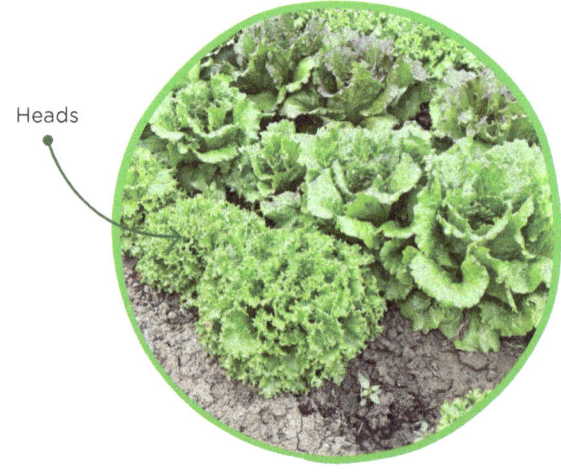

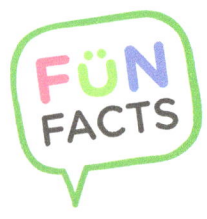 Lettuce varieties come in all different shapes, sizes, colors, and flavors. There are five common types of lettuce: butterhead (Bibb), cos (romaine), crisphead (iceberg), leaf (green leaf), and **stem** (celtuce).

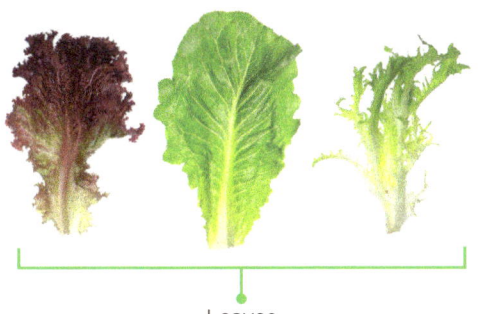
Leaves

PICK
Pick brightly colored, crisp **leaves**. Avoid lettuce with **wilting** leaves. Headed varieties of lettuce should be firm. Colors are different depending on **variety**.

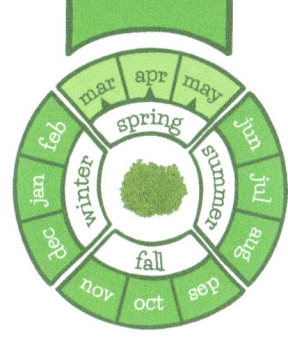

Varieties available year-round

Peak Season
March-May

STORE
Refrigerate unwashed, loosely packed leaves and heads in a closed plastic bag up to 7 days. Lettuce with **roots** still attached may sit on a countertop with roots in water for 5-7 days or per packaging recommendations. For commercially packaged lettuce and salad greens, look at the "Best By" date.

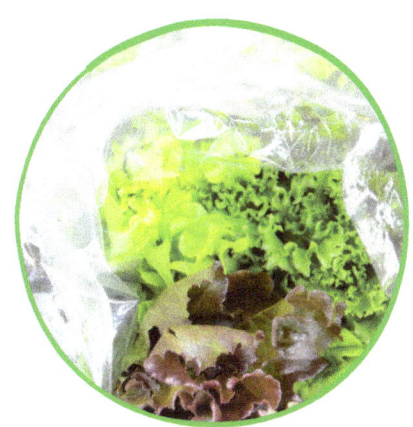

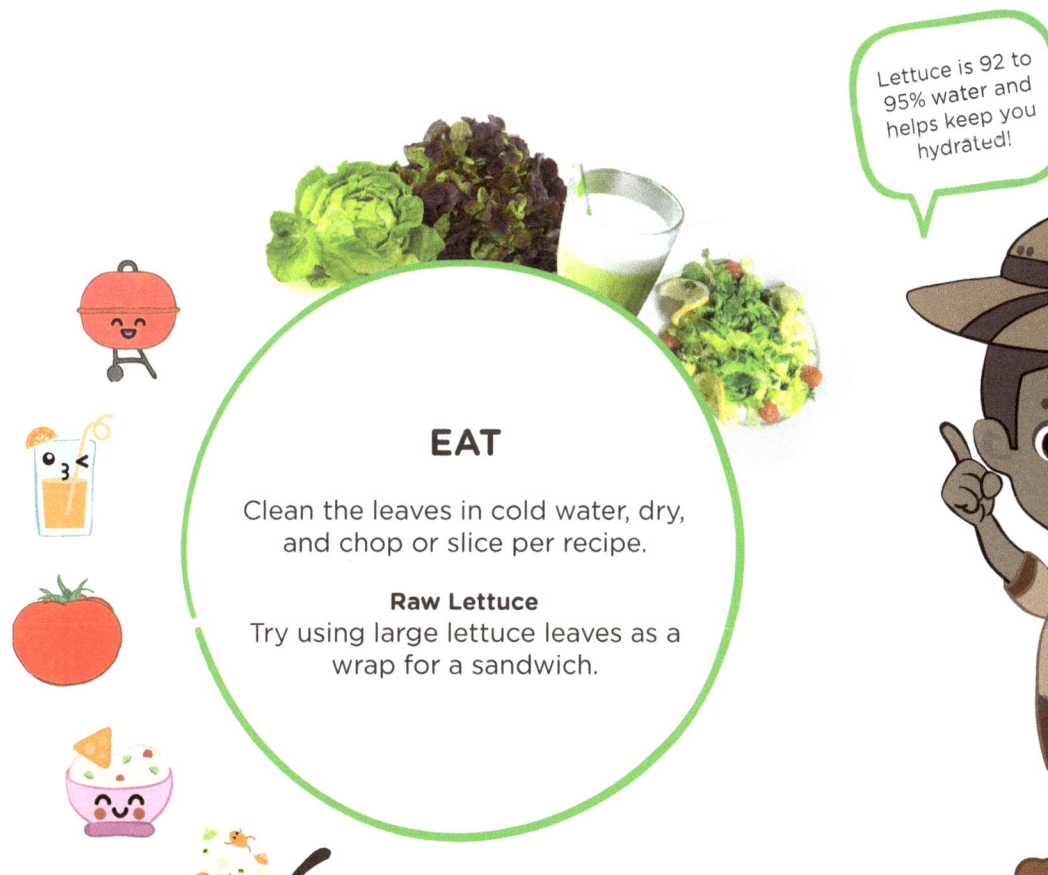

EAT
Clean the leaves in cold water, dry, and chop or slice per recipe.

Raw Lettuce
Try using large lettuce leaves as a wrap for a sandwich.

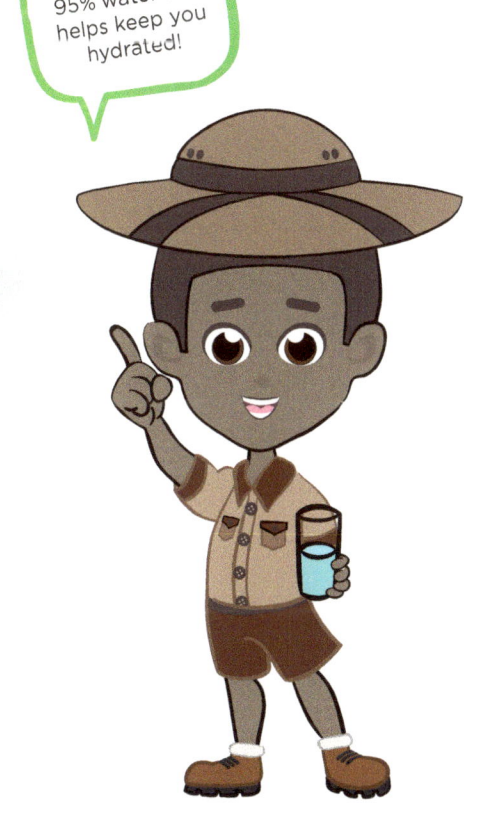

Lettuce is 92 to 95% water and helps keep you hydrated!

A Book of Vegetables 85

LETTUCE VARIETIES

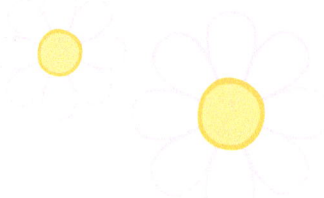

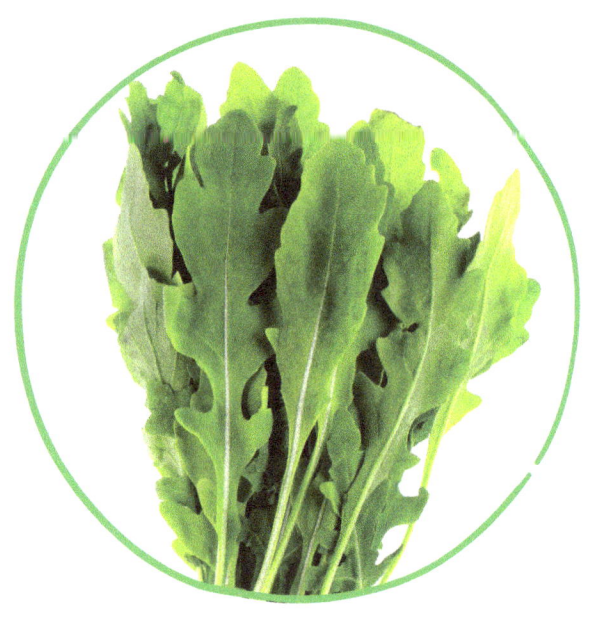

ARUGULA [AROO-GU-LA]

A pungent and peppery salad green that is a perfect addition to sandwiches, pasta, and grains. Other names for this leafy green include rocket and rucola.

BUTTERHEAD (BIBB) [BIB]

A type of head lettuce with soft, tender **leaves**, and a sweet delicate flavor.

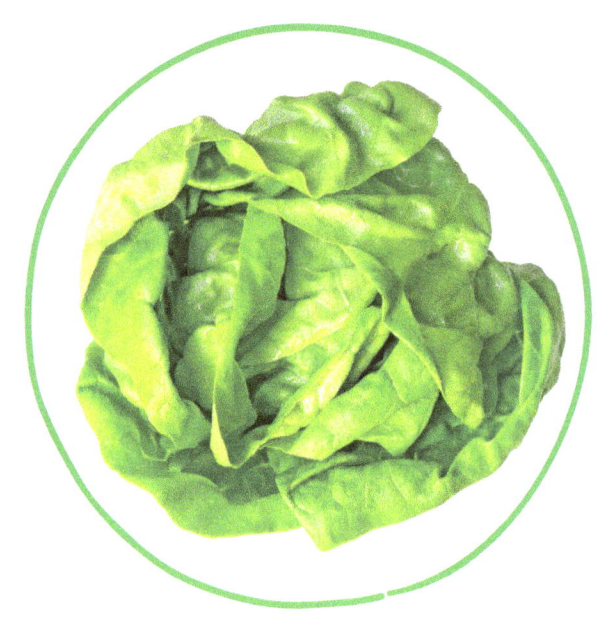

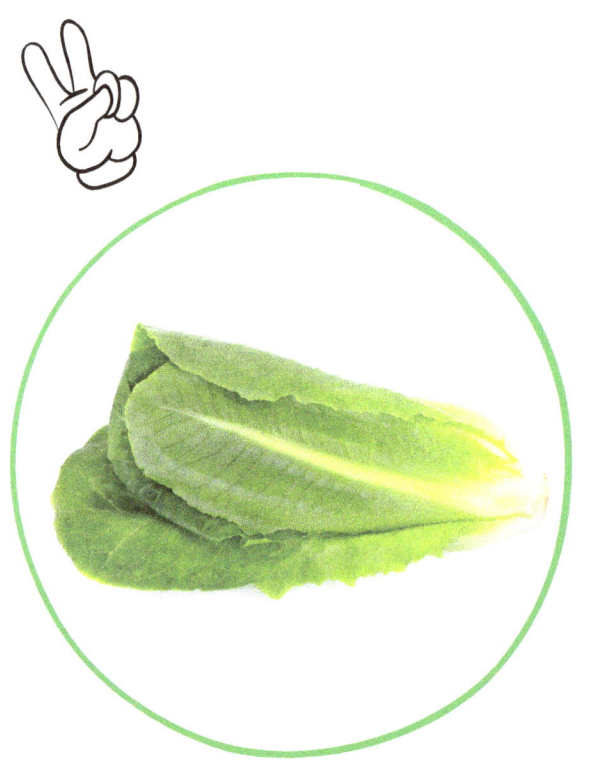

COS (ROMAINE) [RO-MAIN]

Romaine is a hearty leaf lettuce with a thick, slightly bitter, center rib, and a big crunch.

CRISPHEAD (ICEBERG) [AHYS-BURG]

Iceberg lettuce is the most commonly eaten and least nutrient dense lettuce. It is very mild in flavor and has a crisp **texture**.

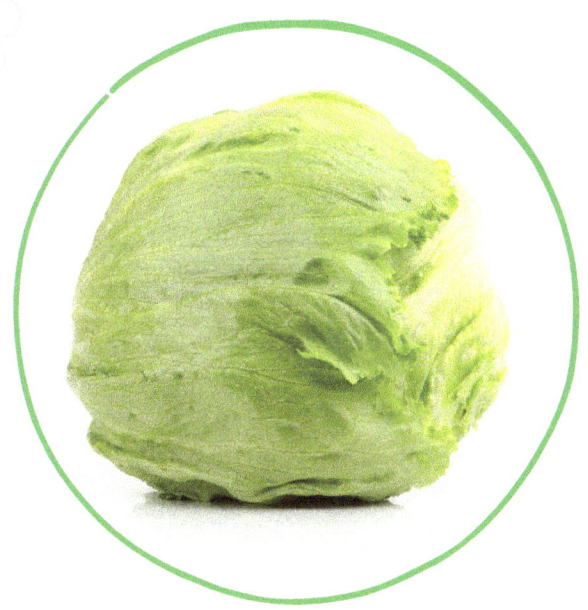

ENDIVE [EN-DIVE]

There are three main **varieties** of the salad green endive:

- Belgian endive is slightly bitter and silky in texture. It's scoop shape makes it perfect for dipping or using like a chip.

- Curly endive or frisée is slightly bitter and peppery in flavor. It's crunchy **stem** makes it a great addition to salads.

- Escarole is mildly bitter, crisp, and often added to soups.

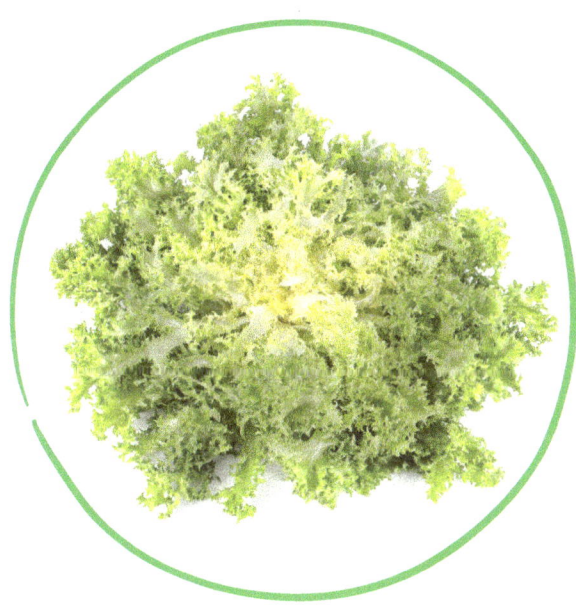

LEAF (GREEN LEAF) [GREEN LEEF]

Green leaf lettuce is the most commonly grown lettuce in home gardens. It is semi-crisp and mild in flavor.

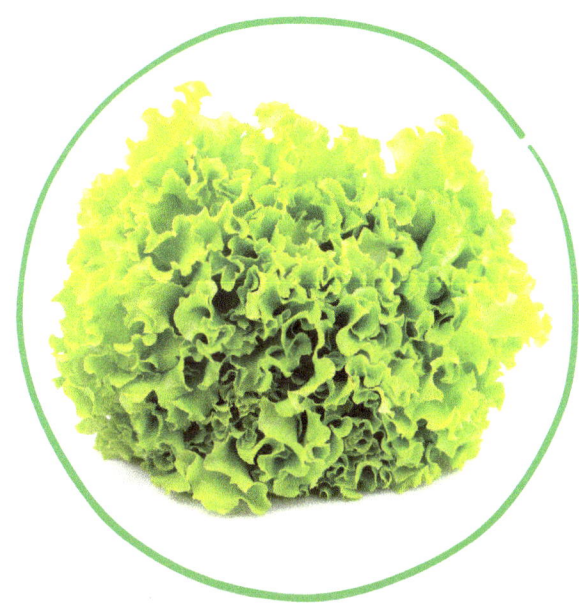

A Book of Vegetables

MUSHROOM

[mush-room]

earthy, meaty, moist, rich, tender

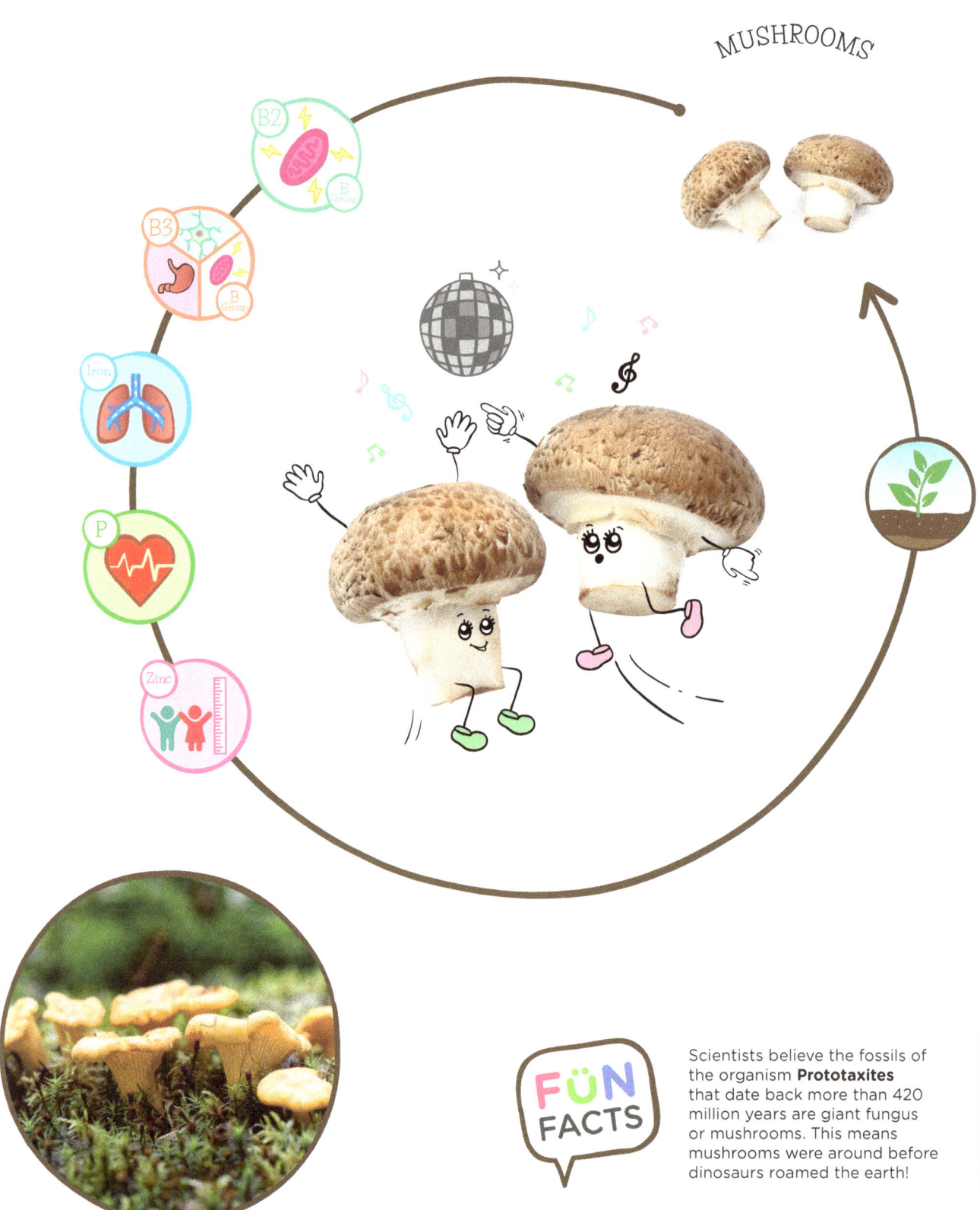

MUSHROOMS

FUN FACTS

Scientists believe the fossils of the organism **Prototaxites** that date back more than 420 million years are giant fungus or mushrooms. This means mushrooms were around before dinosaurs roamed the earth!

Where Does Broccoli Come From?

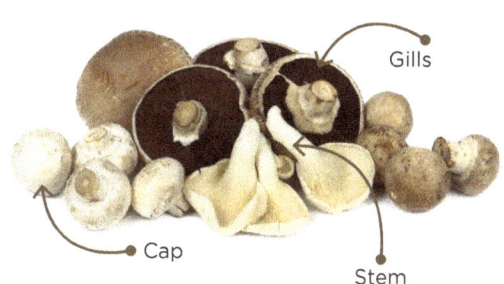

PICK
Pick **plump**, smooth looking caps and **stems**. Avoid **mushrooms** with **bruises**, soft spots, slime and a sour smell.

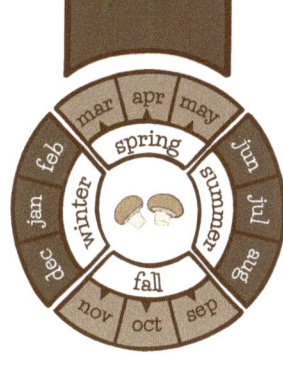

Varieties available year-round

Peak Season
March-May;
September-November

STORE
Remove from plastic packaging and refrigerate unwashed, raw mushrooms in a closed paper bag for up to 7 days and sliced mushrooms for 1-2 days. Refrigerate cooked mushrooms in an airtight container for 3-5 days.

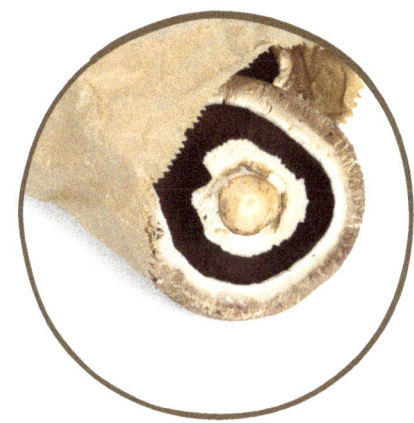

MUSHROOM TIDBITS

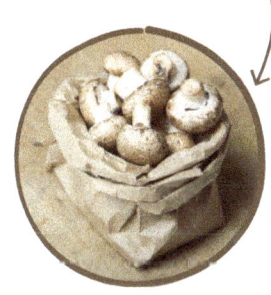

Mushrooms continue to grow after **harvesting** and "sweat" in plastic. Storing mushrooms in brown paper bags help prevent moisture from being trapped and causing them to **spoil**.

Mushrooms make a great replacement for meat.

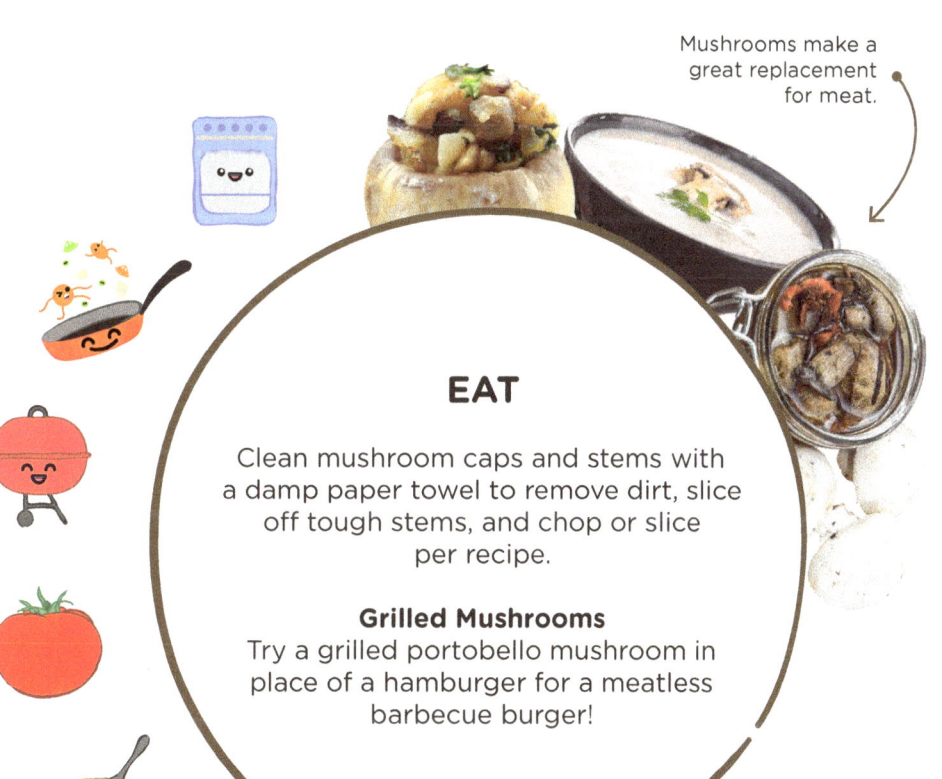

EAT
Clean mushroom caps and stems with a damp paper towel to remove dirt, slice off tough stems, and chop or slice per recipe.

Grilled Mushrooms
Try a grilled portobello mushroom in place of a hamburger for a meatless barbecue burger!

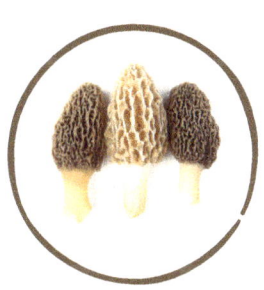

Chanterelle and Morel mushrooms are a good source of **vitamin D** which helps keep bones, teeth and, muscles healthy.

A Book of Vegetables

MUSHROOM VARIETIES

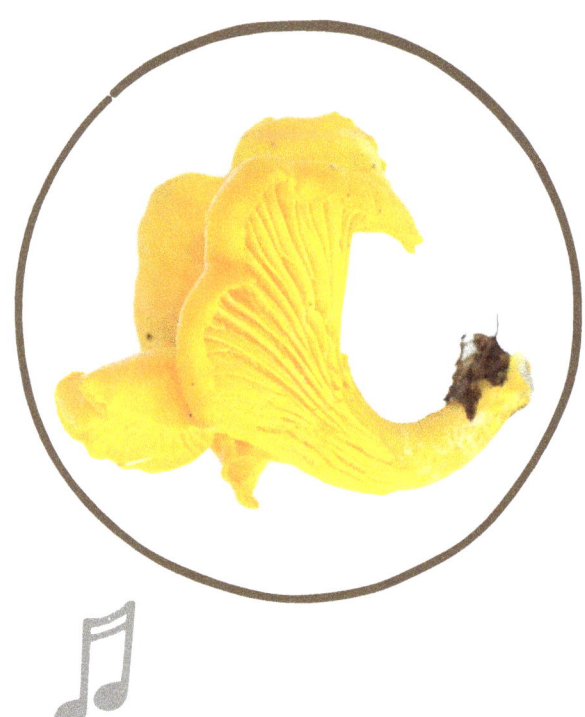

CHANTERELLE [CHAN-TE-RELLE]

Trumpetlike in appearance for both their shape and color, these **fleshy**, firm, mild flavored **mushrooms** have an apricot-like scent.

MOREL [MORE-EL]

Morel mushrooms are honeycomb in appearance, with a chewy, meaty, **texture** and an earthy, nutty flavor. They are **foraged** rather than **farmed**.

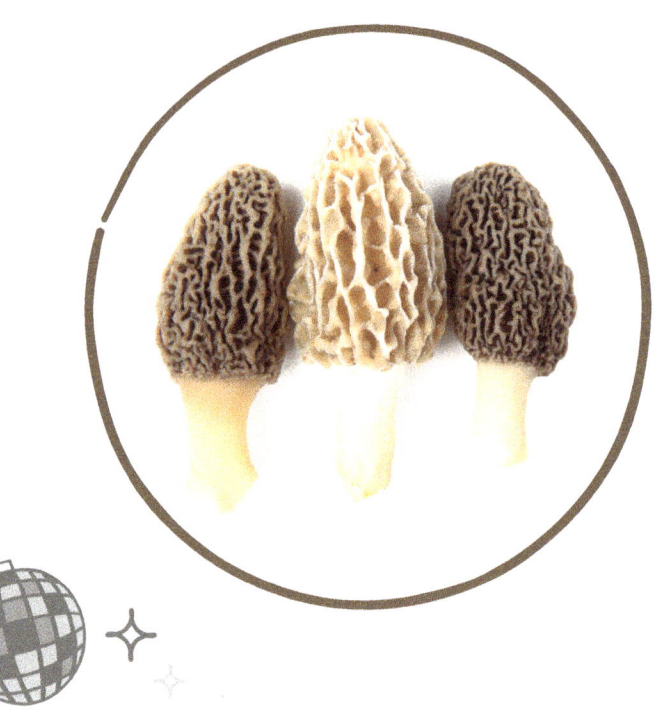

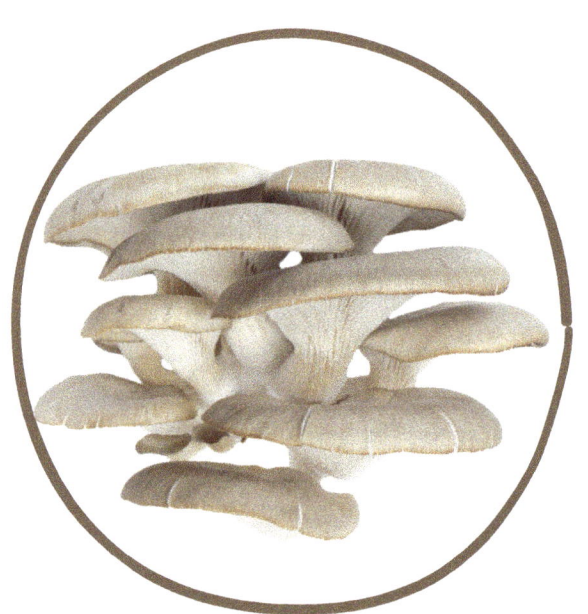

OYSTER [OYS-TER]

Fan-shaped and whitish in color, oyster mushrooms have a delicate odor, sweet flavor, and velvety texture.

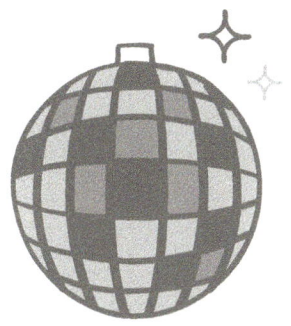

PORTOBELLO [POR-TO-BEL-LO]

Large, fully grown caps of white button mushrooms, these dense mushrooms are meaty, rich, and flavorful.

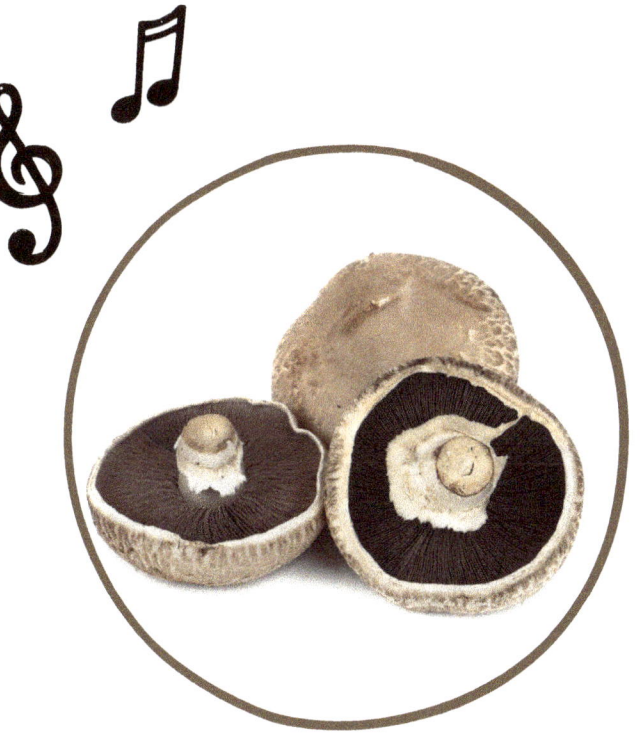

SHIITAKE [SHE-TA-KEY]

Shiitake mushrooms have a woody aroma and earthy umami flavor. Their curved **stems** should be removed before eating.

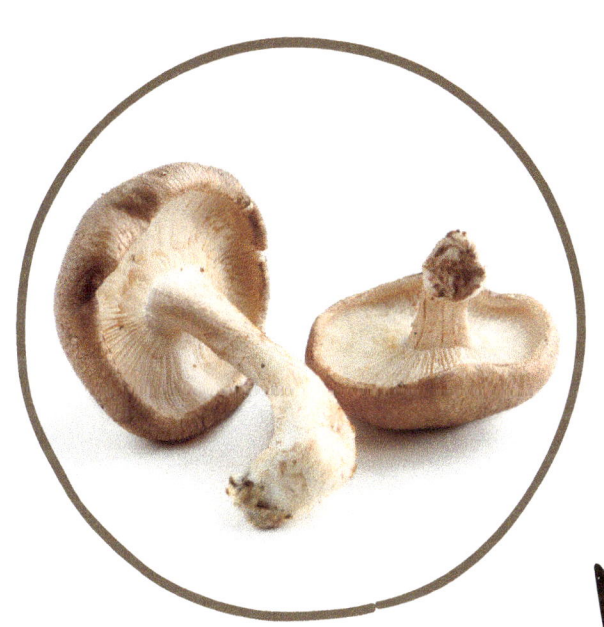

WHITE BUTTON [WAHYT BUHT-N]

Harvested when they are young, white button mushrooms are mild in flavor and are the most commonly consumed mushroom in the United States.

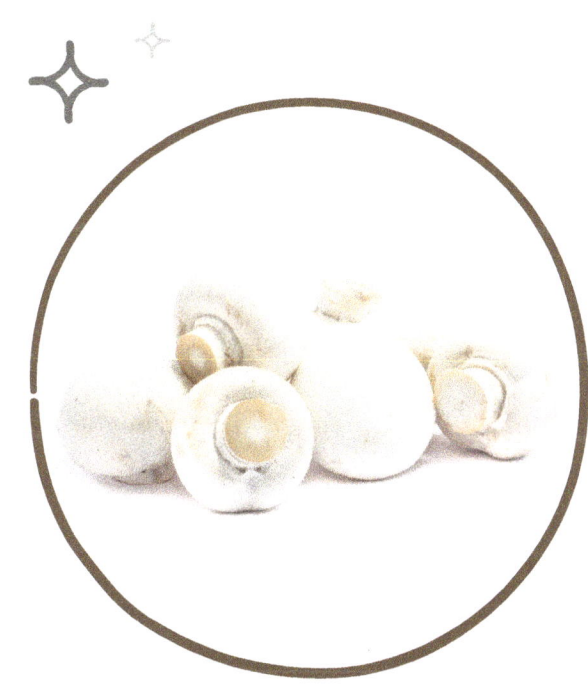

OCA
NEW ZEALAND YAM

[oh-kah] | [noo zee-land yeah-m]

crunchy, lemony, starchy, sweet, tangy

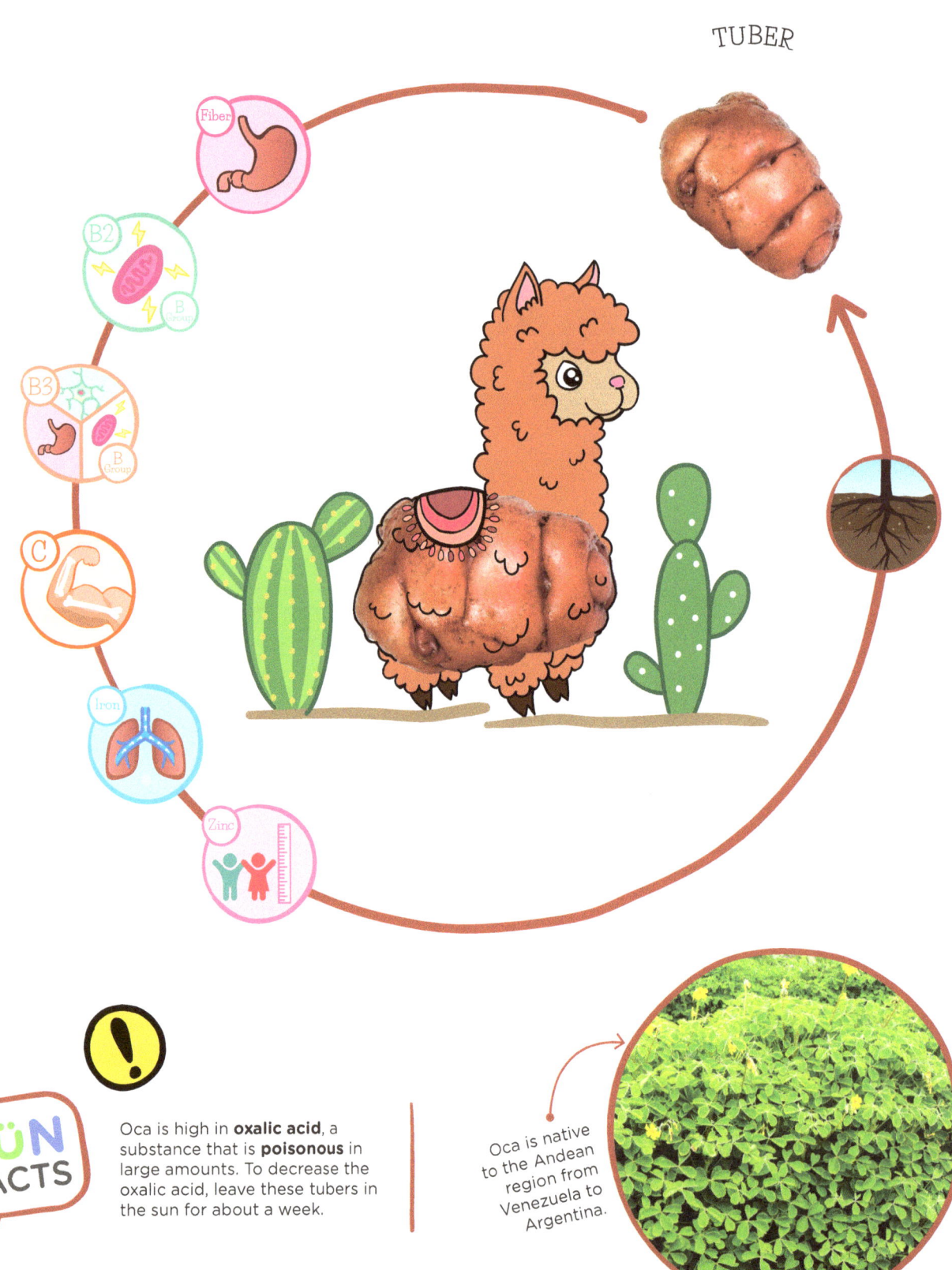

TUBER

FUN FACTS

Oca is high in **oxalic acid**, a substance that is **poisonous** in large amounts. To decrease the oxalic acid, leave these tubers in the sun for about a week.

Oca is native to the Andean region from Venezuela to Argentina.

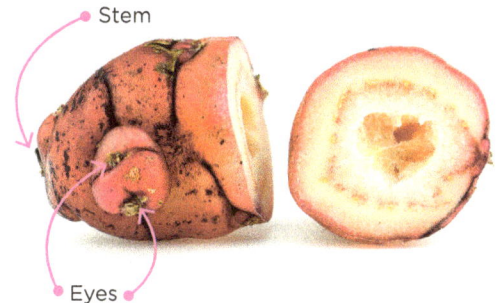

PICK
Pick brightly colored, small, firm, slightly glossy **tubers** with a ribbed surface. Avoid oca with **bruises** and soft spots.

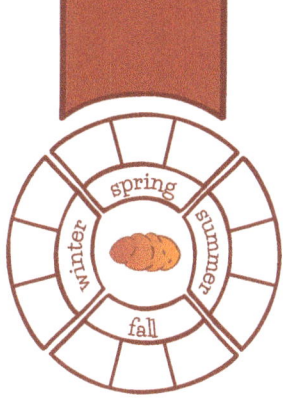

Available imported year-round

STORE
Keep oca in a basket that is well-ventilated and store in a cool, dark place for up to 3 months.

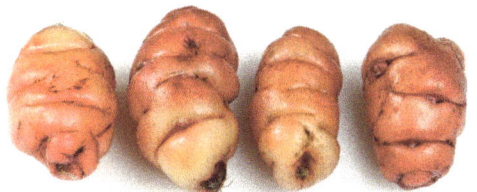

EAT

Clean the skin and scrub with a vegetable brush, then chop or slice per recipe. Oca can be **prepared** the same way you use potatoes!

Roasted Oca
Preheat your oven to 400 degrees F. Chop oca and **root** vegetables such as carrots and parsnips into 1 inch chunks, toss with olive oil, and season with salt and pepper. Spread in a single layer on a **greased**, foil-lined roasting tray, and roast for 15-20 minutes turning occasionally until tender and can be easily **pierced** with a fork.

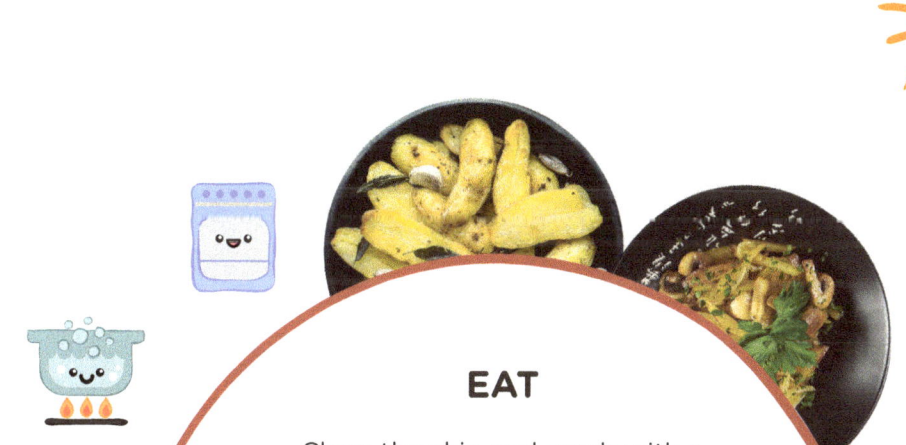

OCA TIDBITS

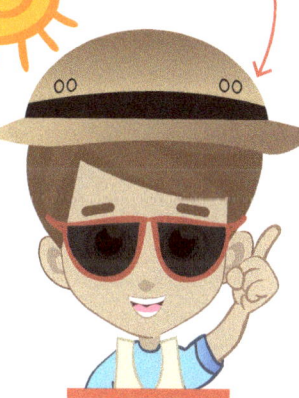

The sun sweetens this tuber.

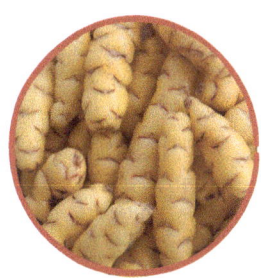

Oca are small and often about the size of a thumb. **Varieties** are pink-orange, yellow, apricot, and golden.

A Book of Vegetables 93

OKRA

[oak-rah]

bitter, crunchy, mild, silky, slimy

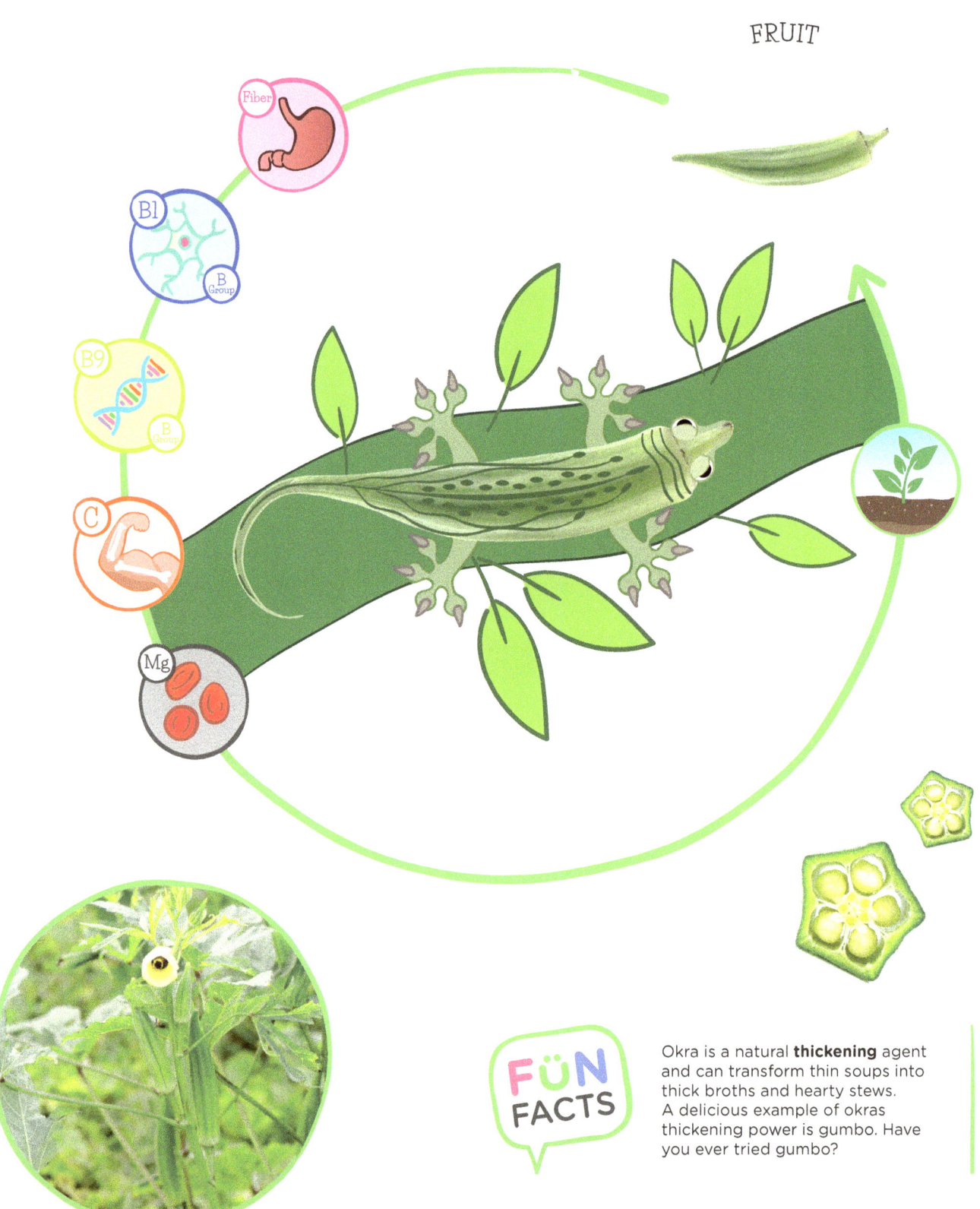

FRUIT

Okra is a natural **thickening** agent and can transform thin soups into thick broths and hearty stews. A delicious example of okras thickening power is gumbo. Have you ever tried gumbo?

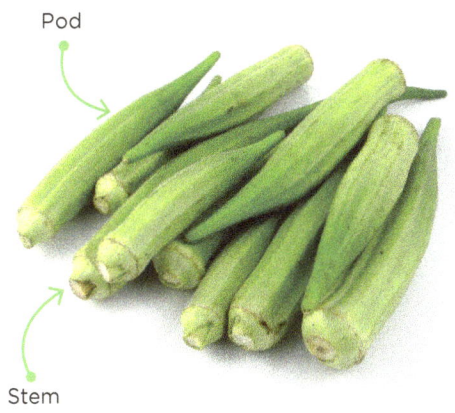
Pod
Stem

PICK
Pick brightly colored, small, young, **fruit** that are less than 3 inches in length, feel tender, and snap when broken in half. Avoid dry and dull okra that are hard and browning.

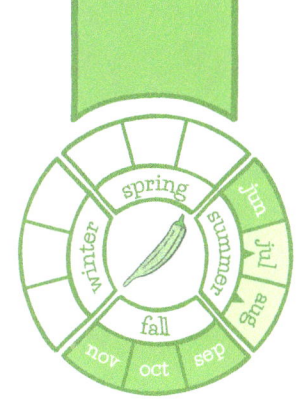

Available June to November; Imported year-round

Peak Season
July-August

STORE
Refrigerate unwashed, raw okra in a dry paper towel in a closed plastic bag for up to 3 days. Refrigerate cooked okra in an airtight container for 3-5 days.

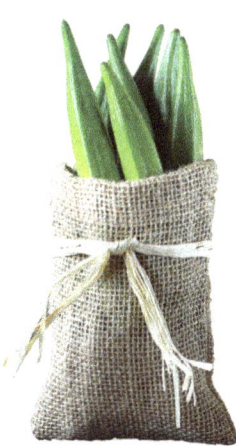

OKRA TIDBITS

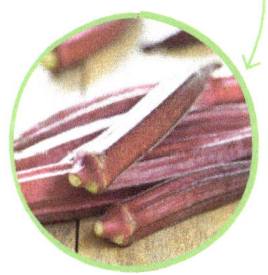

Okra **varieties** are available in red, green, and purple.

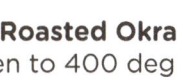

EAT

Clean the skin and scrub with a vegetable brush to remove fuzz on the skin. Slice off **stem** and leave whole or chop pod per recipe.

Roasted Okra
Preheat your oven to 400 degrees F. Slice okra in half-length wise (hotdog style), toss with olive oil, spread in a single layer on a foil-lined roasting tray, and roast for about 25 minutes until the edges are golden brown.

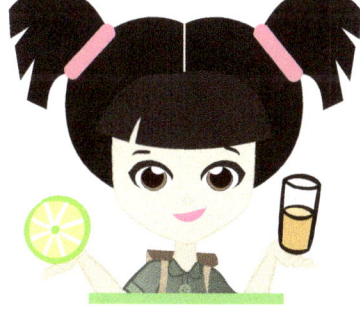

Cooked okra can be slimy! Cook okra in an acid such as lemon or vinegar to minimize the slime.

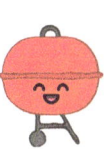
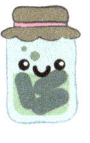
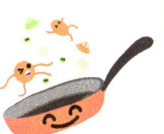
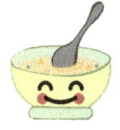
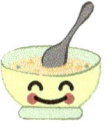

A Book of Vegetables   95

ONION

[on-yon]

astringent, crunchy, pungent, spicy, sweet

BULB

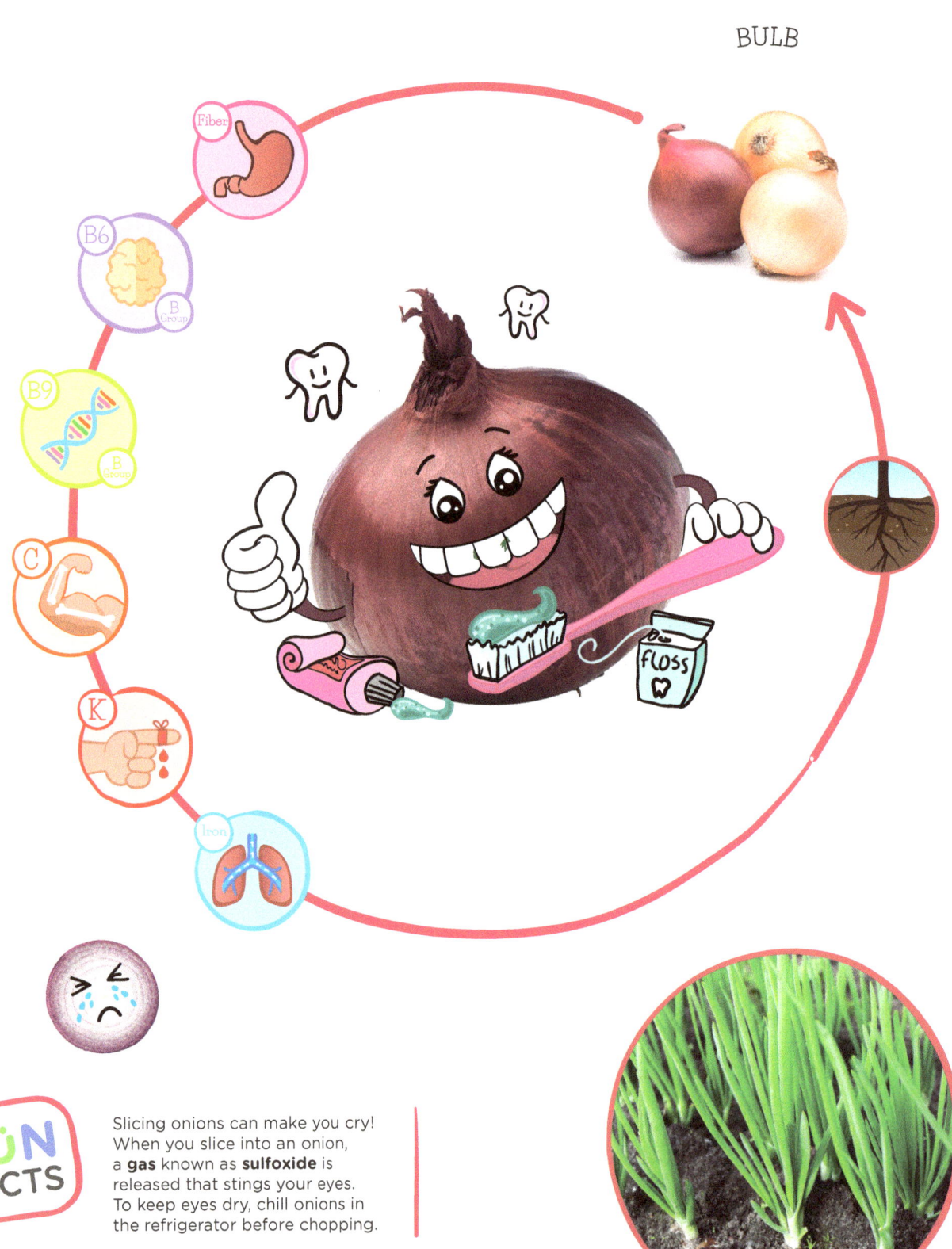

FUN FACTS

Slicing onions can make you cry! When you slice into an onion, a **gas** known as **sulfoxide** is released that stings your eyes. To keep eyes dry, chill onions in the refrigerator before chopping.

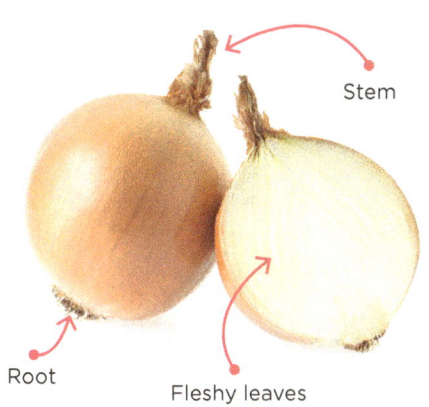

Stem
Root
Fleshy leaves

PICK
Pick firm, well shaped **bulbs**, with dry, paper-like **leaves**. Avoid onions with **sprouts**, **mold**, wet spots, or that smell musty. Scallions should have bright green, crisp tops.

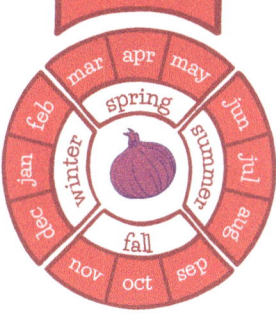

Varieties available year-round

STORE
Keep bulb onions in a basket that is well-ventilated and store in a cool, dry, dark place for up to 3 months. Do not store onions in plastic bags. Refrigerate sliced, raw onions in an airtight container for up to 7 days and cooked onions for 3-5 days.

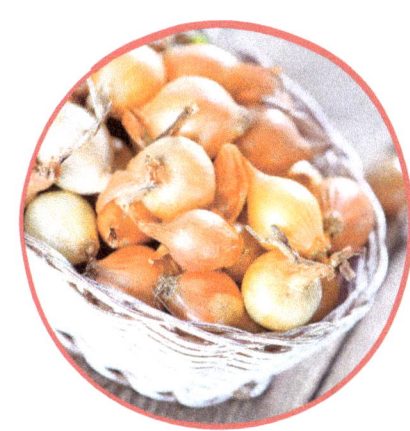

ONION TIDBITS

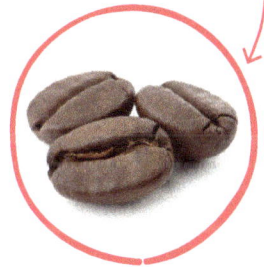

Eating onions can make your breath smell bad. To freshen onion breath, chew a little parsley or a coffee bean.

EAT
Slice off the **stem** end and peel the dry, outside papery layers. Keep the **root** end whole. Then clean the knife and set onion on a clean cutting board. Next, slice the onion in half root to stem, then place cut side down and slice or chop per recipe. Slicing off the hard root end last will make chopping onions easier and your slices more **uniform** in size by keeping the layers together!

Sautéed Onions
Sauté onions in olive oil over medium heat for 5-10 minutes until tender, **translucent**, and golden-brown.

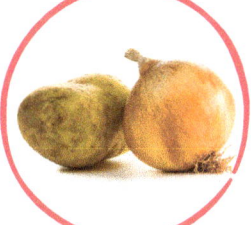

Do not store onions near potatoes because a chemical reaction speeds up how fast they both spoil.

A Book of Vegetables 97

ONION VARIETIES

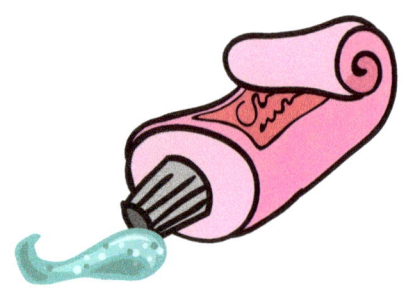

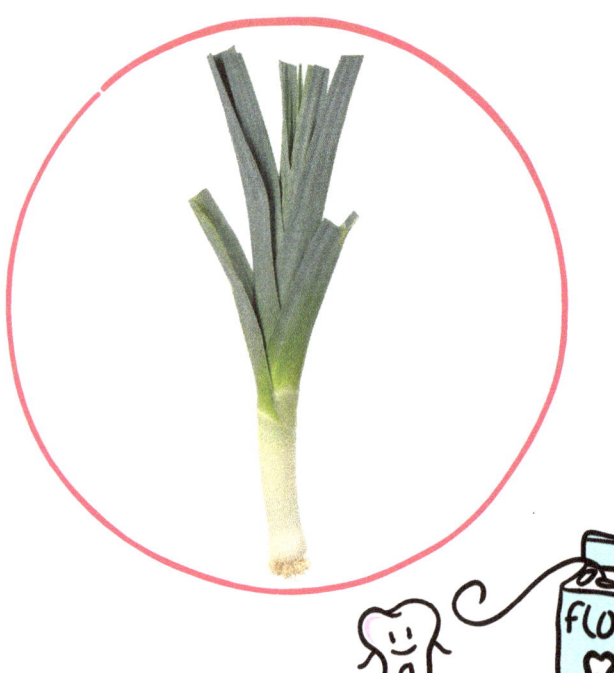

LEEK [LEEK]

Leeks look like overgrown scallions. This **bulb**-less onion **variety** has a subtle, sweet flavor and may substitute for onions in any cooked dish. It is most commonly **prepared** in soups and casseroles.

SCALLION [SCAL-LEON]

Often called "green onions," these fast-growing onions are **harvested** before bulbs form and are used for their green, **cylindrical stalks**. The mild flavor of the greens are perfect as a garnish on salads, soups, and casseroles.

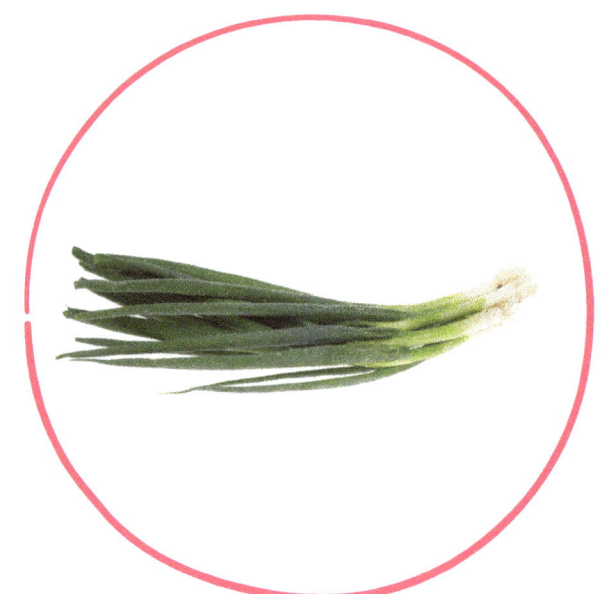

SHALLOT [SHAL-LOT]

Shallots have small clusters of bulbs and look like garlic with their brown-orange papery skin. Shallots have the aroma and flavor of a mild onion, with a hint of garlic, and are often used in sauces and dressings.

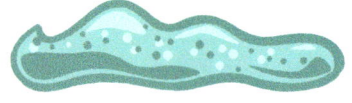

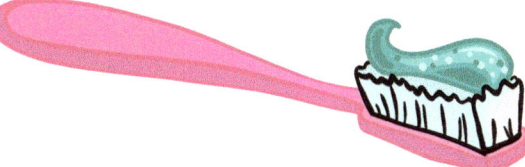

RED ONION [RED ON-YON]

Red onions are purplish in color and, when fresh, they are most often mild, sweet, and eaten raw. Red onions stored for long periods of time may become more pungent and spicy.

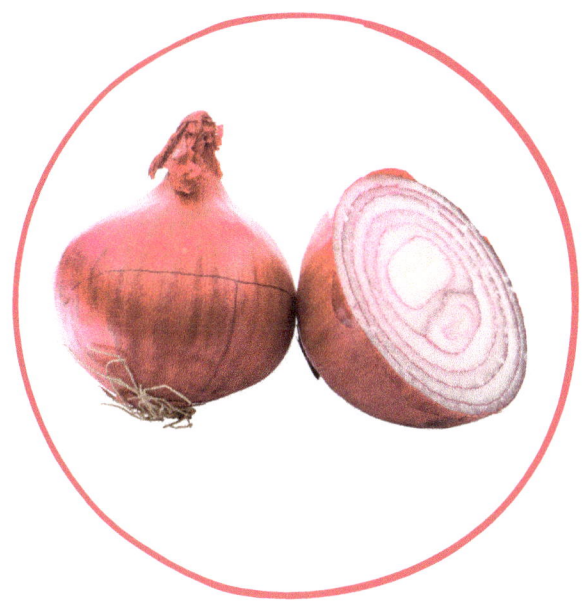

WHITE ONION [WAHYT ON-YON]

White onions are one of the most **versatile** onions. They are known for their mildly sweet flavor. They can be chopped into salsa or chutneys, enjoyed raw, or cooked into any recipe that require an onion.

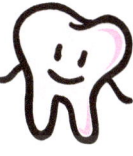

YELLOW ONION [YEL-OH ON-YON]

Yellow onions are the most common, all-purpose cooking onion. They are globe-shaped and have a balance of astringent and sweet flavors. Do not mistake yellow onions with Vidalia or Walla Walla sweet onions which are consumed raw or fried in onion rings!

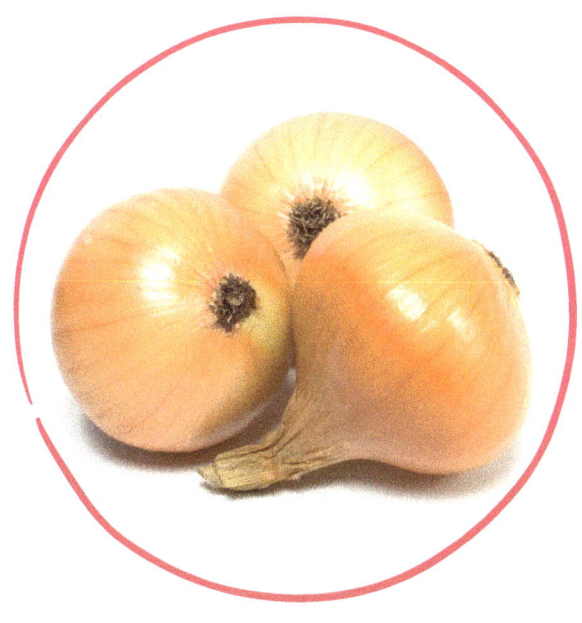

A Book of Vegetables

PARSNIP

[pars-nip]

aromatic, earthy, nutty, starchy, sweet

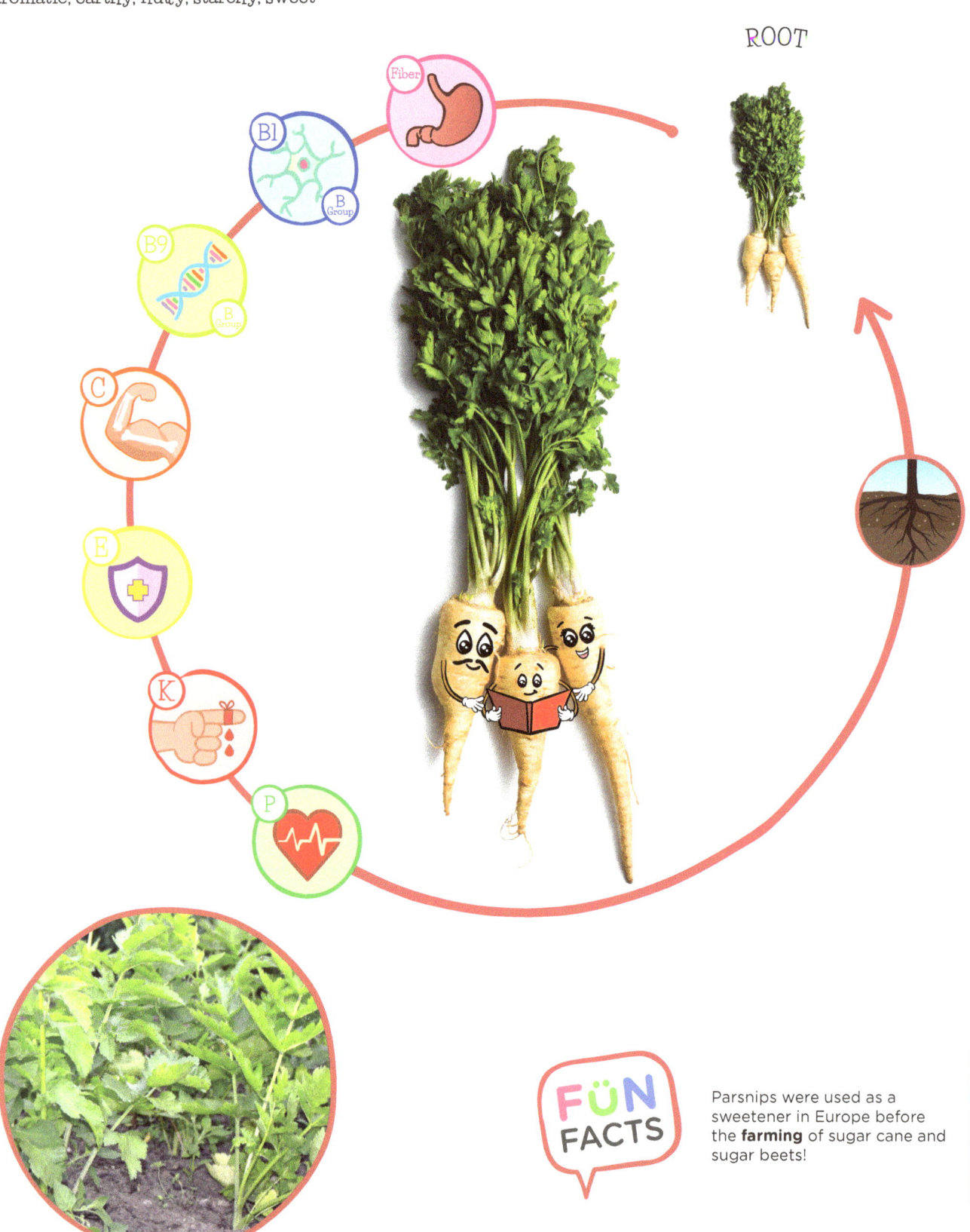

ROOT

FUN FACTS: Parsnips were used as a sweetener in Europe before the **farming** of sugar cane and sugar beets!

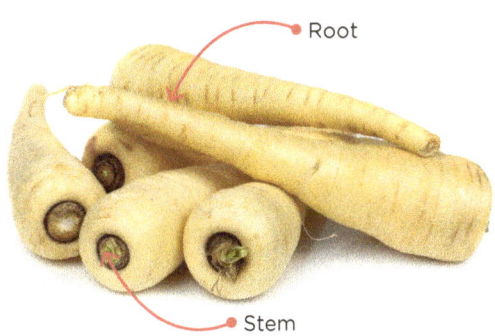
Root
Stem

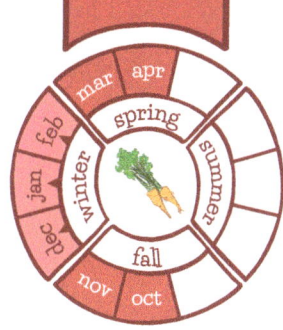

PICK
Pick creamy white, firm, straight, smooth-skinned **roots**. Avoid parsnips with dark or soft spots. Small to medium sized parsnips are best, as large roots may be tough and woody.

Available October to April; Imported year-round

Peak Season
December-February

STORE
Refrigerate unwashed, raw parsnips in a moist paper towel in an open plastic bag for up to 4 weeks. Refrigerate cooked parsnips in an airtight container for 3-5 days.

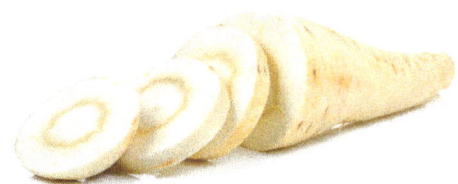

PARSNIP TIDBITS

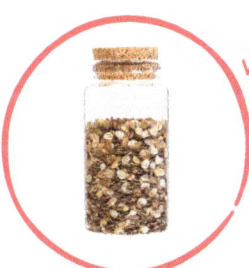

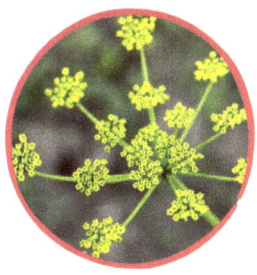

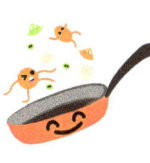
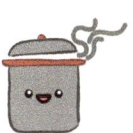
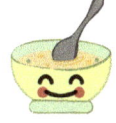

EAT
Clean the skin with a vegetable brush and trim attached **stems**, peel if desired, use whole if small or chop or slice per recipe.

Maple Roasted Parsnip
Preheat your oven to 425 degrees F. Peel and slice 1 pound of parsnips into fry-sized pieces. Boil parsnips for 2 minutes, then drain and toss with 2 tablespoons of melted butter, 2 tablespoons of maple syrup, and season with salt and pepper. Next, spread mixture in a single layer on a **greased**, foil-lined roasting tray, and roast for about 30 minutes. Turn frequently until tender and parsnip slices are golden brown.

Parsnip **seeds** are collected from small yellow **flowers** that form when plants are left unharvested and grow into a second season. The roots will become woody and inedible, but you can collect the seeds to grow parsnip the following season.

A Book of Vegetables 101

PEPPER

[pep-per]

crisp, juicy, refreshing, spicy, sweet

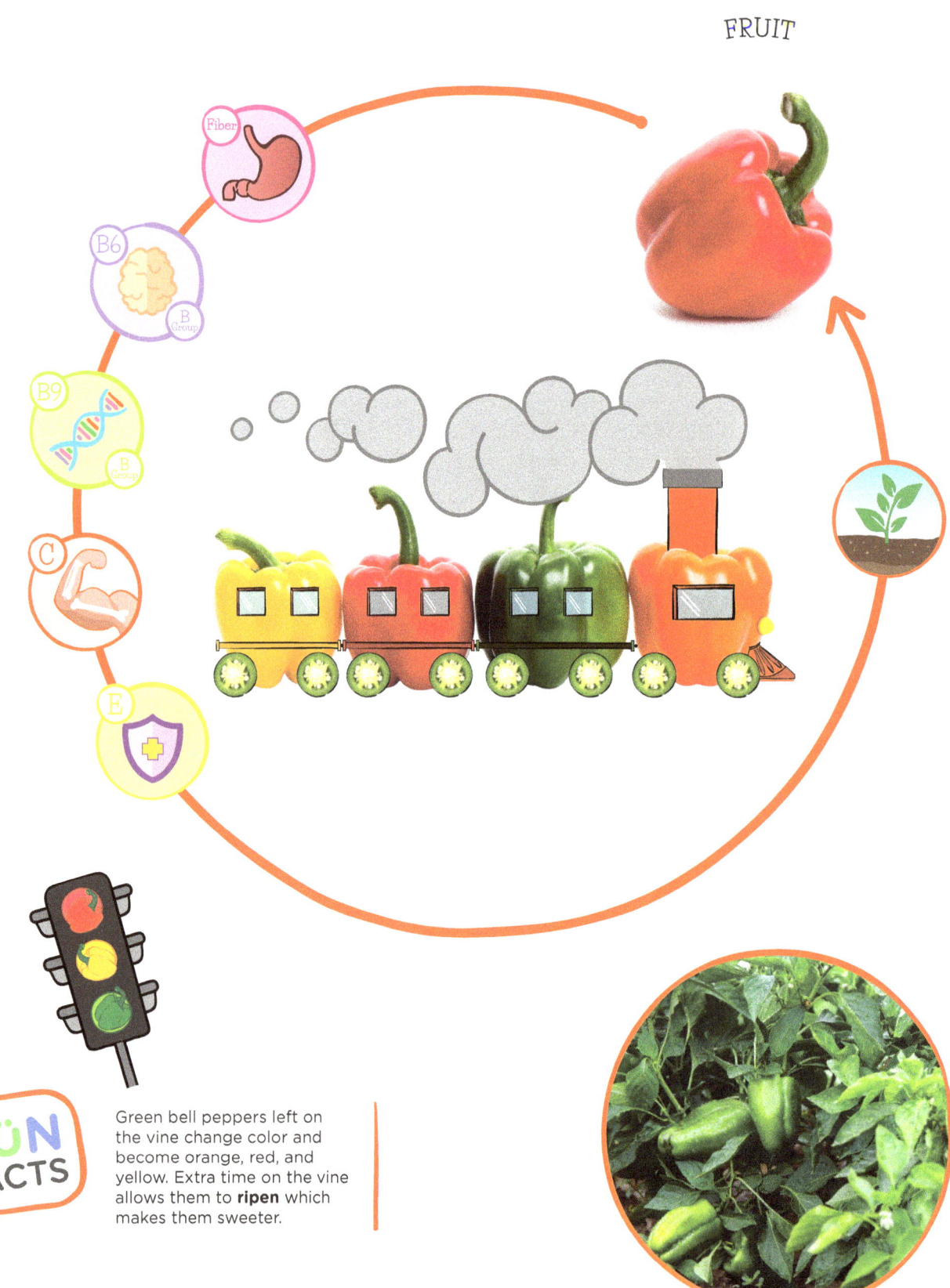

FRUIT

FUN FACTS

Green bell peppers left on the vine change color and become orange, red, and yellow. Extra time on the vine allows them to **ripen** which makes them sweeter.

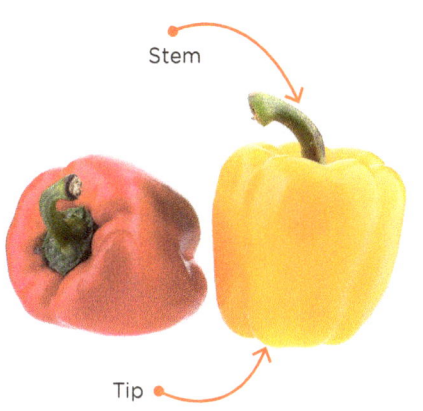

Stem

Tip

PICK
Pick shiny, firm, well-shaped, thick-**fleshed fruit**. Avoid peppers with soft spots or are shriveled in appearance.

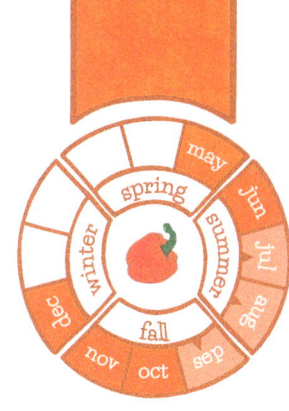

Available May to December; Imported year-round

Peak Season
July-September

STORE
Refrigerate unwashed, raw peppers in an open plastic bag for up to 2 weeks. Refrigerate raw sliced or chopped peppers in an airtight container for 2-3 days and cooked peppers in an airtight container for 3-5 days.

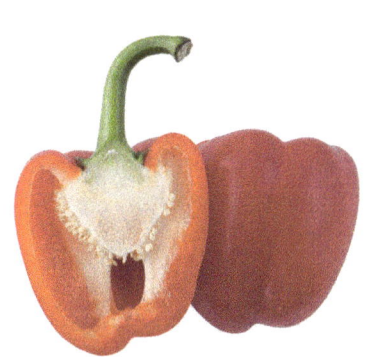

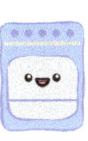

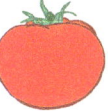

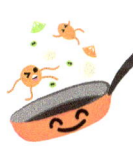

EAT
Clean the skin, slice the pepper in half from **stem** to tip (hotdog style), remove the stem, **seeds**, and whiteish ribs with a knife or your fingers. Tap any remaining seeds out of the pepper, and chop or slice per recipe.

Roasted Peppers
Preheat your oven to 450 degrees F. Place halved peppers in a single layer on a foil-lined roasting tray in the top third of the oven for about 25 minutes or until the skins are wrinkled and the peppers are black on top. Allow the peppers to cool, then peel the skin off the pepper and eat or add to a recipe with roasted peppers.

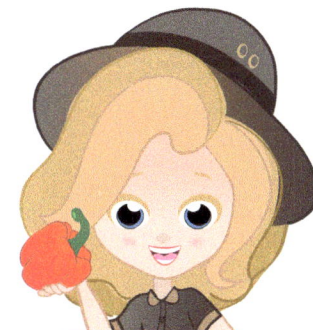

PEPPERS TIDBITS

Peppers are a good source of **Vitamin B12** which helps the body make red blood **cells** and keep the **nervous system** healthy.

A Book of Vegetables

PLANTAIN

[plan-tin]

bland, earthy, firm, mild, starchy, sweet

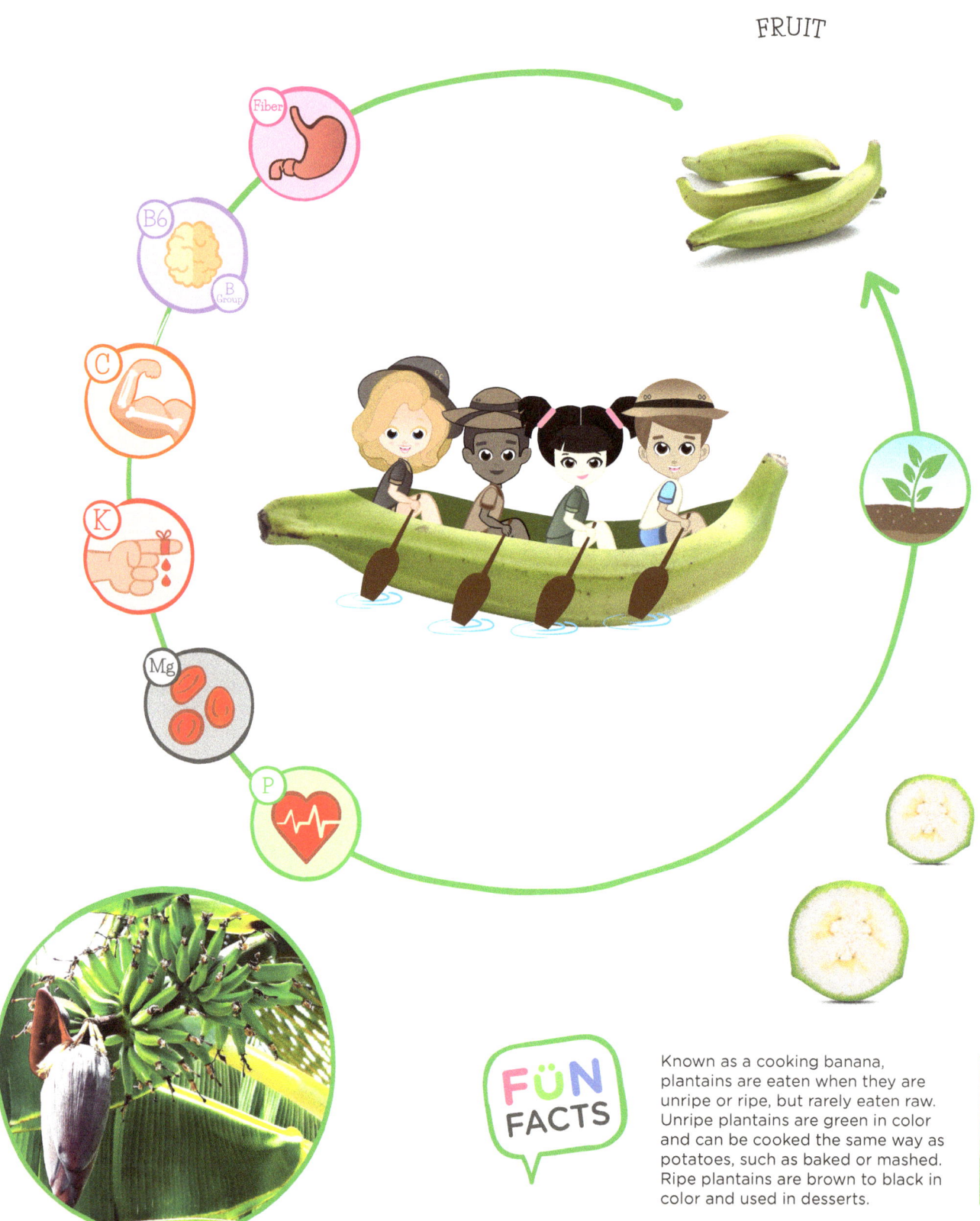

FRUIT

FUN FACTS

Known as a cooking banana, plantains are eaten when they are unripe or ripe, but rarely eaten raw. Unripe plantains are green in color and can be cooked the same way as potatoes, such as baked or mashed. Ripe plantains are brown to black in color and used in desserts.

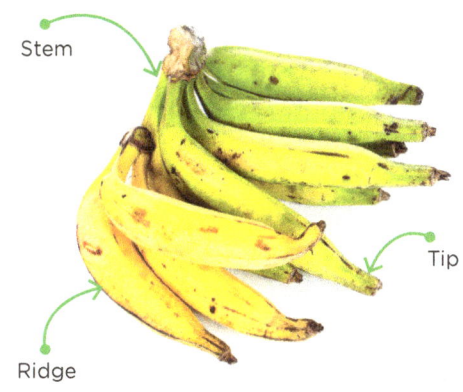

Stem · Tip · Ridge

PICK

UNRIPE: Pick green, firm **fruit**. Avoid unripe plantains with cracks and soft spots.

RIPE: Pick yellow with brown spots, brown, to black firm fruit (the darker in color, the sweeter the fruit). Avoid **ripe** plantains with cracks and soft spots.

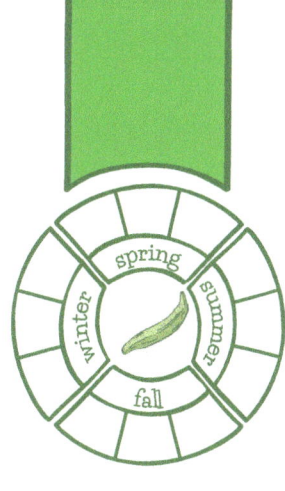

Available imported year-round

STORE

Keep plantain on the countertop at room **temperature** until desired ripeness is achieved. Refrigerate ripe fruit and cooked plantains in an air tight container for 3-5 days.

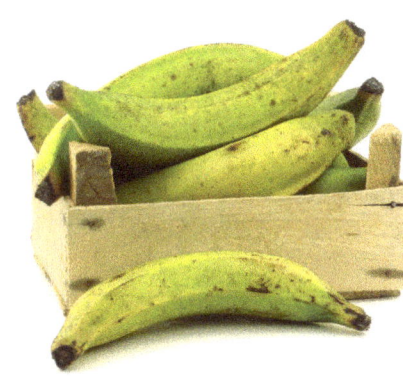

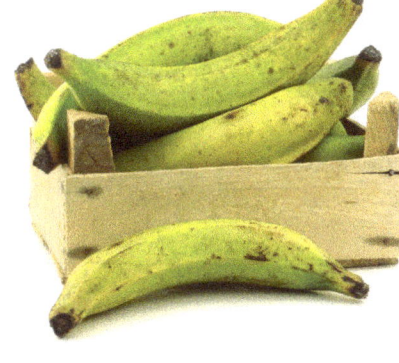

EAT

Clean the skin and slice off the **stem** and tip. Lightly cut the surface of the plantain on the four ridges of skin being careful not to cut into the fruit. Peel the skin away from the **flesh** and chop or slice per recipe.

Fried Plantains

Slice plantains into 1/2 inch coins. Fry pieces in coconut oil over medium-high heat for about 3 minutes, until they are light golden and semi-soft. Place plantains on a paper towel to cool and then smash fruit into flat rounds with the bottom of a water glass. Next, place plantains back in hot oil for another 3 minutes until crisp and golden brown. Cool on new paper towels to remove excess oil, squeeze fresh lime juice over the top, and sprinkle with salt.

PEELING PLANTAIN

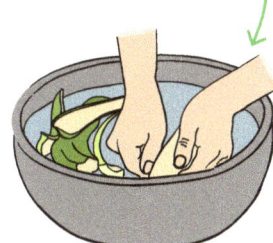

Green plantain skin may be peeled underwater to minimize bruising.

A Book of Vegetables 105

POTATO

[po-tate-o]

buttery, creamy, earthy, nutty, sweet

TUBER

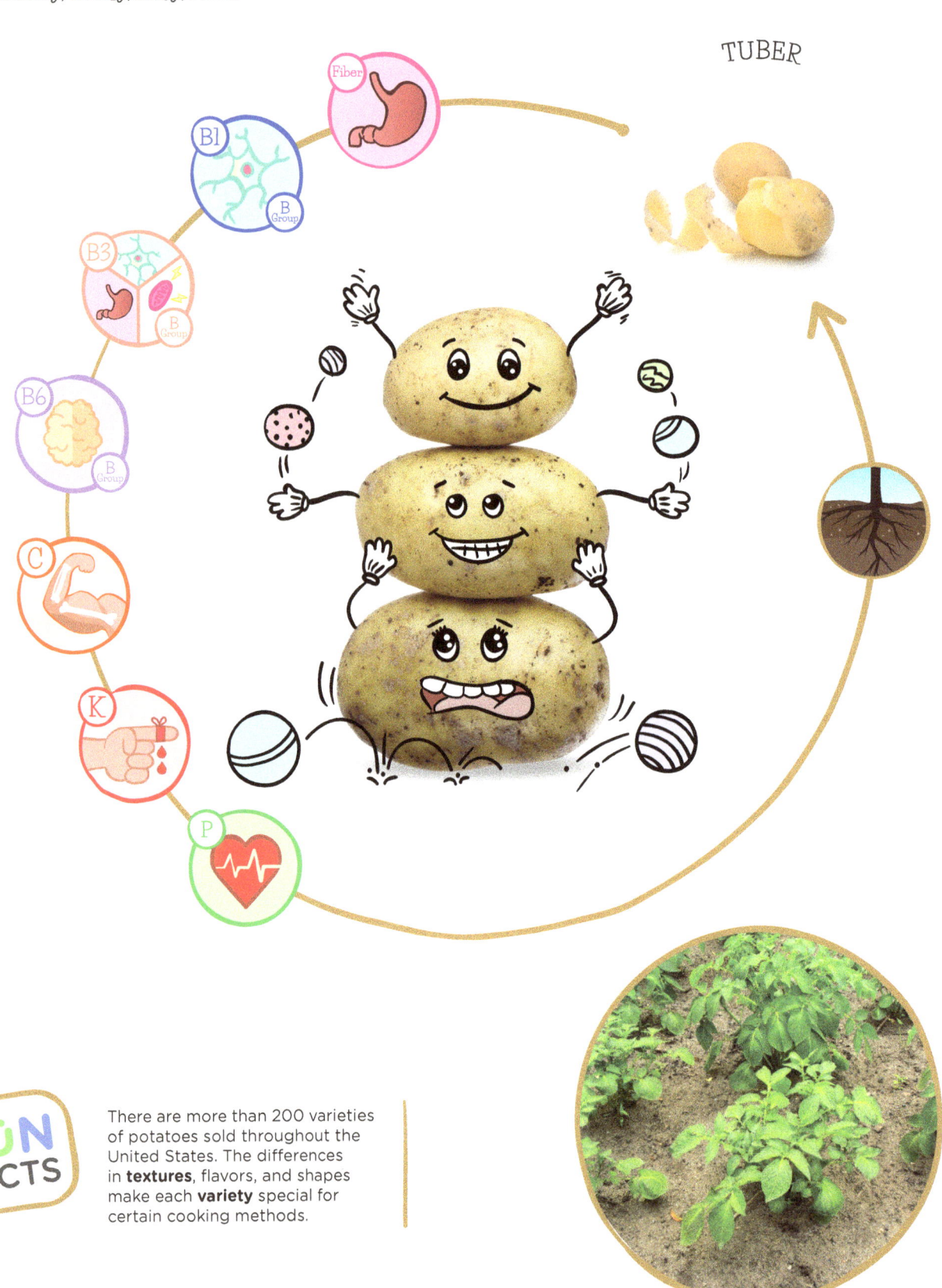

FUN FACTS

There are more than 200 varieties of potatoes sold throughout the United States. The differences in **textures**, flavors, and shapes make each **variety** special for certain cooking methods.

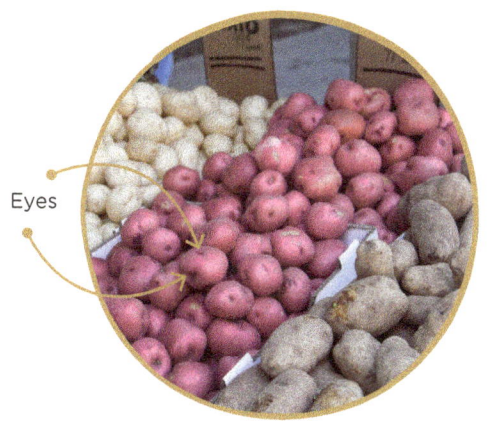
Eyes

PICK
Pick firm **tubers**. Avoid potatoes with green, wrinkled skin, soft spots, cuts, and **sprouts**.

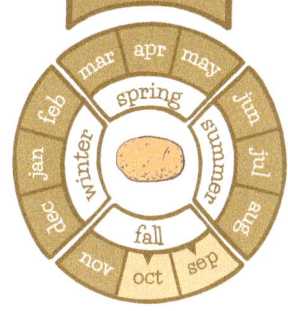

Varieties available year-round

Peak Season
September-October

STORE
Keep potatoes well-ventilated in a basket and store in a cool, dark place for up to 3 months. Do not store potatoes near onions because they cause each other to **spoil** faster. Refrigerate raw sliced potatoes in a bowl of cold water for up to 24 hours and cooked potatoes in an airtight container for 3-5 days.

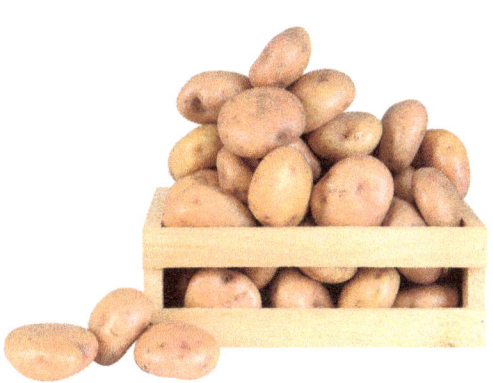

EAT
Clean the skin with a vegetable brush, peel if desired, then chop or slice per recipe. Potatoes should be cooked or placed in cold water with vinegar or lemon juice immediately after peeling to prevent browning.

Baked Potato
Preheat your oven to 425 degrees F. Coat potatoes with olive oil, place on a foil-lined roasting tray, stab them with a fork 3-4 times and bake for about 45 minutes until tubers are tender and can be easily **pierced** with a fork.

In 1995, the potato became the first vegetable to be grown in space.

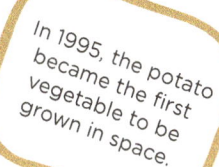

A Book of Vegetables 107

POTATO VARIETIES

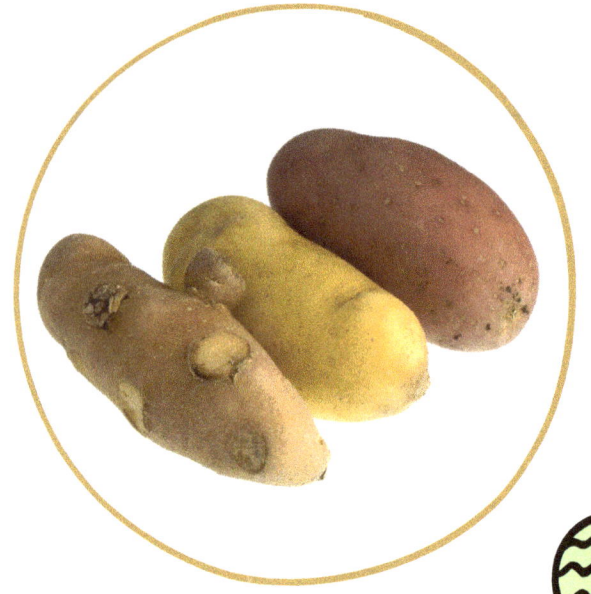

FINGERLING [FIN-GER-LING]

Finger-shaped in appearance, the skins and **flesh** come in orange-yellow, purple, red and white. These firm, waxy potatoes are buttery, nutty, and perfect for roasting or using in potato salads.

PURPLE POTATO [PUR-PUHL PO-TAT-O]

Purple potatoes are small to medium in size with purple-blue skin and blue, lavender, pink, purple, or white flesh. These firm and moist potatoes are earthy and nutty, and great in salads or roasted vegetable mixes.

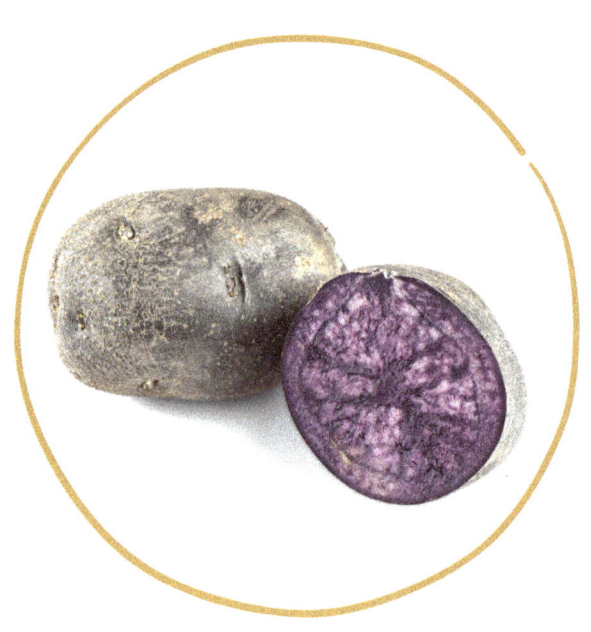

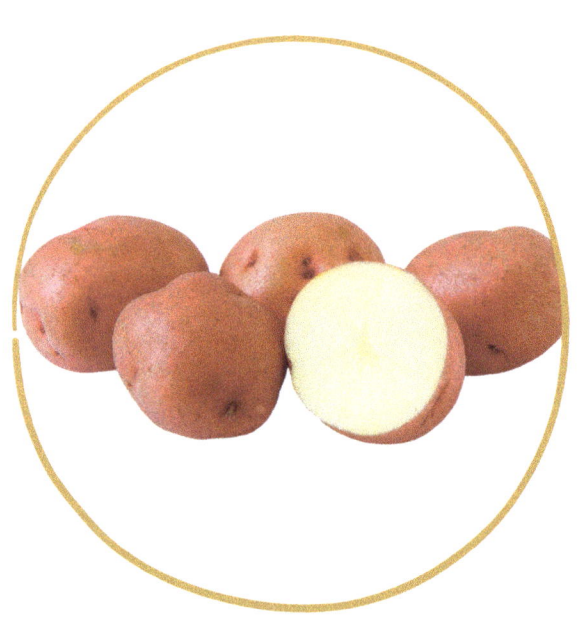

RED POTATO [RED PO-TAT-O]

Red potatoes have smooth red skin and white flesh. These small to medium potatoes are waxy, creamy, and sweet. They are great in stews, roasted, fried, and in potato salads.

RUSSET [RUS-SET]

Russet potatoes are oval in shape with light brown, netted skin and white to yellow flesh. These medium to large potatoes are dry, light, and fluffy with a mild, earthy flavor. Russet potatoes are the potato of choice for baking, frying, and mashing.

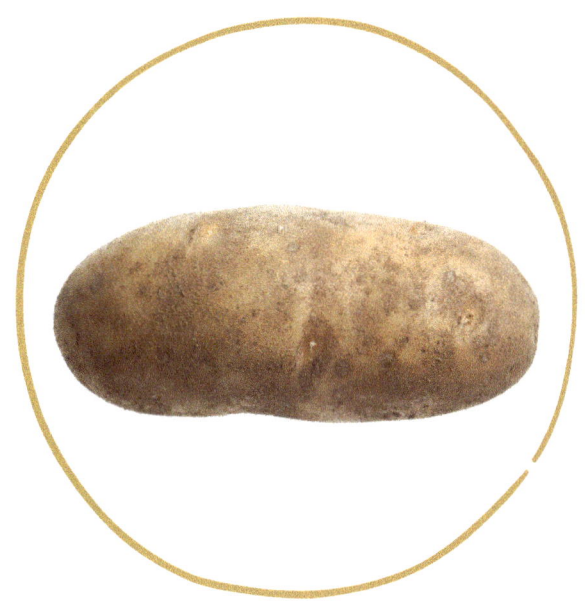

WHITE POTATO [WAHYT PO-TAT-O]

White potatoes are small to medium in size and round to long in shape. They have thin white or tan skin with white flesh. Their dense, creamy **texture** is sweet and mild. Skip peeling this potato and grill, mash, or use them for potato salads.

YELLOW POTATO [YEL-OH PO-TAT-O]

Yellow potatoes have tan to yellow skin and golden flesh. They range in size from very small and round to large and oval shaped. Their waxy, velvety texture, and sweet buttery flavor is best **prepared** baked, mashed, and roasted.

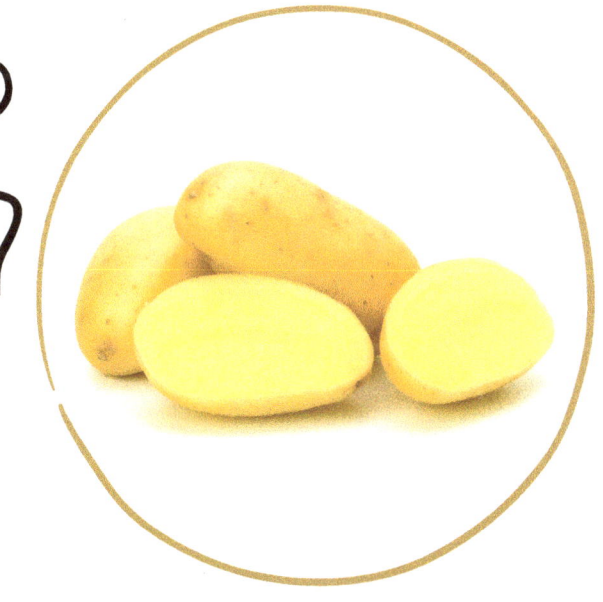

A Book of Vegetables

RADISH AND GREENS

[rad-ish]

crisp, mild, peppery, spicy, zesty

ROOT | STEM | LEAVES

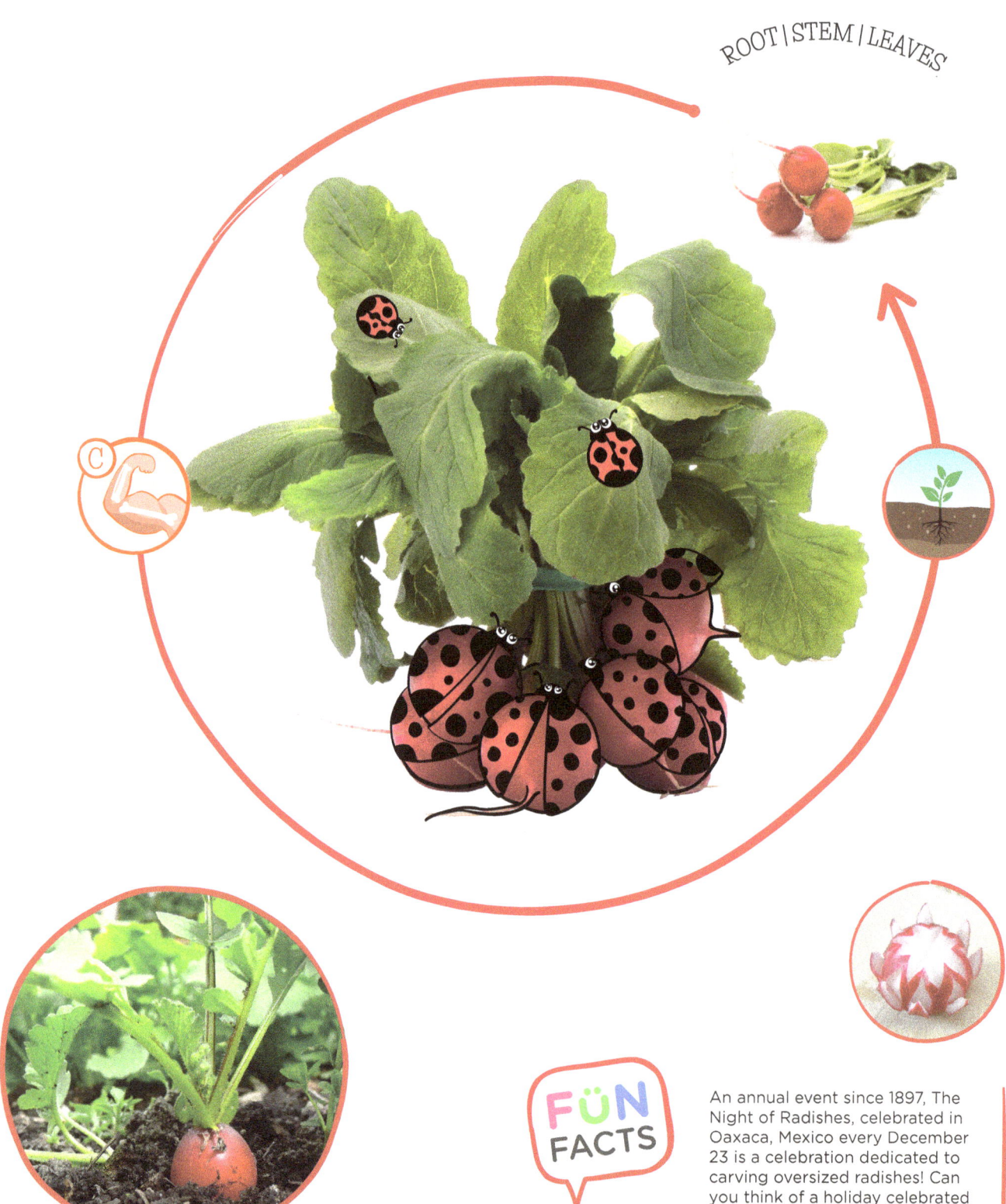

FUN FACTS

An annual event since 1897, The Night of Radishes, celebrated in Oaxaca, Mexico every December 23 is a celebration dedicated to carving oversized radishes! Can you think of a holiday celebrated in the United States that involves carving a vegetable?

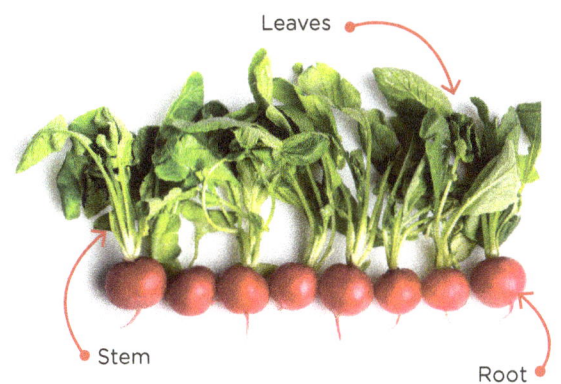

Leaves · Stem · Root

PICK
Pick brightly colored, firm, smooth **roots**. Avoid radishes with cracks, cuts, and soft centers. Attached greens should be bright green and crisp.

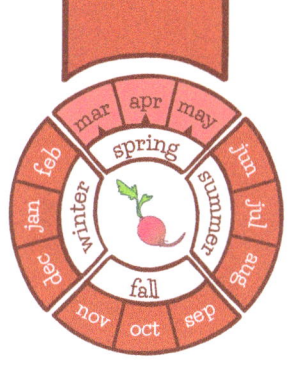

Varieties available year-round

Peak Season
March-May

STORE
Refrigerate unwashed, raw radish in an open plastic bag for up to 14 days. Refrigerate cooked radishes in an airtight container for 3-5 days. Raw radish greens should be refrigerated separately in an airtight container for 2-3 days.

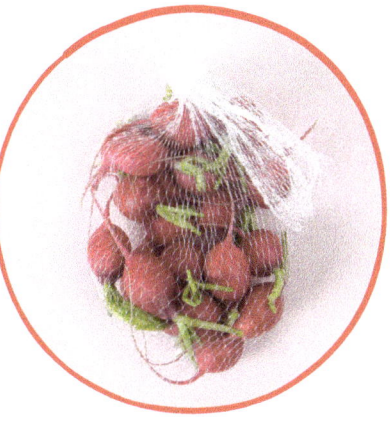

RADISH VARIETIES

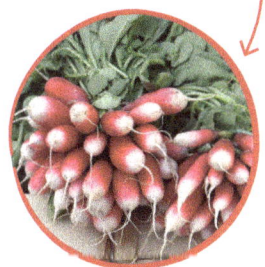

French Breakfast Radish

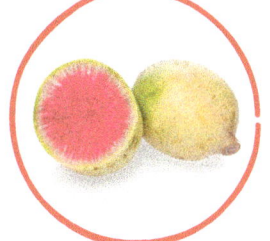

Watermelon Radish

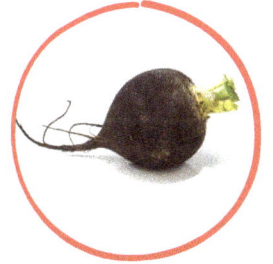

Black Radish

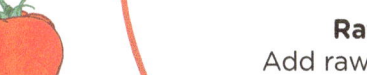
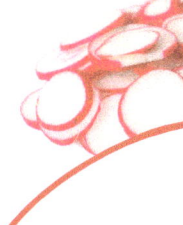

EAT
Clean the skin with a vegetable brush, trim attached **stems**, and eat whole or chop or slice per recipe.

Raw Radishes
Add raw radishes to your veggie tray!

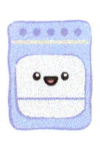
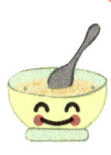

A Book of Vegetables 111

RHUBARB

[ru-barb]

acidic, sour, sweet-tart, tangy, tender

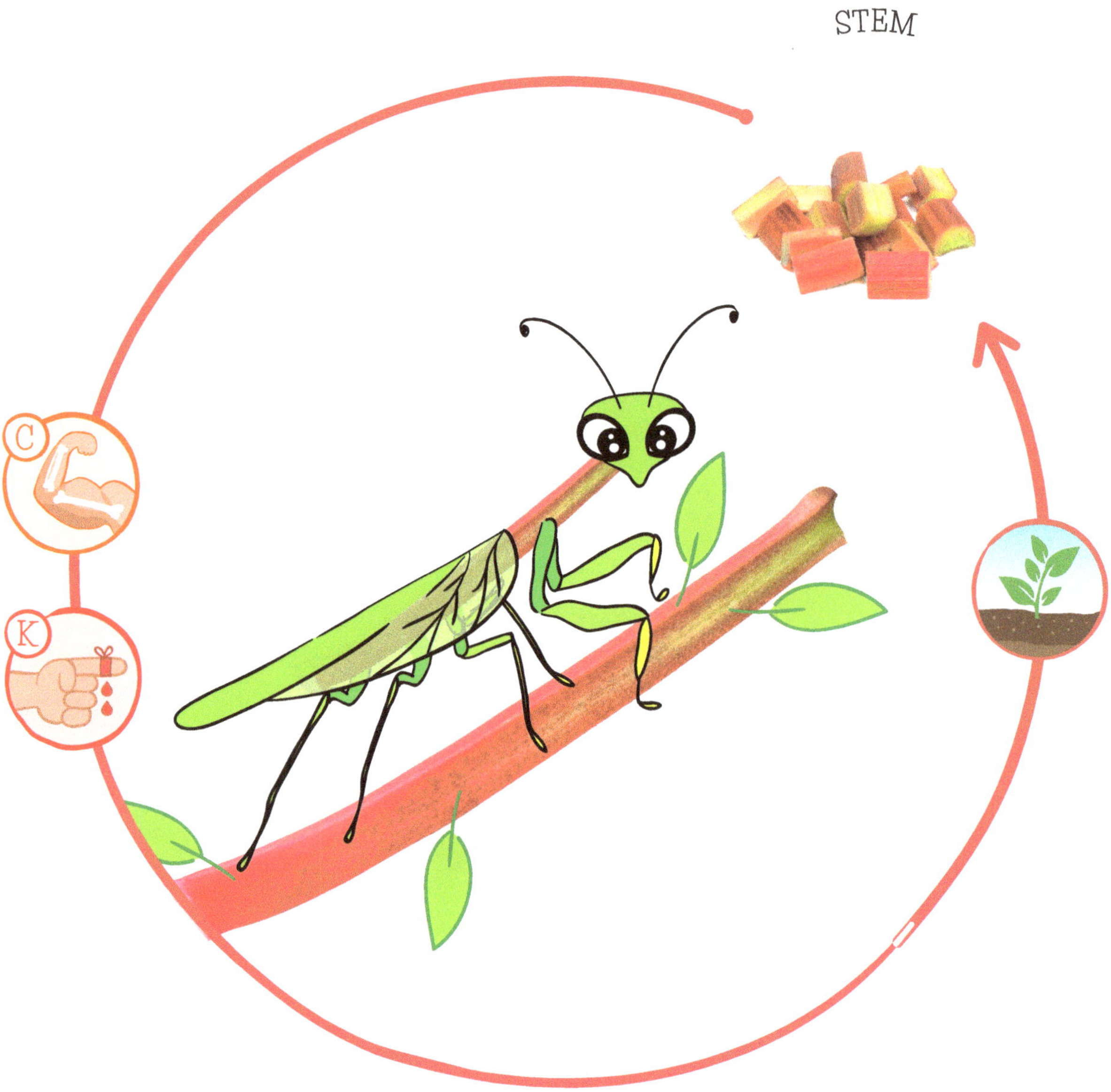

STEM

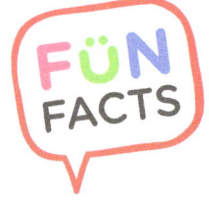

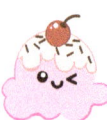
Although rhubarb is a vegetable, it is often thought of as a **fruit** because they are typically eaten in jams and pies!

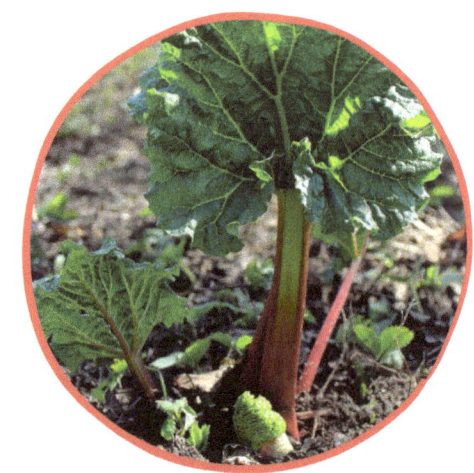

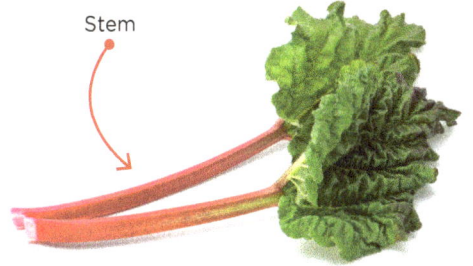

PICK
Pick pink or red, thin **stems**. Avoid rhubarb with many cuts and **bruises**. Thick or green rhubarb tend to be more stringy and sour.

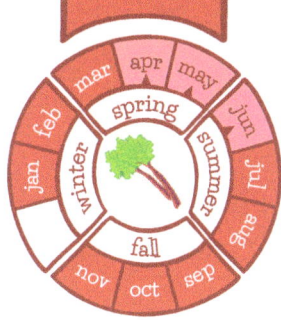

Available January to November

Peak Season
April - June

STORE
Refrigerate raw rhubarb in a closed plastic bag for up to 7 days. Refrigerate baked rhubarb wrapped in plastic or foil for 3-5 days.

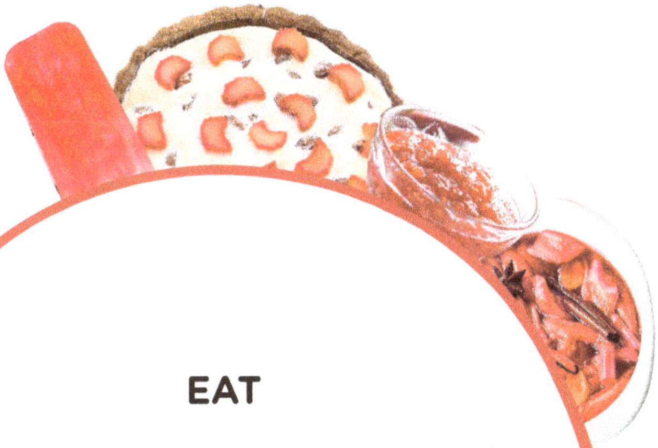

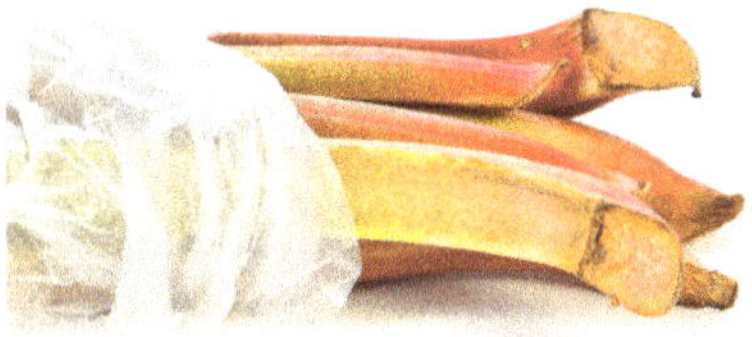

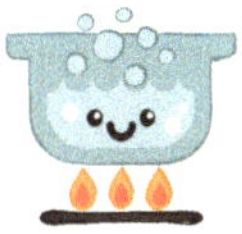

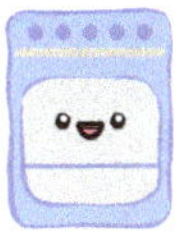

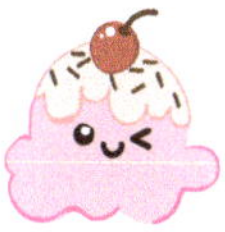

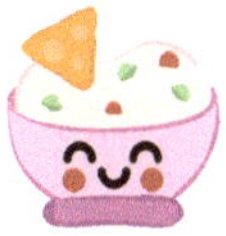

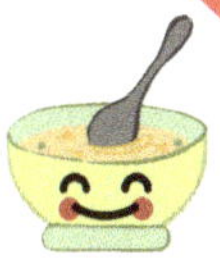

EAT
Clean the skin, slice off the **leaves** and ends, then chop or slice per recipe.

Rhubarb Sauce
Combine 1/4 cup sugar and 1/4 cup of water in a small saucepan and bring to a boil. Add about 2 cups of chopped rhubarb and cook for 5-10 minutes stirring occasionally until rhubarb is tender and sauce has thickened. Serve over pancakes or ice cream!

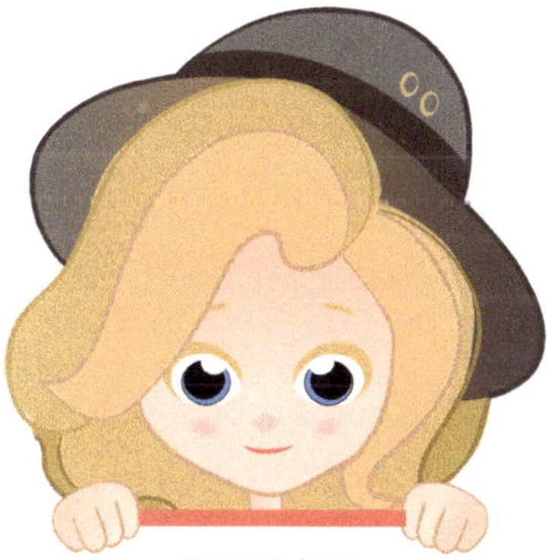

RHUBARB LEAVES

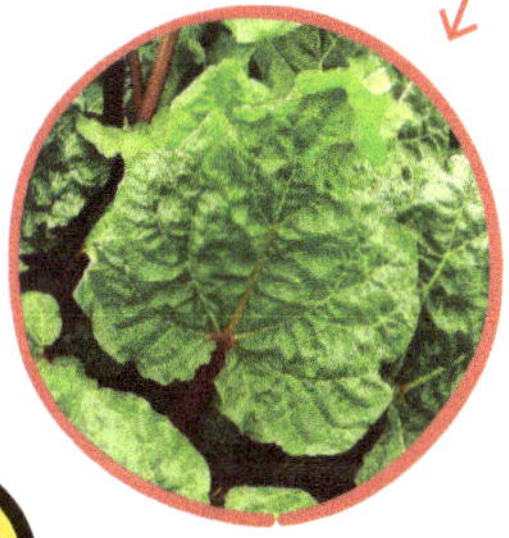

Never eat rhubarb leaves because they are **poisonous** and may make you sick.

A Book of Vegetables

RUTABAGA
SWEDE

[root-a-bay-ga] | [sweed]

crisp, juicy, mild, rich, sweet

ROOT

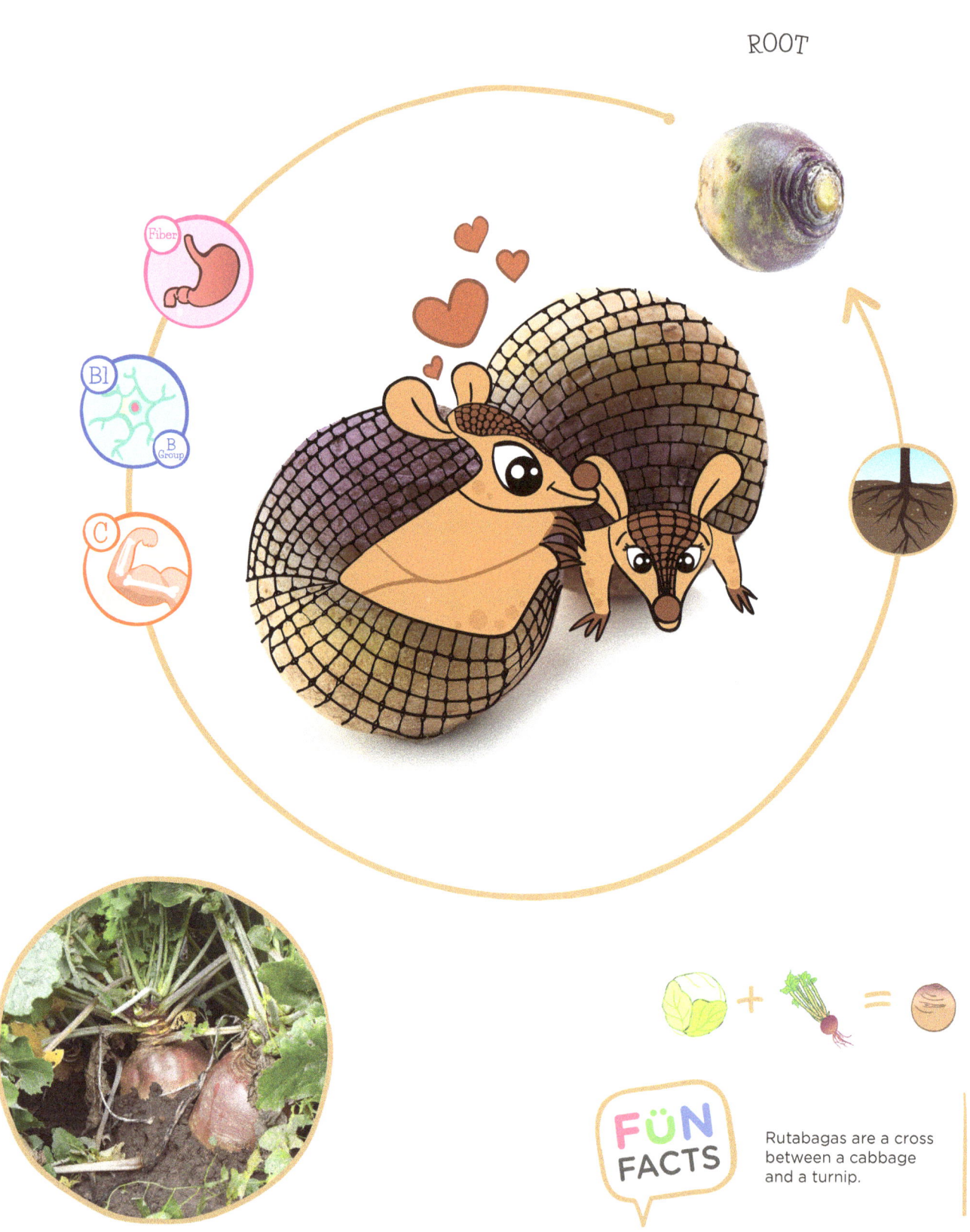

Rutabagas are a cross between a cabbage and a turnip.

FUN FACTS

114 | Where Does Broccoli Come From?

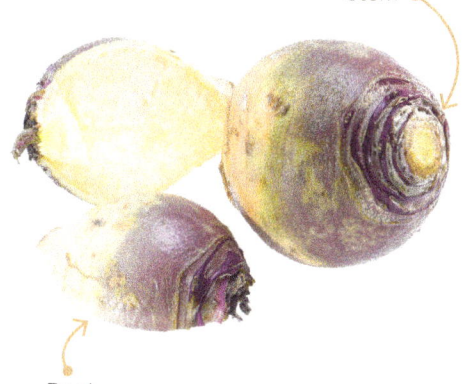

Stem

Root

PICK
Pick firm, round, smooth **roots** that feel heavy for their size. Avoid rutabaga with many cuts or cracks in the skin and soft spots.

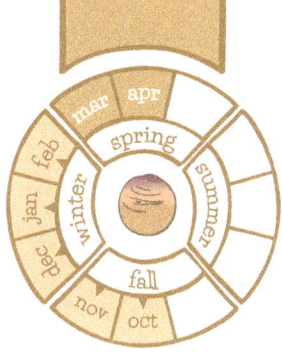

Available October to April; Imported year-round

Peak Season
October-February

STORE
Refrigerate raw rutabaga in an open plastic bag for up to 3 weeks. Refrigerate cooked rutabagas in an airtight container for 3-5 days.

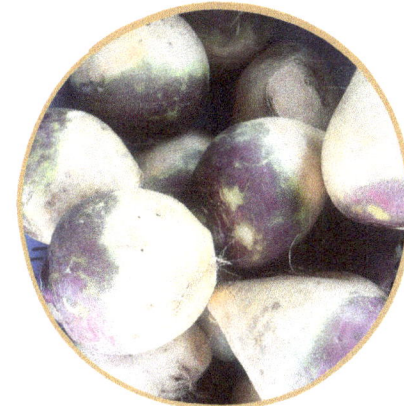

RUTABAGA TIDBITS

Rutabaga and turnip look very similar. Can you spot the differences?

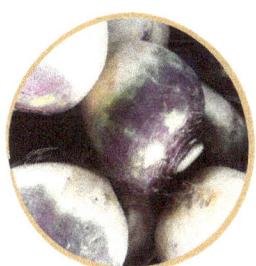

Rutabaga

EAT

Clean the skin with a vegetable brush, slice off **stem** end, peel, and chop or slice per recipe.

Raw Rutabaga Slaw
Make a sweet and savory veggie slaw with equal parts rutabaga, celeriac, and carrot. Add raisins, toss with olive oil and honey, then season with salt and pepper.

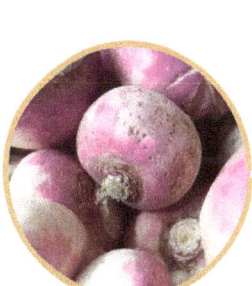

Turnip

A Book of Vegetables 115

SALSIFY
SCORZONERA

[sal-suhf-e] | [scor-zo-ne-ra]

crunchy, earthy, nutty, oyster-like, sweet

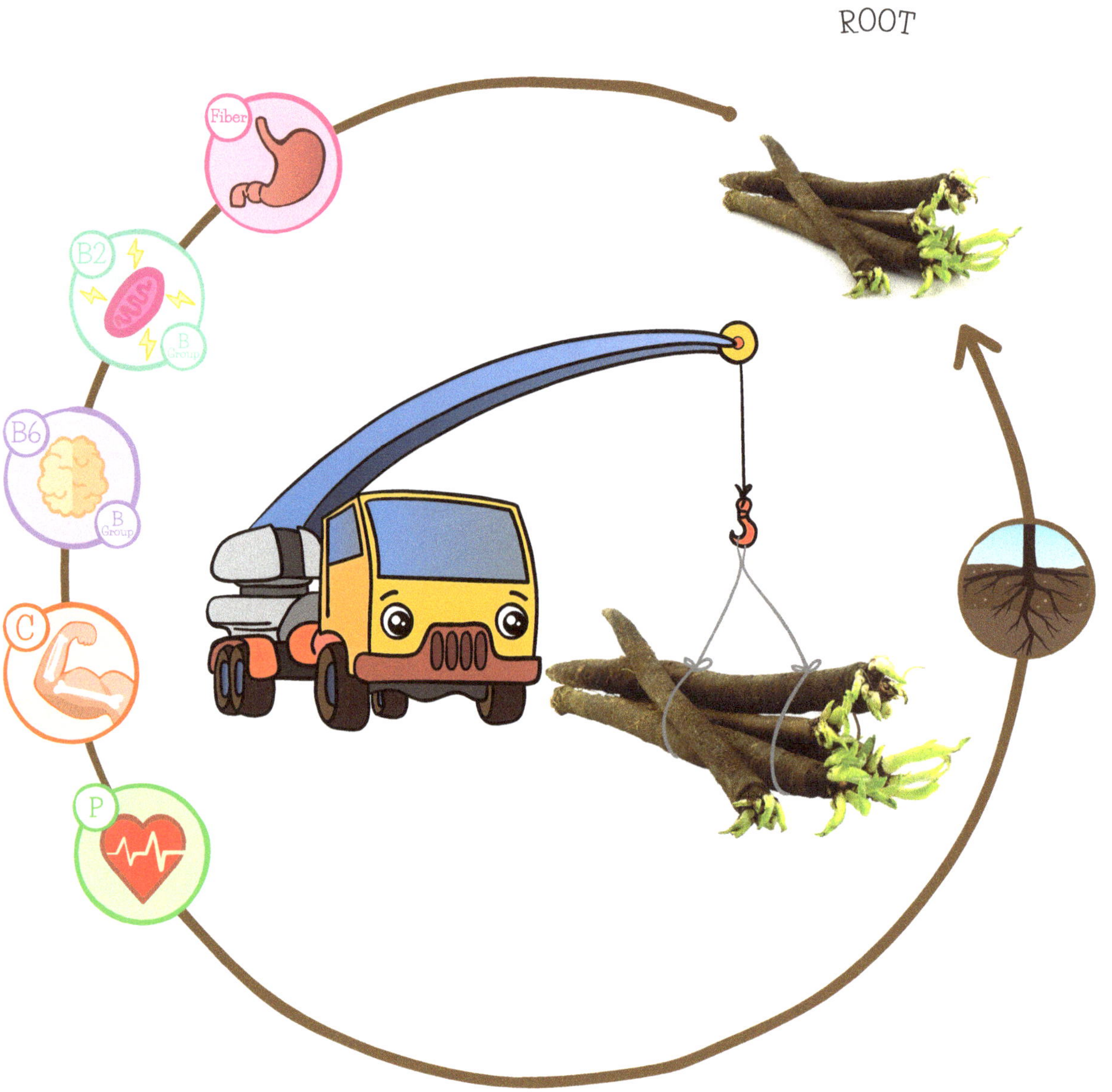

ROOT

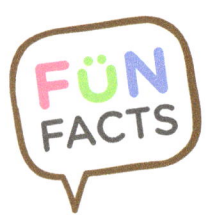

Sometimes salsify is called the "oyster plant," "oyster root," or "vegetable oyster" because of its earthy, sweet, oyster-like flavor. It can be cooked in many of the same ways as asparagus and artichoke.

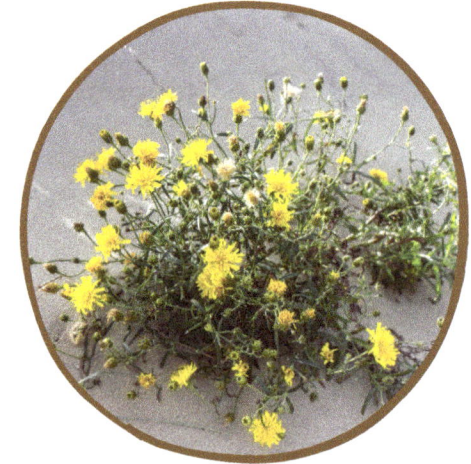

116 | Where Does Broccoli Come From?

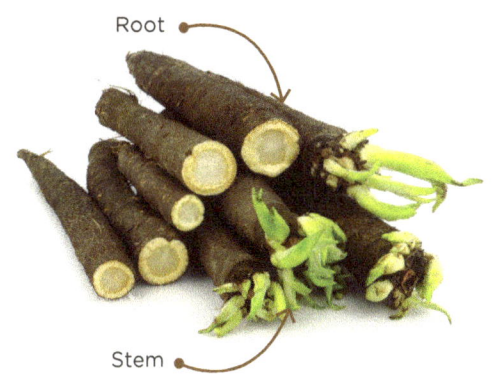
Root
Stem

PICK
Pick firm, well-formed, medium sized **roots** that are about the size of a large carrot and feel heavy for their size. Avoid salsify with cuts.

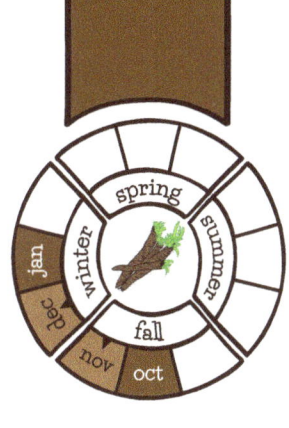

Available October to January; Imported year-round

Peak Season
November-December

STORE
Refrigerate raw salsify in a closed plastic bag for up to 14 days. Refrigerate cooked salsify in an airtight container for 3-5 days.

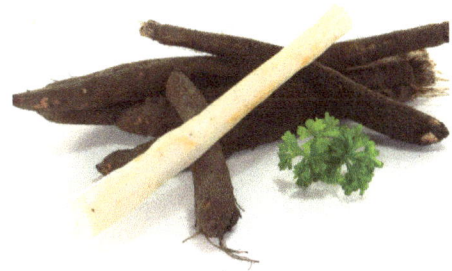

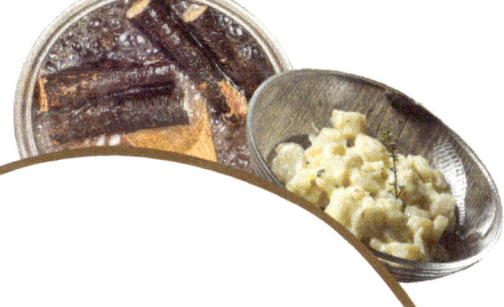

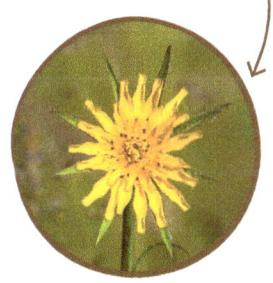

SALSIFY FLOWERS

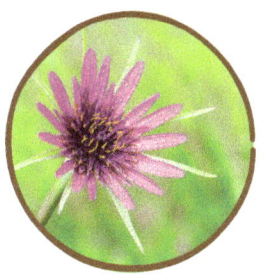

EAT
Clean the skin, scrub with a vegetable brush, and peel. If salsify is difficult to peel, try soaking the root in water for one hour first or peeling after it has been cooked. Chop or slice per recipe. Salsify should be cooked or placed in cold water with vinegar or lemon juice immediately after peeling to prevent browning.

Steamed Salsify
Steam salsify for 10-15 minutes until tender and serve with garlic butter.

There are two **varieties** of salsify, black salsify, also known as scorzonera, and white salsify. Both varieties have **edible flowers** that look like dandelions! Black salsify have bright yellow flowers and white salsify have bright purple flowers.

A Book of Vegetables

SEA VEGETABLES

[see vej-tuh-buhls]

chewy, crunchy, salty, sweet, umami

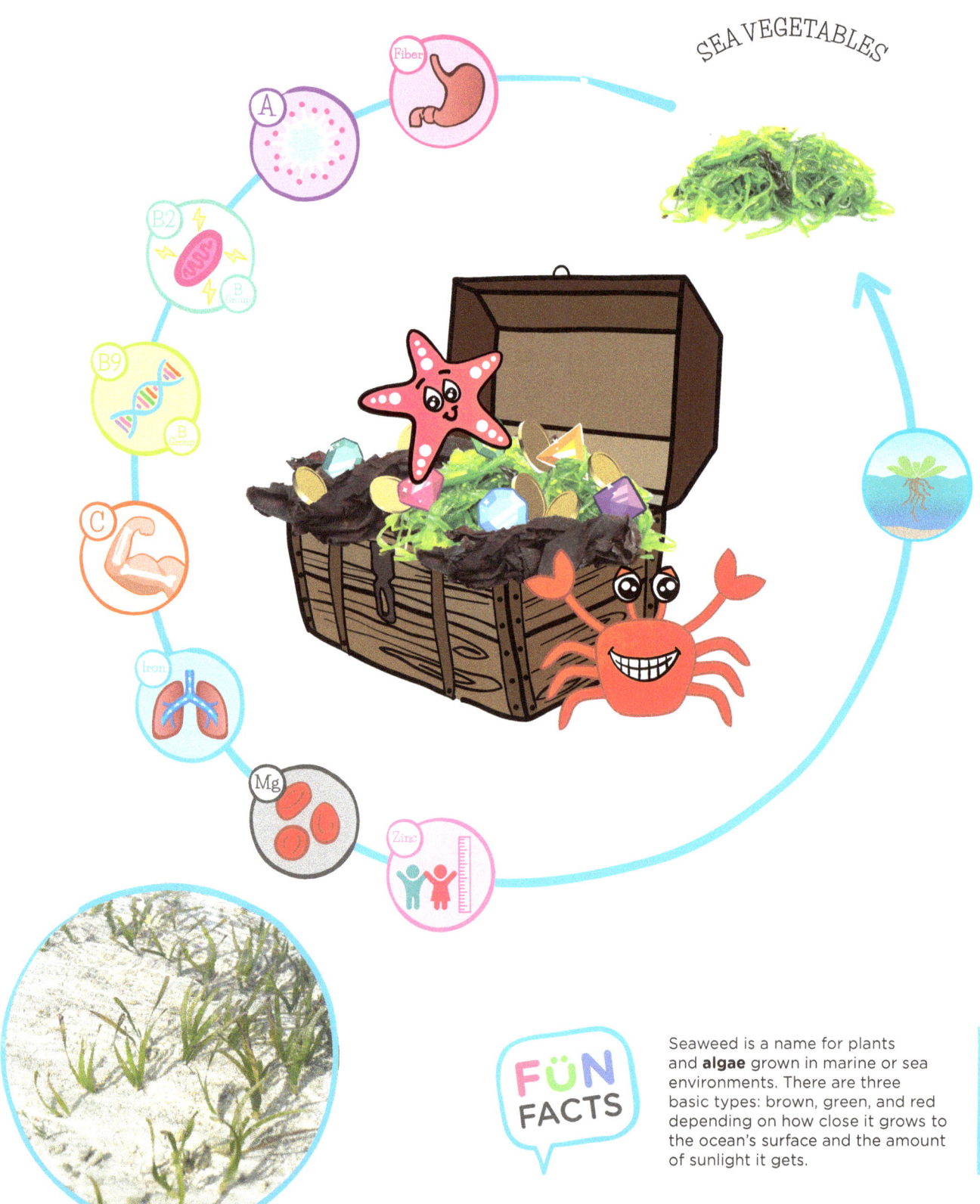

FUN FACTS

Seaweed is a name for plants and **algae** grown in marine or sea environments. There are three basic types: brown, green, and red depending on how close it grows to the ocean's surface and the amount of sunlight it gets.

118 | Where Does Broccoli Come From?

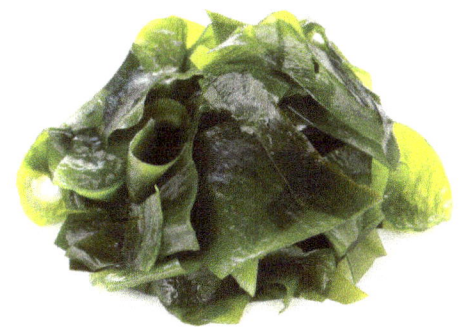

PICK
Most **sea vegetables** are sold prepackaged and dried within the United States in sheets, strips, flakes, or powder form. Fresh seaweed can be **foraged**. Be sure to talk to a local sea vegetable expert to ensure seaweed is safe to eat.

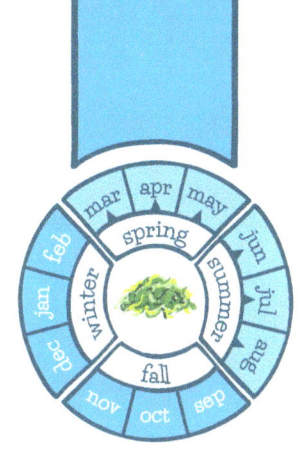

Varieties available year-round; Imported year-round

Peak Season
March-August

STORE
Refrigerate dried sea vegetables for up to 6 months or store in the pantry for 2-4 months. Look for a "Best By" date on prepackaged sea vegetables.

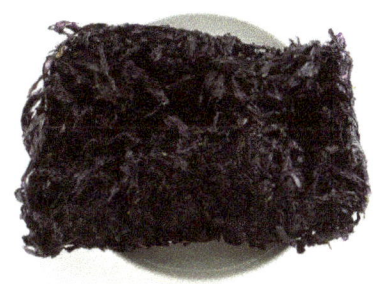

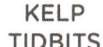

KELP TIDBITS

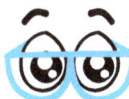

Sea veggies are naturally high in a mineral called **iodine** which is important for growth and development.

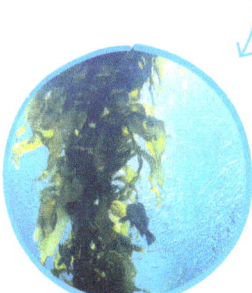

Kelp is a type of seaweed that grows to be very large. In fact, kelp is the fastest growing plant on land or sea and can grow up to two feet a day!

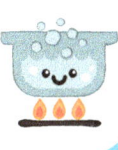

EAT
To rehydrate dried sea vegetables, fill a bowl with water and allow them to soak for 10-15 minutes until soft. Drain and then chop or slice per recipe.

Garnish with Sea Vegetables
Add dried kombu to soup broth for a salty, umami flavoring or sprinkle dulse granules as a seasoning in place of salt on your roasted vegetables.

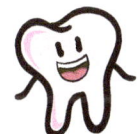

Kelp is a good source of **calcium** which helps build strong bones and teeth and keeps your heart beating strong.

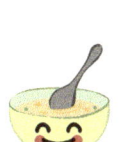
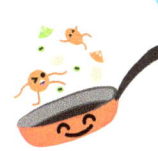

A Book of Vegetables

SEA VEGETABLE VARIETIES

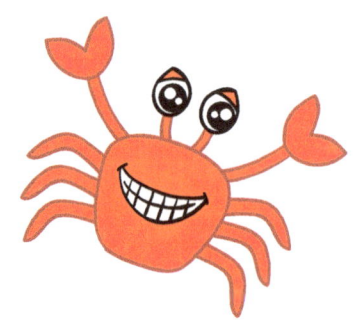

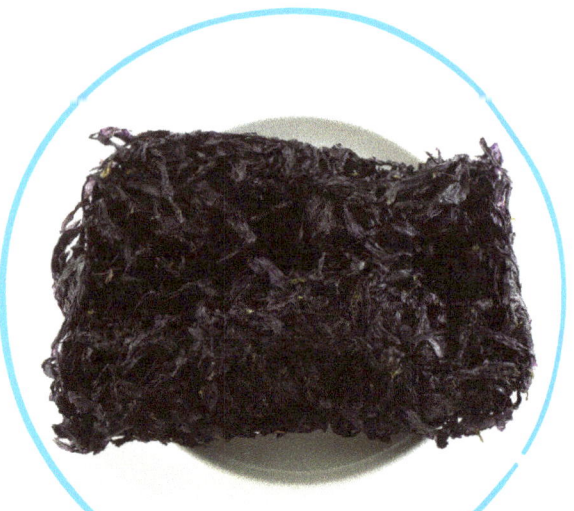

ARAME [ARA-MAE]

Arame is a type of kelp that is available dried in dark brown strands. It has a mild, sweet flavor and firm **texture**. It can be added to salads, soups, or sautéed with other vegetables.

DULSE [DUHLS]

Dulse is a salty, red seaweed with flat, fan-shaped **fronds**. It is often referred to as the "beef jerky of the sea" for its chewy texture. When fried, it is said to taste like bacon.

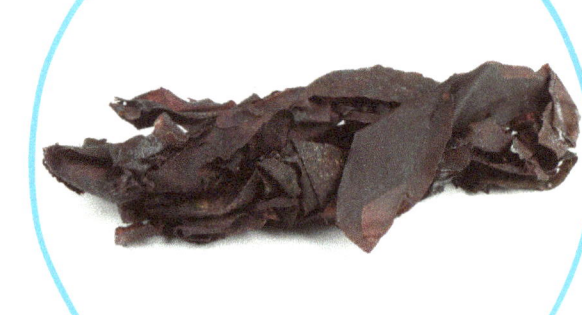

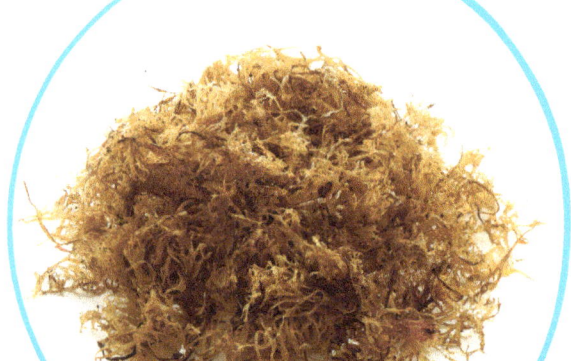

IRISH MOSS [AHY-RISH MAWS]

Have you ever tried a **sea vegetable** before? You probably have and didn't know it! **Carrageenan** is a substance found in Irish moss that is used as a natural **stabilizing** or **thickening** agent in foods and beauty products. Look at the ingredient list on the nutrition facts label of yogurt and see if you can find it!

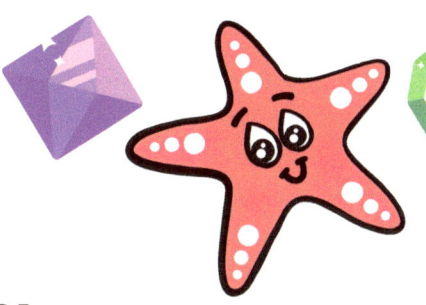

KOMBU [KOM-BOO]

Kombu is a brown seaweed most often used to make dashi, flavorful Japanese broths or cooking **stocks** such as miso soup. It is also used to soften and flavor pots of beans.

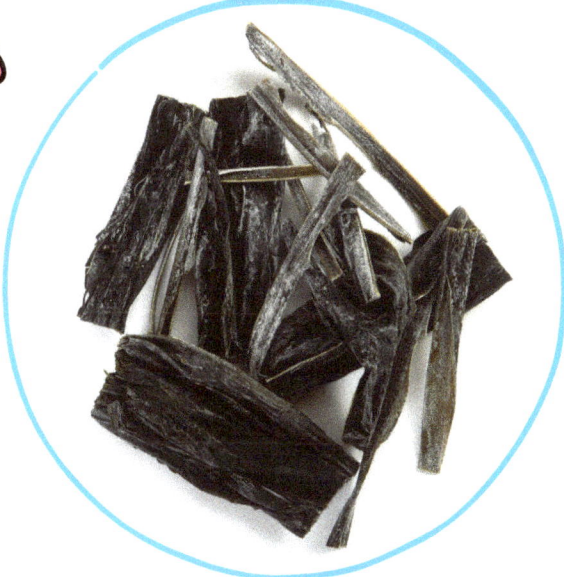

NORI [NOR-EE]

Nori is a red seaweed typically sold in dried sheets. It is commonly found wrapped around sticky rice in sushi, crumbled over savory dishes as a crispy topping, or eaten as a dried snack chip.

WAKAME [WAH-KA-MEH]

Wakame is a sweet tasting, chewy, brown seaweed. However, when wakame is cooked it turns green. It is often served fresh or rehydrated and tossed with sesame oil over salads.

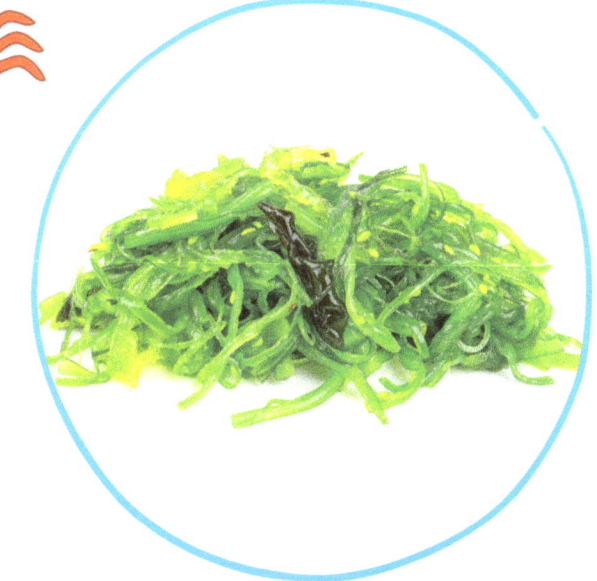

A Book of Vegetables

SPINACH

[spin-ach]

bitter, crisp, delicate, earthy, nutty

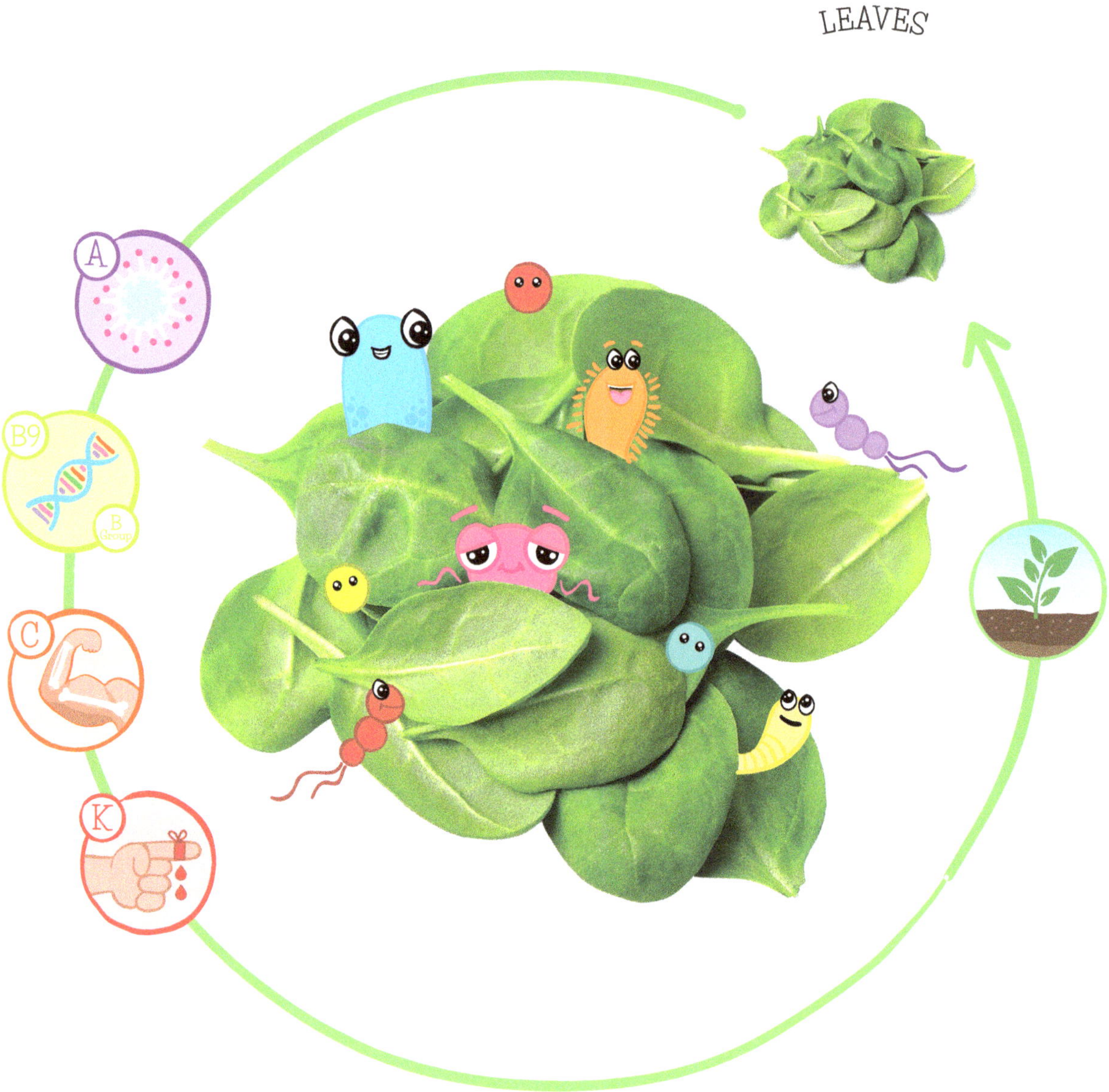

LEAVES

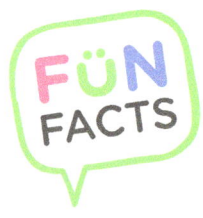

Spinach shrinks when cooked. While fresh spinach may fill an entire bowl, cooked spinach takes up very little space. You need about 2 pounds of spinach to make 4 cooked servings or about 3 cups.

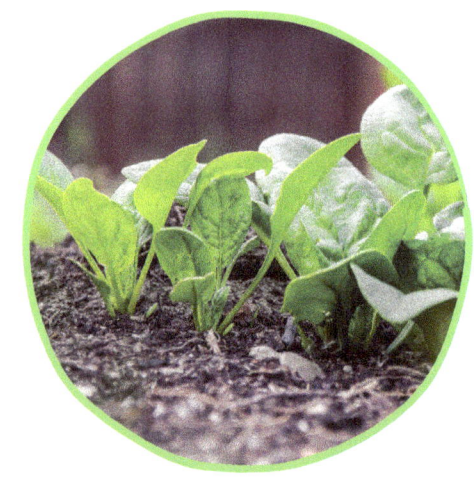

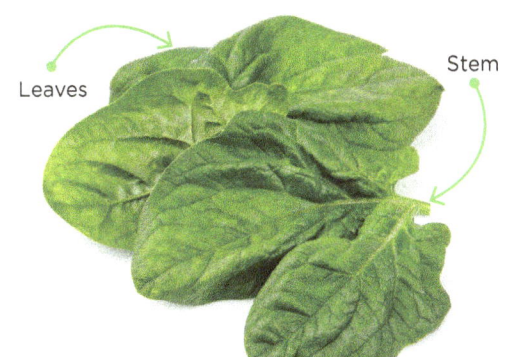
Leaves · Stem

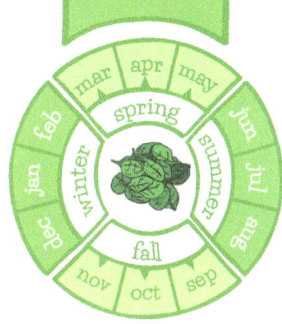

Varieties available year-round

Peak Season
March-May;
September-November

PICK
Pick dark green, crisp **leaves**. Avoid spinach that is **wilting**, yellowing, or slimy.

STORE
Refrigerate unwashed, raw spinach in an open plastic bag for up to 7 days. Refrigerate cooked spinach in an airtight container for 3-5 days.

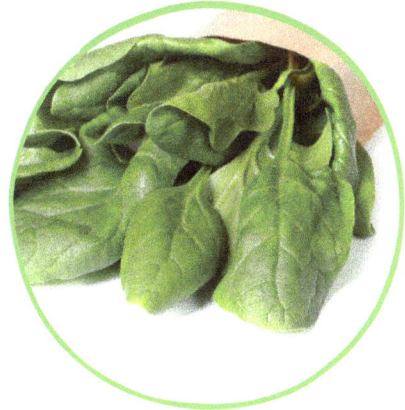
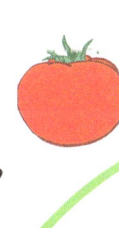
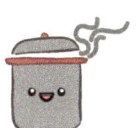
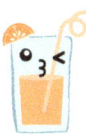

EAT
Clean spinach in a bowl of cold water, stirring leaves around with clean hands and drain. Repeat if leaves still look or feel gritty, then dry on a clean dish towel. If eating raw mature leaves, slice or tear off tough **stems**. Chop or slice per recipe. Bags of pre-washed greens do not need to be cleaned again.

Green Spinach Smoothie
Make a "Monster Smoothie" by grabbing a handful of clean spinach leaves and adding it to your favorite smoothie recipe.

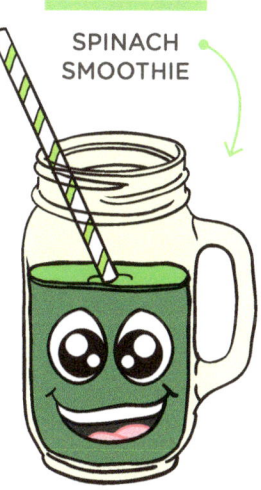

SPINACH SMOOTHIE

Spinach is the perfect addition to smoothies! It has a very mild flavor that is masked by **fruit** and a delicate **texture** that easily liquifies when blended.

A Book of Vegetables 123

SPROUT

[sp-rout]

crisp, crunchy, sweet, tangy, tender

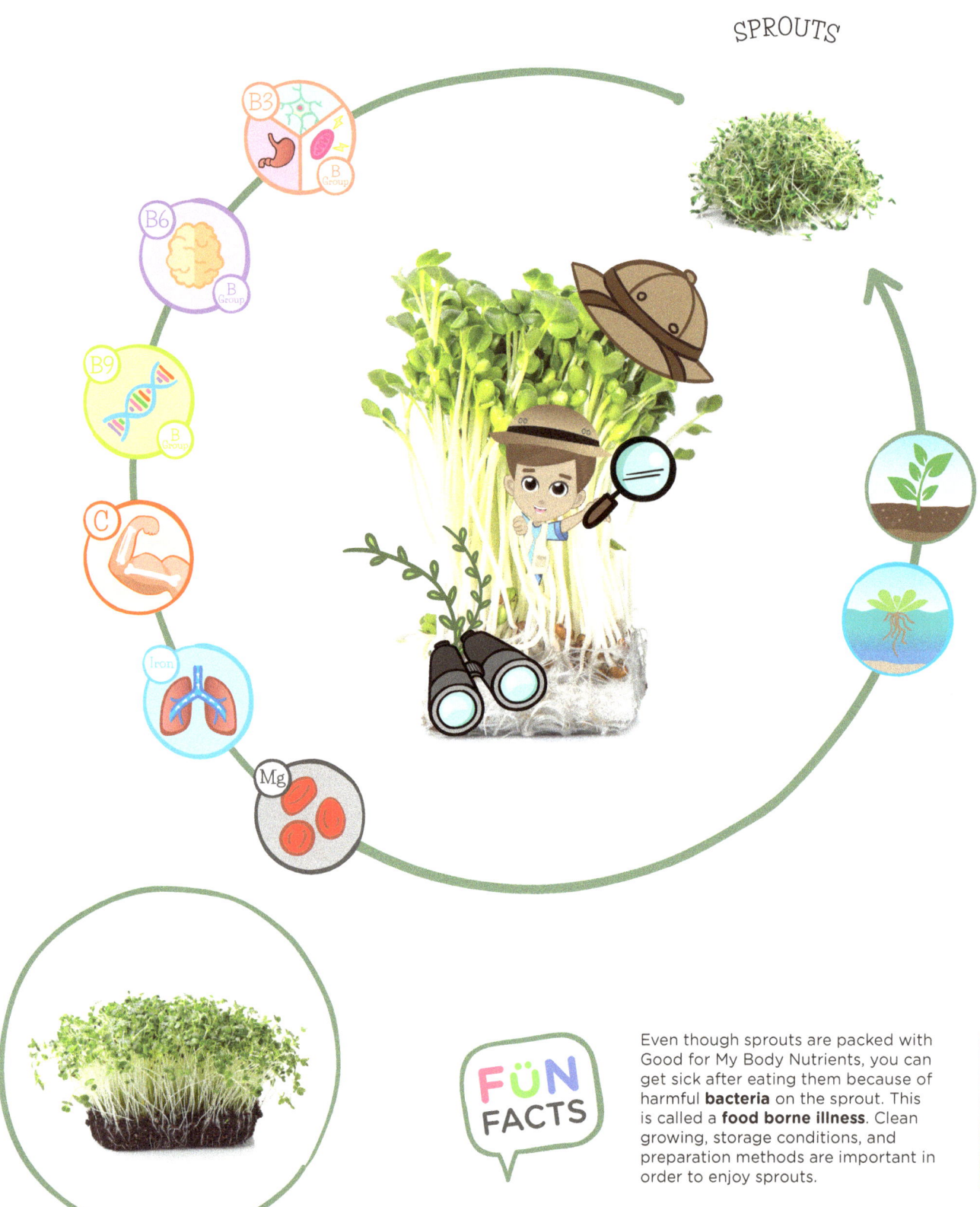

SPROUTS

FUN FACTS

Even though sprouts are packed with Good for My Body Nutrients, you can get sick after eating them because of harmful **bacteria** on the sprout. This is called a **food borne illness**. Clean growing, storage conditions, and preparation methods are important in order to enjoy sprouts.

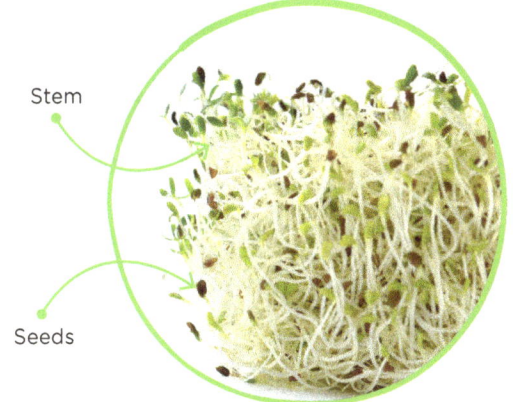
Stem
Seeds

PICK
Pick clean, crisp **sprouts**. Avoid sprouts with dark spots, appear slimy, and have a musty smell.

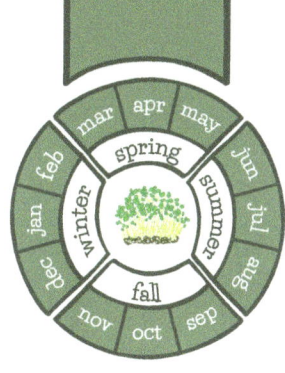

Varieties available year-round

STORE
Refrigerate sprouts in a well-ventilated plastic container for 5-10 days.

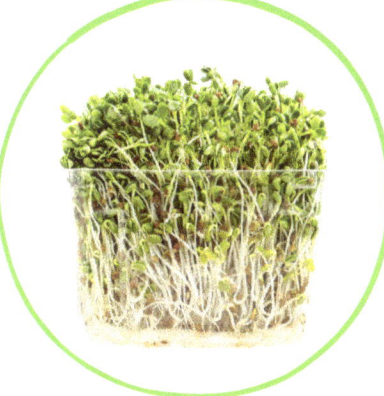

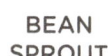
BEAN SPROUT

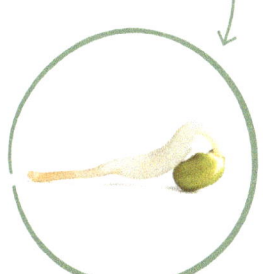

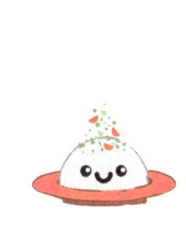

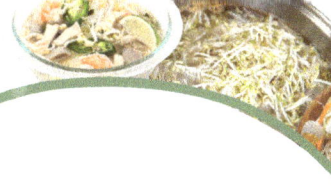

EAT
Clean sprouts thoroughly under cold running water, tossing as you rinse so all sprouts are evenly rinsed, then drain and dry them on a clean dish towel.

Raw Sprouts
Add raw sprouts to sandwiches or cold pasta salad for a flavorful crunch.

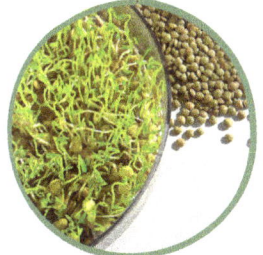

Almost all beans, grains, or **seeds** allowed to soak overnight and grow can sprout tiny plants!

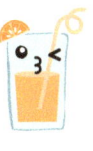
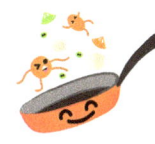

A Book of Vegetables 125

SPROUT VARIETIES

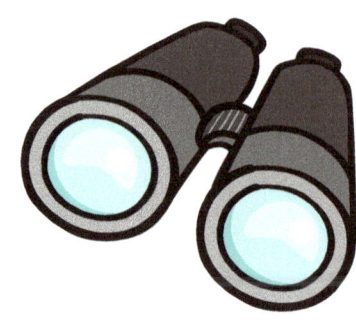

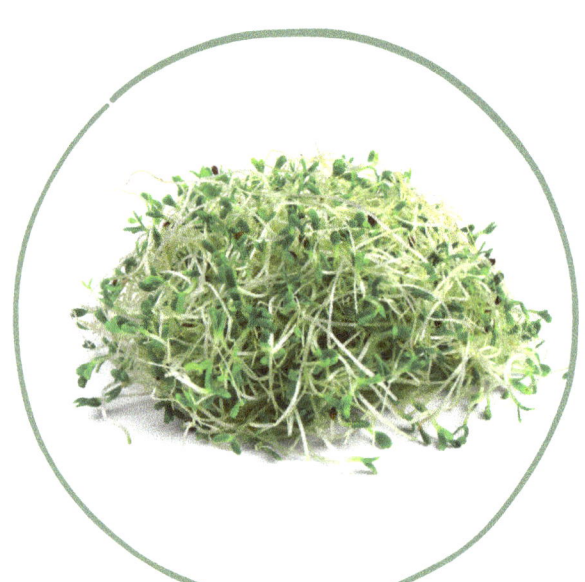

ALFALFA [AL-FAL-FA]

Alfalfa **sprouts** are white and thread-like with tiny green tips. They have a mild, nutty flavor and are typically eaten raw on salads and sandwiches.

BROCCOLI [BROC-CO-LEE]

Broccoli sprouts have thin white **stalks** with light green **leaves** and dark red **seeds**. These mildly spicy, nutty sprouts are typically eaten raw on salads and sandwiches.

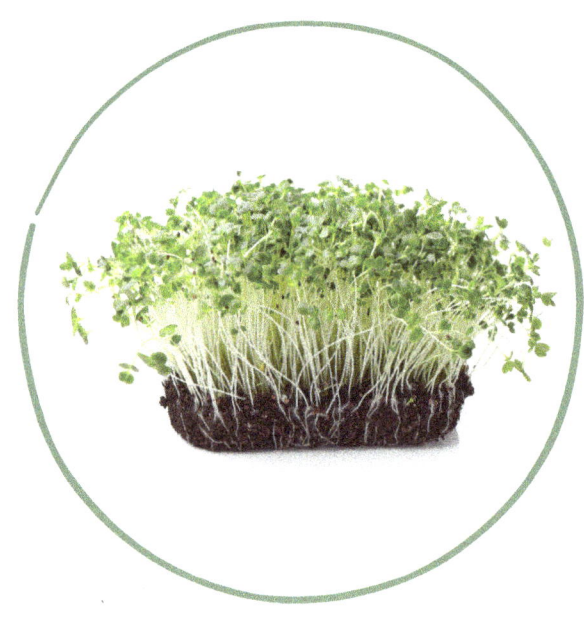

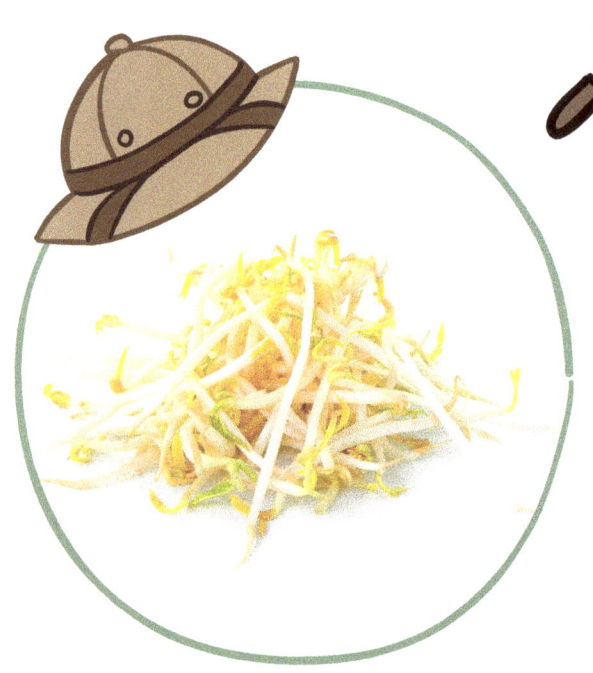

MUNG BEAN [MUHNG BEAN]

The most widely consumed sprouts in the world, mung bean sprouts have thick white stalks with narrowing yellow ends. These large, bland, and crunchy sprouts are a popular addition to Asian dishes, stir-fry, soups, and salads.

RADISH [RAD-ISH]

With several different peppery, zesty, and crunchy **varieties**, radish sprouts are multicolored, from light green, to purple and white, and are typically eaten raw on salads and sandwiches.

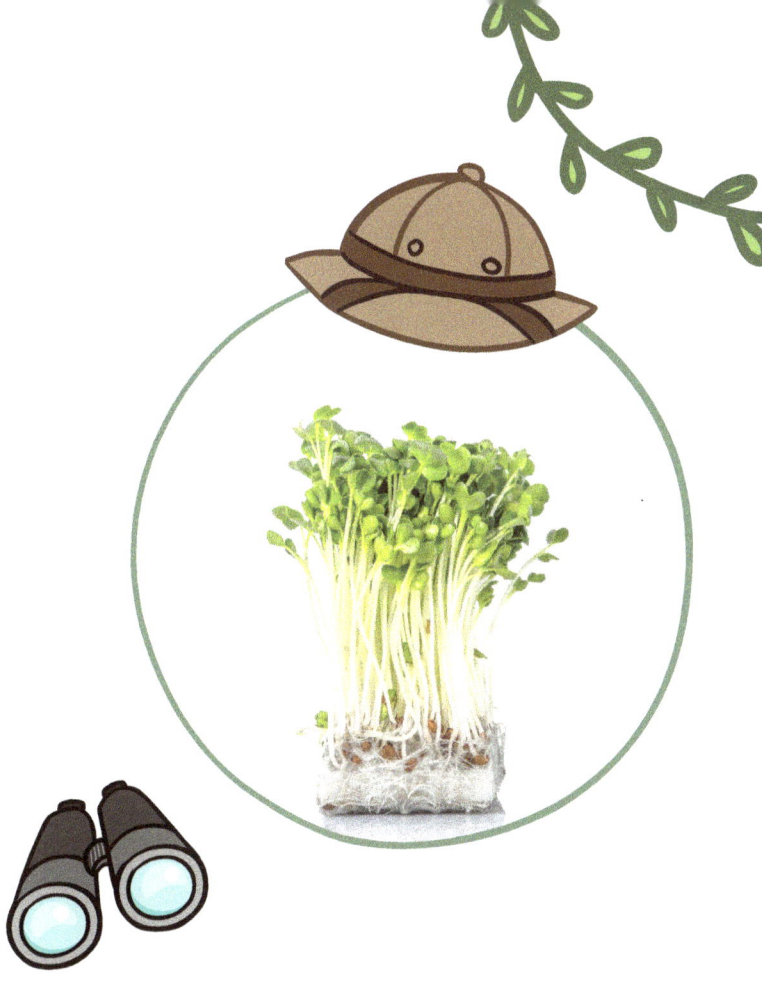

RED CLOVER [RED KLOH-VER]

Red clover is similar to alfalfa sprouts in both taste and appearance. These crisp, mild, and sweet sprouts are typically eaten raw on salads and sandwiches.

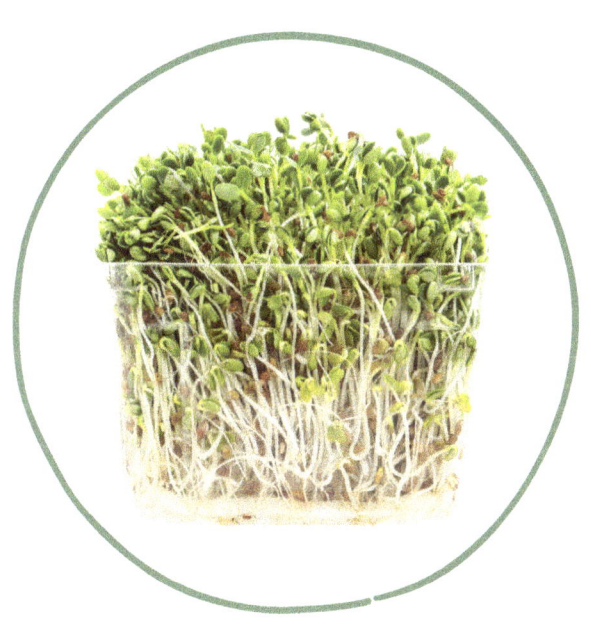

WHEAT GRASS [WEET GRASS]

Wheat grass is in the same family as other **edible** sprouts. It is the early sprouted growth from wheat plant seeds but is typically grown in soil rather than water. This bitter, fibrous sprout is most often added to smoothies or dried into a powdered form to add into other foods.

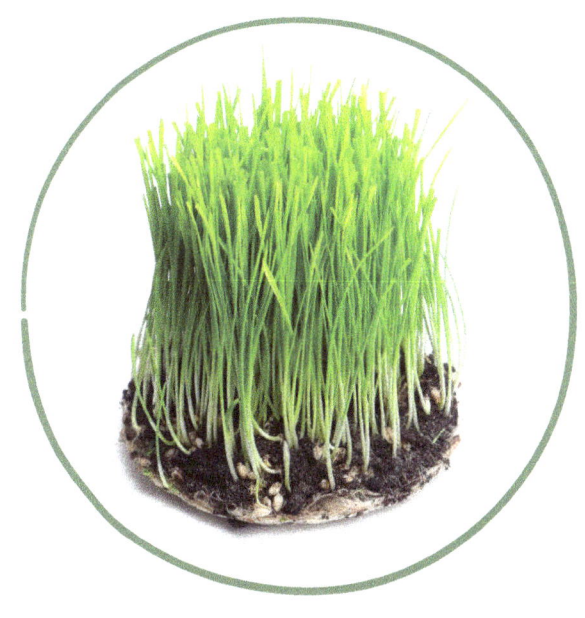

SQUASH, SUMMER

[ska-wash]

mild, nutty, sweet, tender, watery

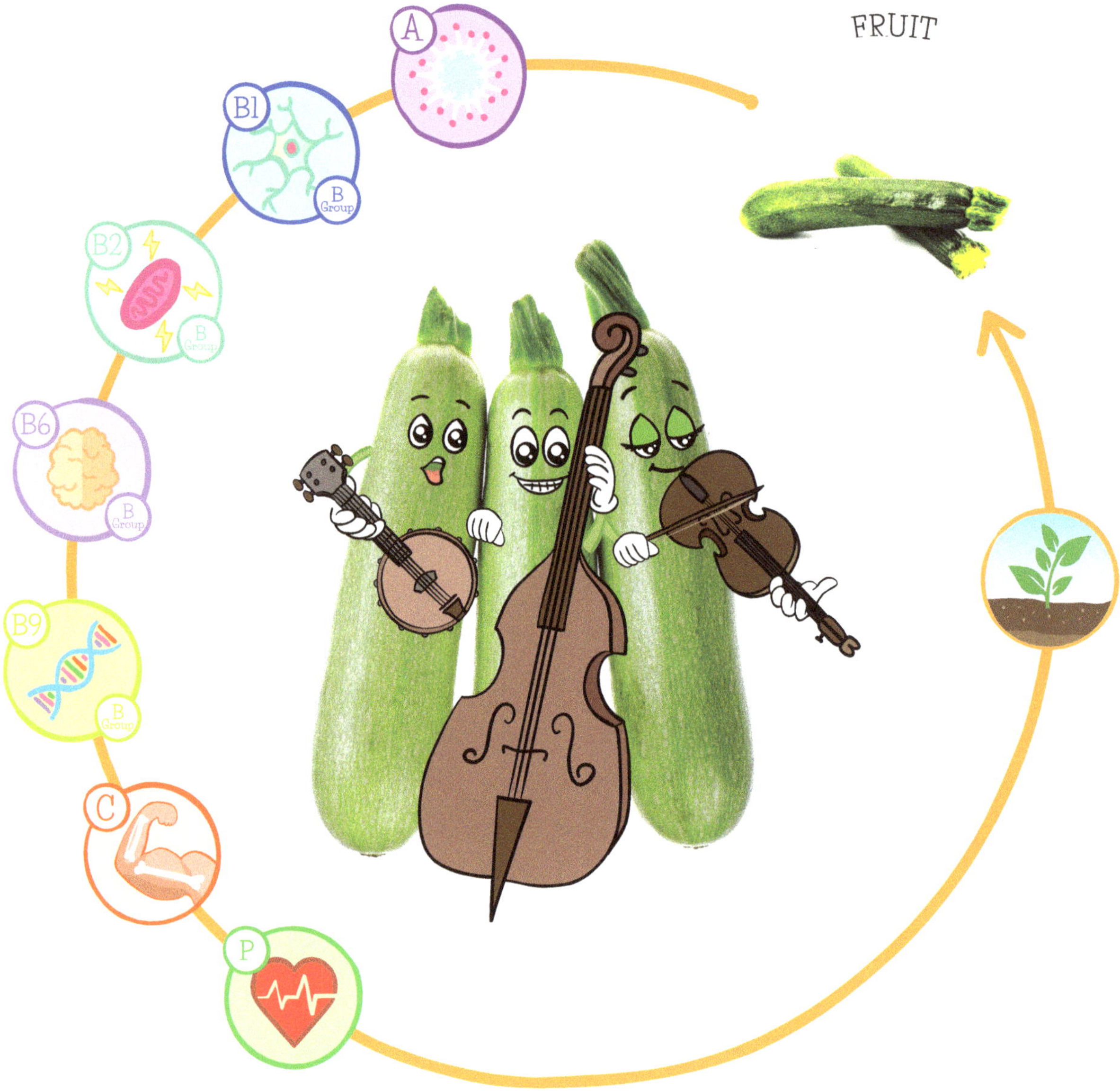

FRUIT

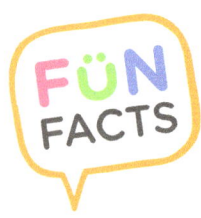

Squash come in many different shapes, sizes, and colors. Summer squash grows rapidly and is usually ready to eat 4-8 days after flowering. They have soft, thin skin, **edible seeds**, and tender, moist **flesh** that cooks quickly.

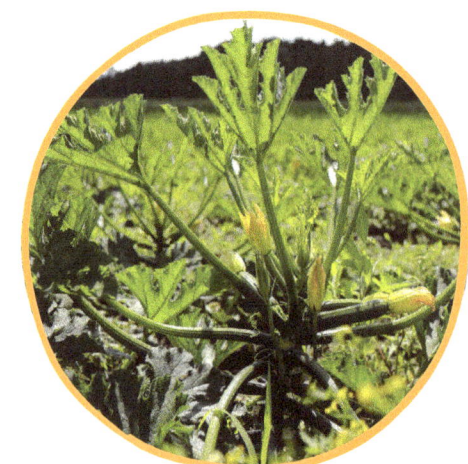

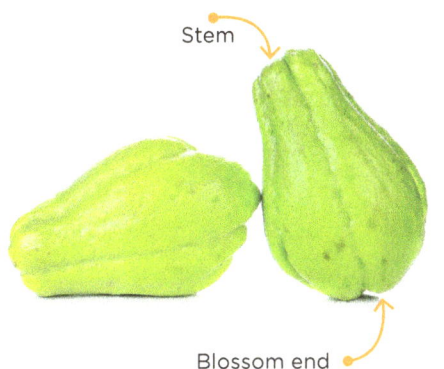
Stem
Blossom end

PICK
Pick vibrantly colored, firm, crisp **fruit** with skin that is soft enough to cut with a fingernail. Avoid summer squash with wrinkled skin, soft spots, and wet spots.

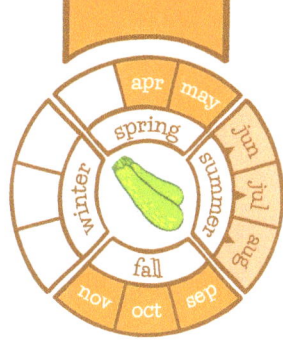

Available April to November; Imported year-round

Peak Season
June-August

STORE
Refrigerate unwashed, raw squash in a closed plastic bag for up to 5 days. Refrigerate cooked squash in an airtight container for 3-5 days.

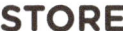

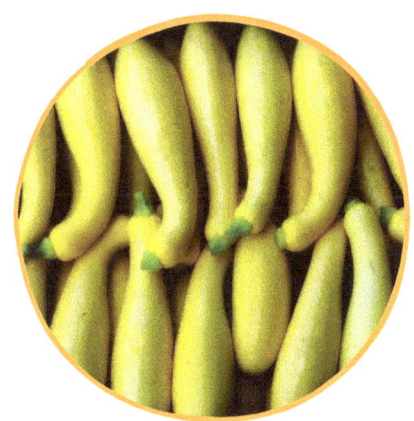

SQUASH BLOSSOMS

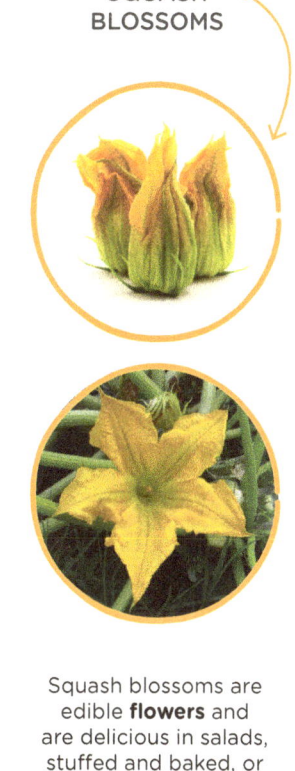

Squash blossoms are edible **flowers** and are delicious in salads, stuffed and baked, or battered and fried.

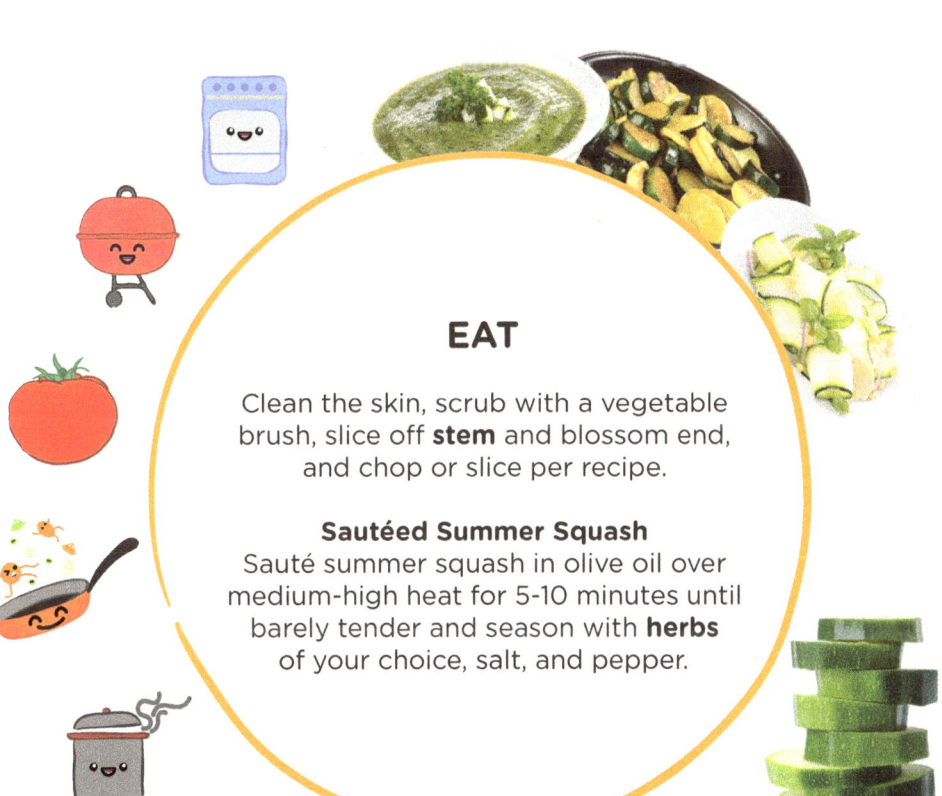

EAT
Clean the skin, scrub with a vegetable brush, slice off **stem** and blossom end, and chop or slice per recipe.

Sautéed Summer Squash
Sauté summer squash in olive oil over medium-high heat for 5-10 minutes until barely tender and season with **herbs** of your choice, salt, and pepper.

A Book of Vegetables 129

SQUASH, SUMMER VARIETIES

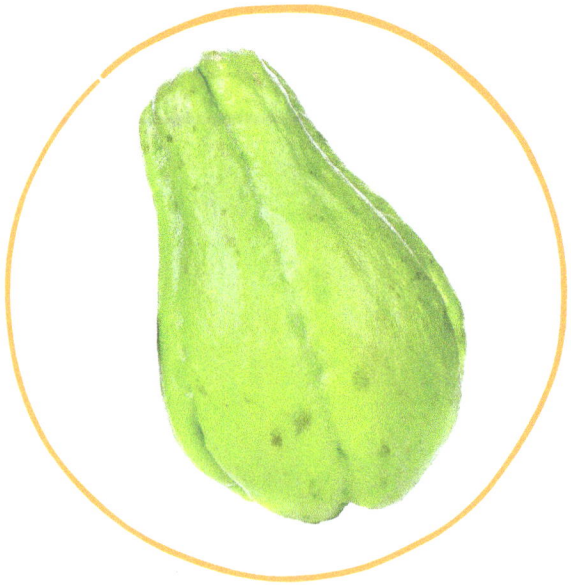

CHAYOTE [CHAY-OH-TEE]

Chayote is a light green, pear-shaped, squash with a single large pit and bland **flesh**. The **texture** is a cross between a cucumber and a potato. Chayote is used in cuisine around the world because it complements a **variety** of flavors while adding great texture.

COUSA [COO-SA]

Shorter and wider than zucchini, cousa squash is often used in Middle Eastern cuisine. It is known for being light, sweet, and tender. The thick width of cousa makes it perfect for stuffing!

PATTY PAN [PAT-EE PAN]

Patty pan squash is very often compared to a flying saucer. It is small, round, and flat with scalloped edges. Patty pan squash have a mild, buttery, grassy flavor when cooked. Use them for decoration, try them sliced raw on a salad, or sauté them with **herbs** and olive oil.

YELLOW SQUASH
[YEL-OH SKA-WASH]

Yellow squash is similar to zucchini in flavor, but looks very different. It has a narrow curved or straight neck, round **bulb**-shaped blossom end, and mildly sweet seeded flesh. Try substituting yellow squash in zucchini recipes.

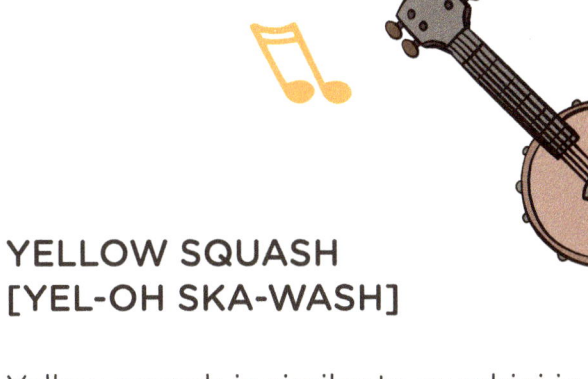

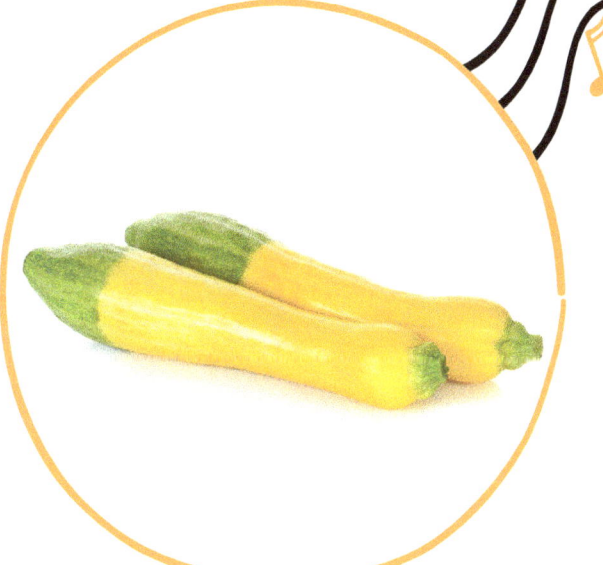

ZEPHYR [ZEF-ER]

Zephyr squash is a hybrid of hybrids. It is a hybrid of yellow crookneck squash and another hybrid squash that is a cross between acorn squash and delicata squash. Zephyr is a two-tone, yellow and green squash that is tender, sweet, and nutty.

ZUCCHINI | COURGETTE
[ZOO-KEY-NI] | [COR-JETTE]

Straight and **cylindrical** with varieties that range from yellow to green, Zucchini is the most popular summer squash in the United States. The longest zucchini recorded by the Guinness Book of World Records measured 8 feet 3.3 inches in Niagara Falls, Canada, 28 August 2014!

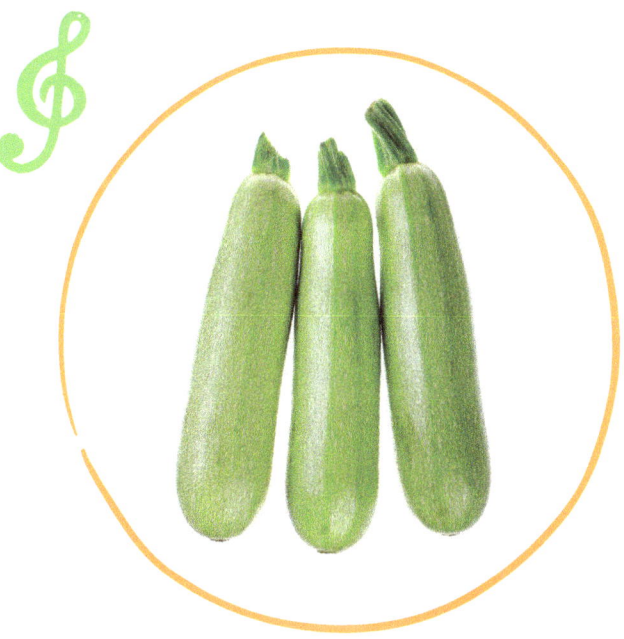

A Book of Vegetables

SQUASH, WINTER

[ska-wash]

earthy, firm, nutty, sweet, tender

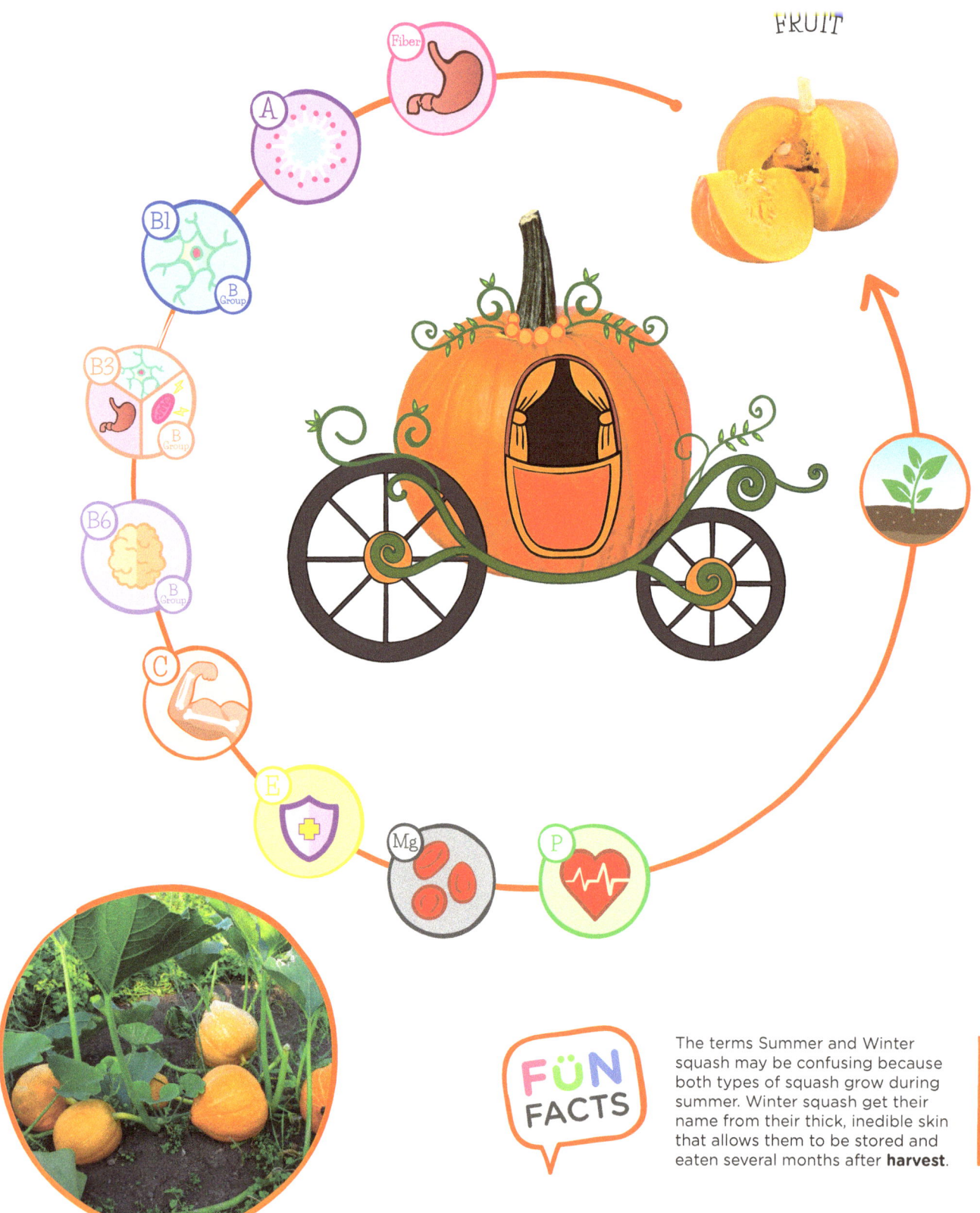

Fun Facts: The terms Summer and Winter squash may be confusing because both types of squash grow during summer. Winter squash get their name from their thick, inedible skin that allows them to be stored and eaten several months after **harvest**.

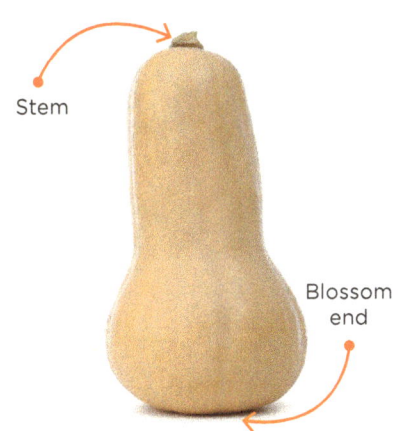

Stem

Blossom end

PICK
Pick richly colored, firm **fruit** with hard, tough skin, that are heavy for their size. Avoid winter squash with cuts, cracks, soft spots, **mold**, or look sunken.

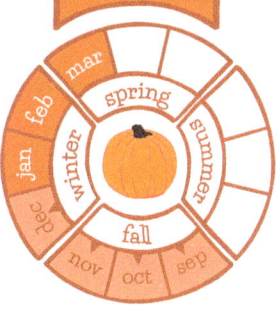

Available September to March; Imported year-round

Peak Season
September-December

STORE
Keep squash in a basket that is well-ventilated and store in a cool, dark place for up to 3 months. Refrigerate raw sliced or chopped winter squash in an airtight container for up to 4 days and cooked in an airtight container for 3-5 days.

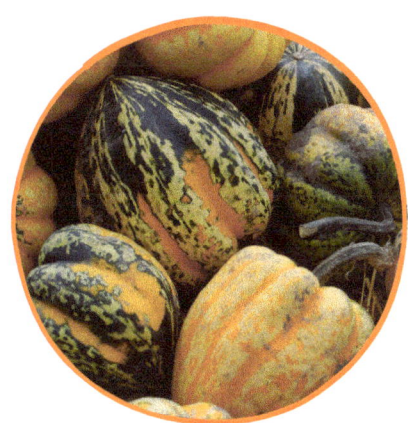

EAT
Clean the skin, slice off **stem** and blossom end or slice in half from stem to blossom end (hotdog style). This may take a bit of muscle! Scoop out the stringy **flesh** and **seeds** and leave halved or slice per recipe.

Roasted Winter Squash
Preheat your oven to 400 degrees F. Slice winter squash in half and coat with olive oil, then place on a foil-lined roasting tray, and roast for 25-30 minutes until squash is tender and lightly browned or can be easily **pierced** with a fork.

SQUASH SEEDS

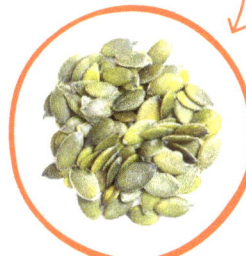

You can eat the seeds! Rinse the seeds until they are clean and free of stringy flesh; dry thoroughly on a clean kitchen towel; coat with olive oil and season as desired; then spread on a foil-lined baking sheet. Bake seeds for 1 hour at 250 degrees F or until light brown and toasted.

A Book of Vegetables 133

SQUASH, WINTER VARIETIES

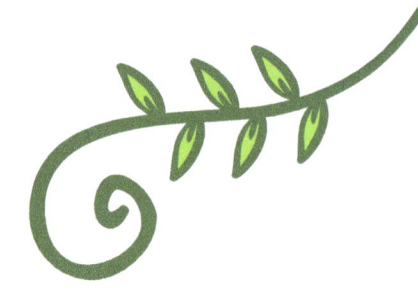

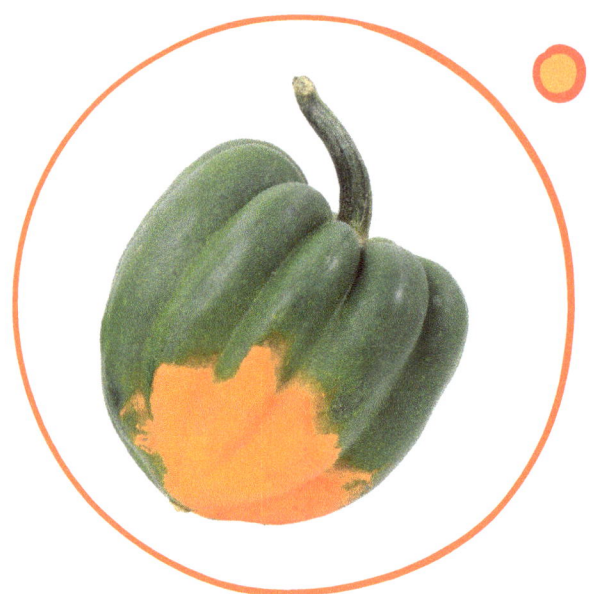

ACORN [A-CORN]

Shaped like a giant ribbed acorn, this blackish-green to golden-yellow squash has **edible** skin and sweet, nutty orange-yellow flesh. Roast acorn squash in half and use them as edible bowls!

BUTTERNUT [BUT-TER-NUT]

Butternut squash is a long-necked squash with a round, **bulb**-shaped, seeded blossom end. It has creamy, beige-colored skin and bright orange **flesh** that tastes sweet and nutty. Butternut squash is delicious as a soup.

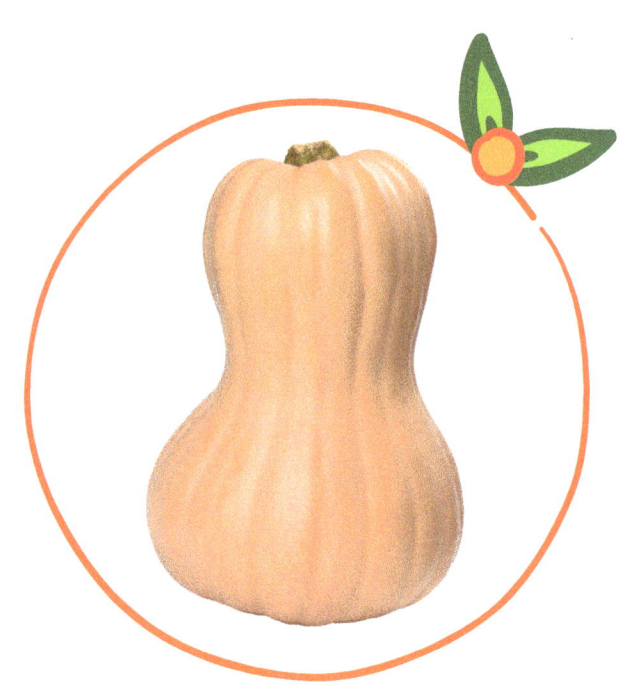

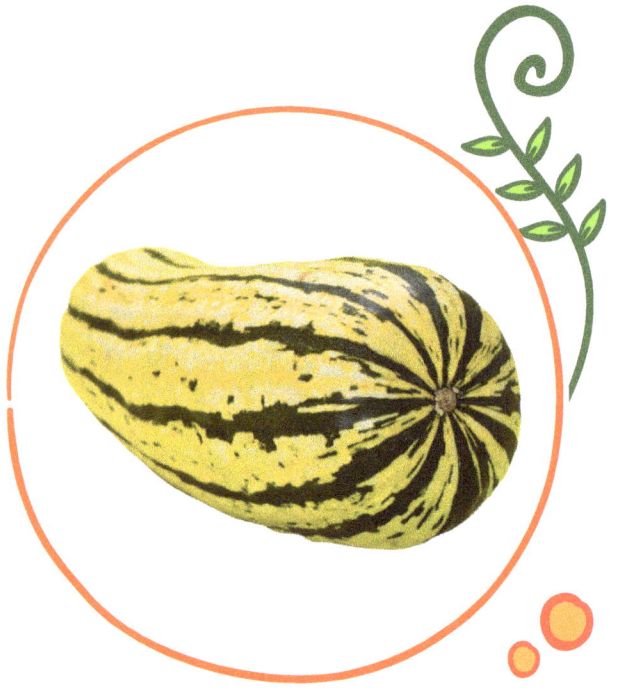

DELICATA [DEL-I-CATA]

Delicata is a small **cylindrical** squash with yellow skin and green stripes. The flesh is orange-yellow and it is often compared in flavor to an earthy mixture of corn and sweet potato. Delicata squash are great roasted with maple syrup.

HUBBARD [HUB-BARD]

Hubbard squash are one of the largest winter squash varieties. They are round with a narrow neck. They have dark green to blue-gray, thick, bumpy skin and firm, sweet orange flesh. This **variety** is similar in flavor to pumpkin and makes a great pie filling.

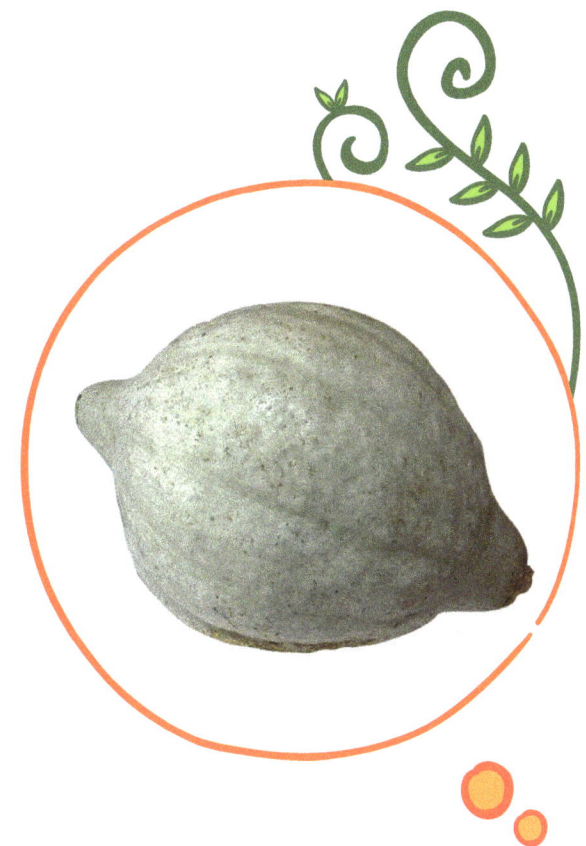

PUMPKIN [PUMP-KIN]

Widely known for jack-o-lantern carving on Halloween and famous for festive pies, there are hundreds of pumpkin varieties differing in color, use, and size. The heaviest pumpkin recorded by the Guinness Book of World Records weighed in at 2,624.6 pounds in Ludwigsburg, Germany, 9 October 2016.

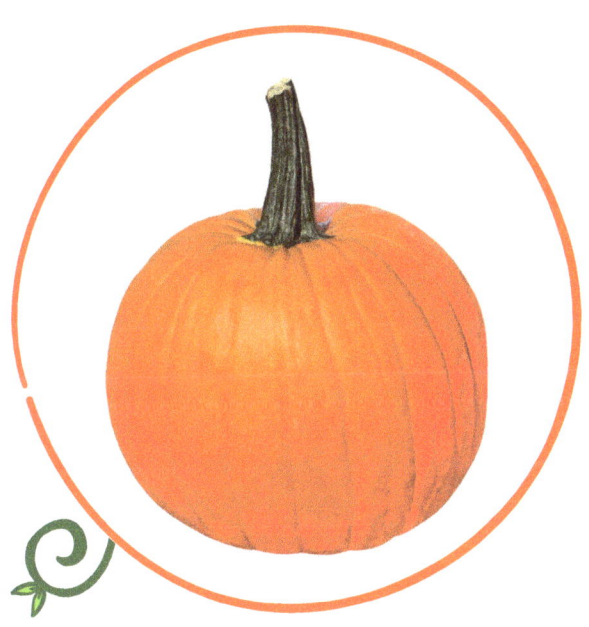

SPAGHETTI [SPA-GET-TI]

Take your fork to the inside flesh of a cooked spaghetti squash and you will know how it got its name. The stringy, sweet, crisp, and tender spaghetti-like strands of this golden yellow squash is perfect tossed with your favorite pasta sauce and topped with parmesan cheese.

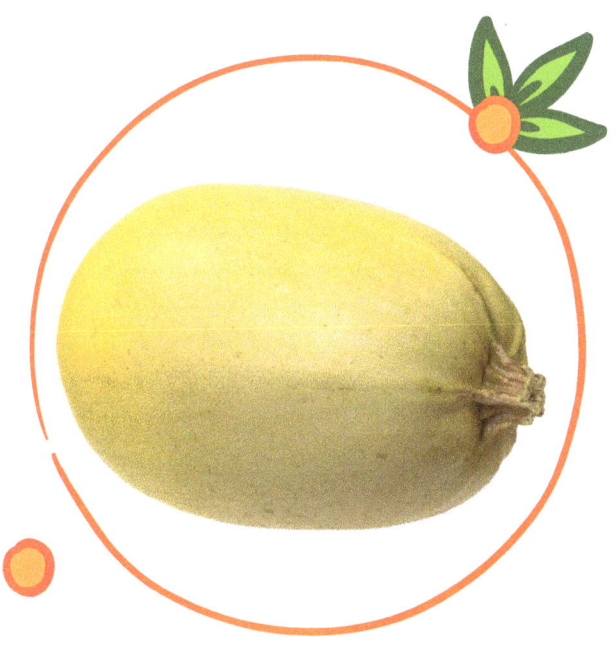

SWEET POTATO

[sweet po-tate-o]

creamy, mealy, moist, sweet, tender

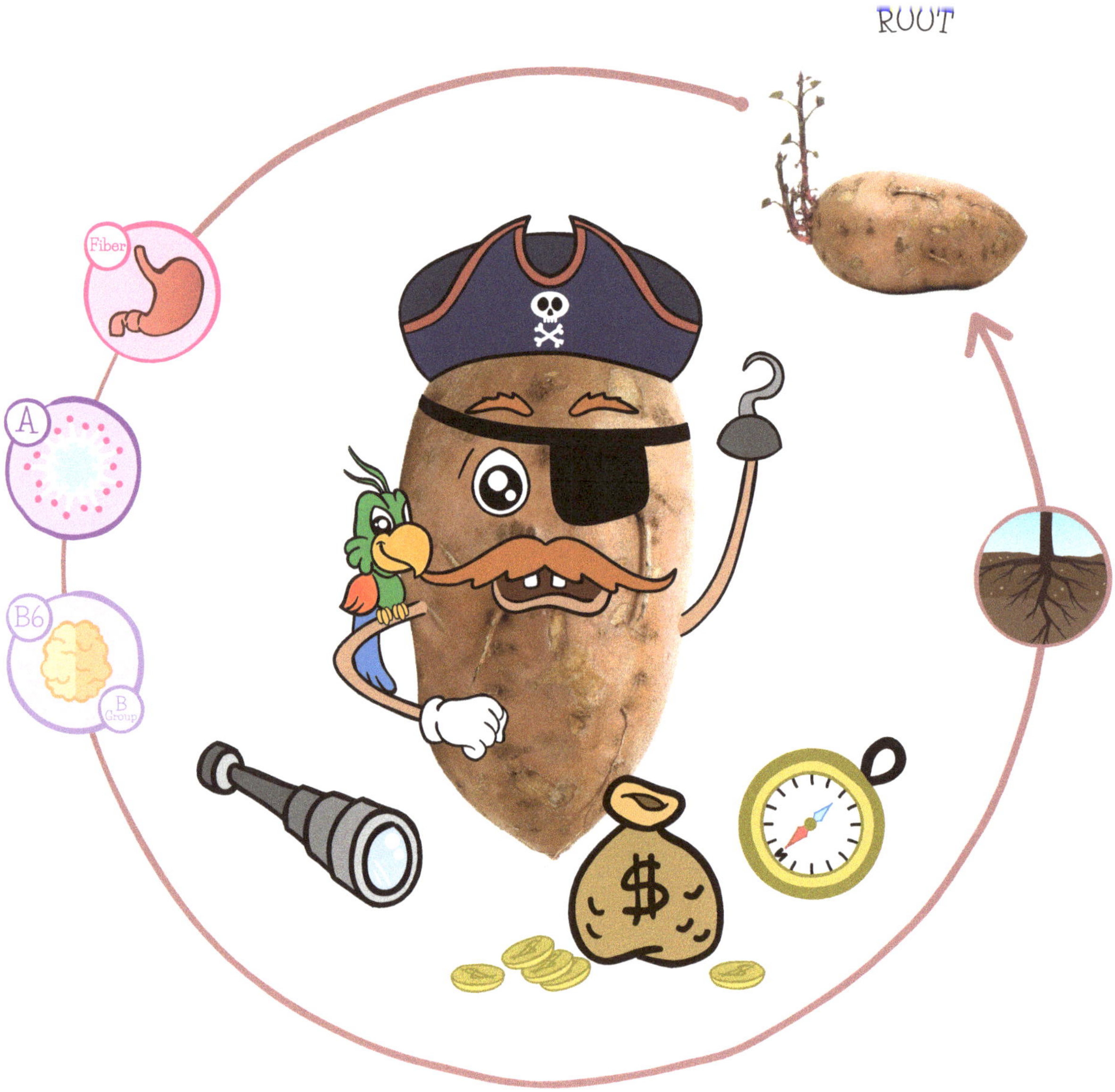

ROOT

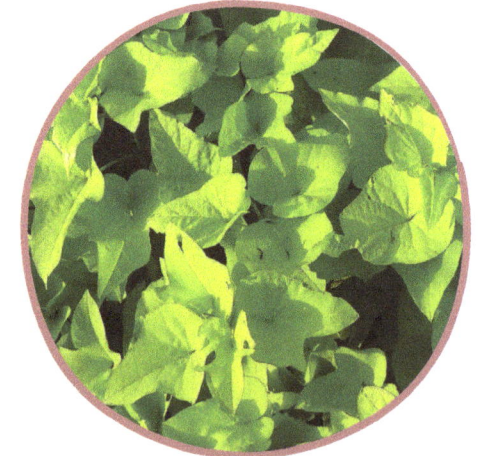

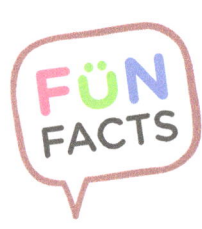

FUN FACTS

While the names are often used interchangeably, yams and sweet potatoes are not even the same type of vegetable. Sweet potatoes are roots and yams are **tubers**. It is believed that the confusion began in the 1700's when people from Africa were brought to the Americas as slaves. At that time, they began calling sweet potatoes yams because they were similar to the vegetable yams they knew from Africa.

136 | Where Does Broccoli Come From?

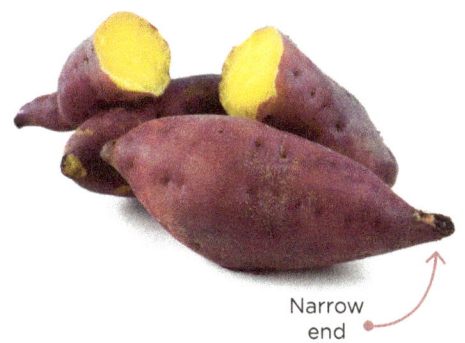

PICK
Pick firm **roots** with thin, smooth skin and narrow ends. Avoid sweet potatoes with cuts, soft spots, and **mold**.

Narrow end

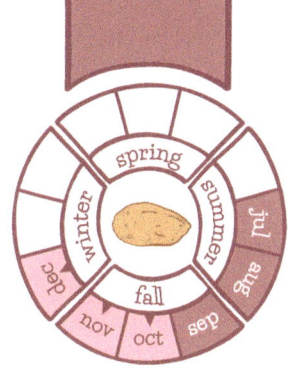

Available July to December; Imported year-round

Peak Season
October-December

STORE
Keep sweet potato in a basket that is well-ventilated and store in a cool, dark place for up to 3 months or at room **temperature** on the countertop for 1-2 weeks. Do not store sweet potatoes near potatoes or onions because they cause each other to **spoil** faster. Refrigerate cooked sweet potatoes in an air tight container for 3-5 days.

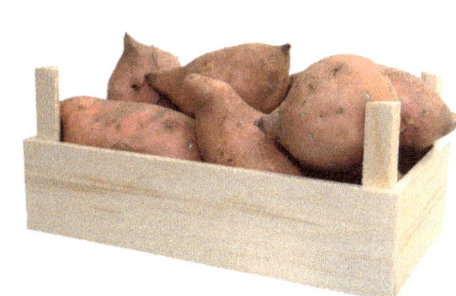

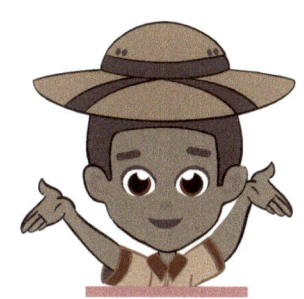

SWEET POTATO TIDBITS

Sweet potatoes are not true potatoes because they are roots and not tubers.

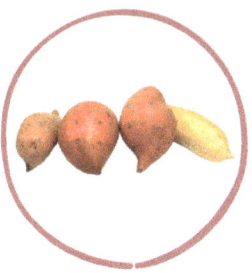

EAT
Clean the skin and scrub with a vegetable brush, peel if desired, then chop or slice per recipe. Potatoes should be cooked or placed in cold water immediately after peeling to prevent browning.

Baked Sweet Potato Fries
Preheat your oven to 425 degrees F, chop sweet potatoes into fry-sized pieces, toss in a bowl with olive oil, cinnamon, and salt then place in a single layer on a **greased** foil-lined roasting tray in the top third of the oven until tender and golden brown, 20-25 minutes, turning occasionally.

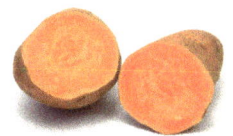

Sweet potato skin color can be white, yellow, red, purple, or brown and the **flesh** can be white, yellow, orange, or even orange-red.

A Book of Vegetables 137

SWISS CHARD
CHARD

[swiss shard]

bitter, earthy, fibrous, tender, tough

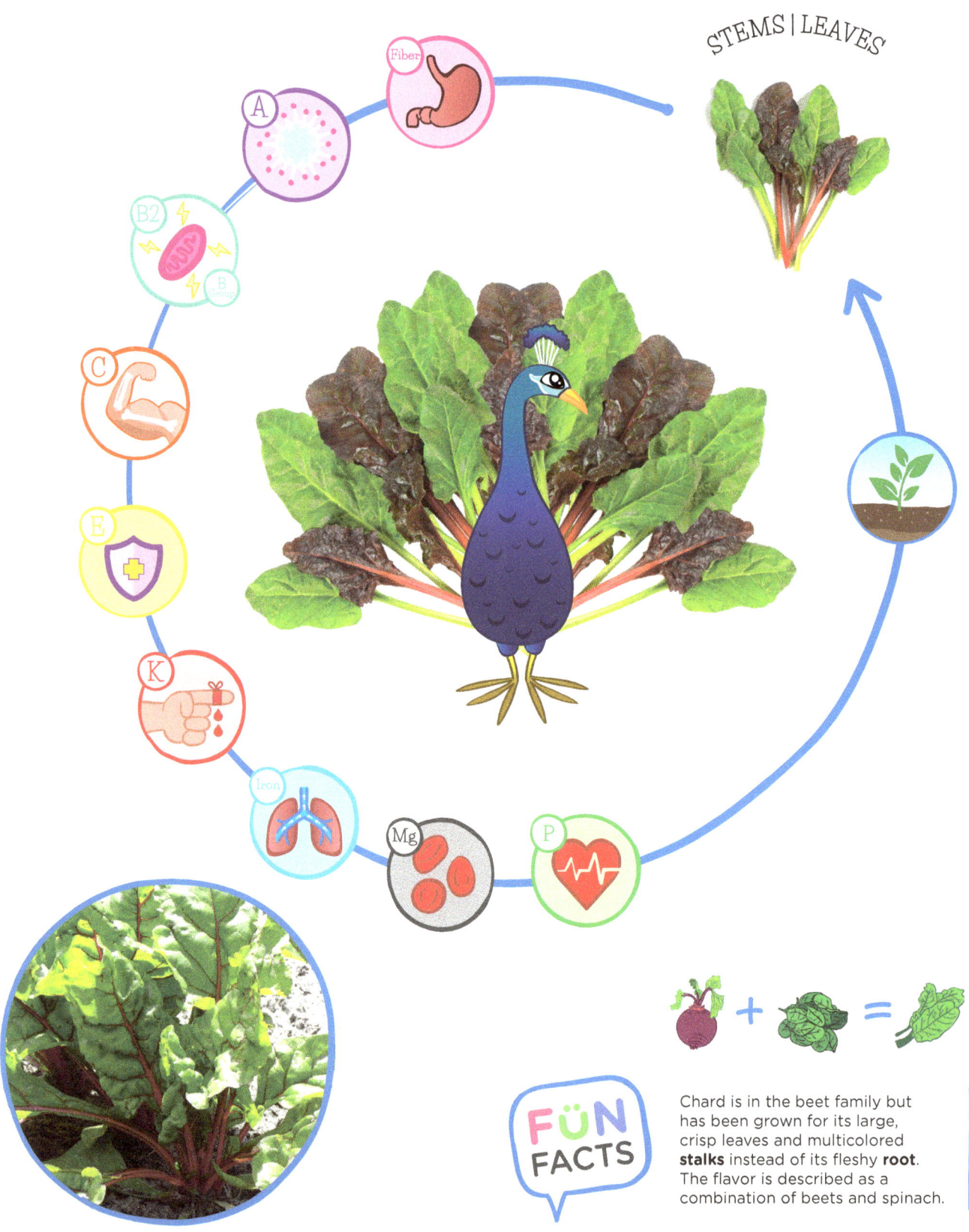

STEMS | LEAVES

FUN FACTS

Chard is in the beet family but has been grown for its large, crisp leaves and multicolored **stalks** instead of its fleshy **root**. The flavor is described as a combination of beets and spinach.

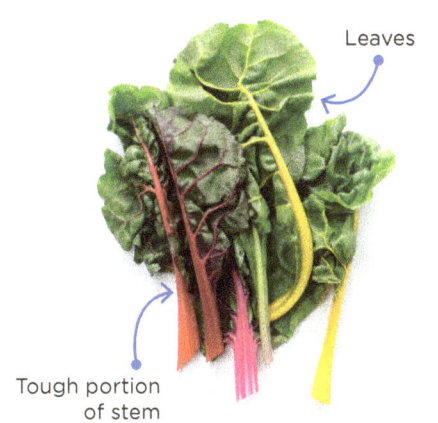

Leaves

Tough portion of stem

PICK
Pick vibrantly colored, crisp **leaves** and **stems**. Avoid Swiss chard that is **wilted** and **bruised**.

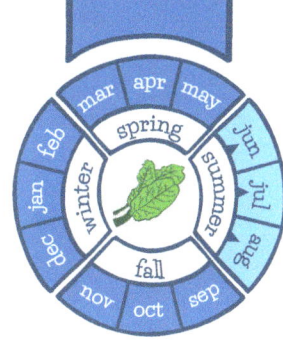

Varieties available year-round

Peak Season
June-August

STORE
Refrigerate unwashed, raw swiss chard in a closed plastic bag for up to 5 days. Refrigerate cooked chard in an airtight container for 3-5 days.

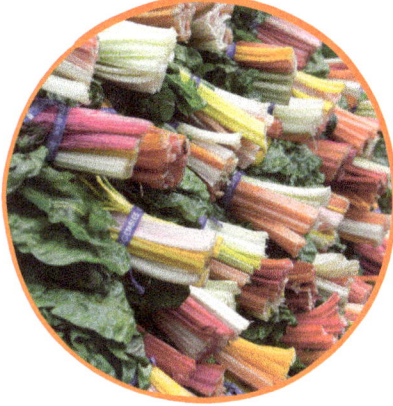

Check out page 61 (Collard Greens) for tips on how to remove the tough portion of the stem.

CHARD TIDBITS

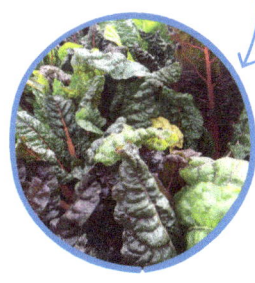

EAT
Clean the leaves several times to remove all dirt and shake off the excess water. Chop off the bottom of the stem, fold each leaf in half lengthwise (hotdog style) and slice the tough portion of the stem from the leaf. Then, stack several of the leaves on top of each other, roll into a large bunch, and chop leaves into thick slices or chop per recipe.

Soup, Stews, and Sautéed Swiss Chard
Add swiss chard to soups and stews. Swiss chard stems may be sautéed on medium-high heat in olive oil and garlic for 8 to 10 minutes until tender.

Chard leaves vary in color from yellow to dark green to red. They have flat, colorful stalks that look similar to celery.

Both the stems and leaves can be used together in a recipe. However, the stems take longer to cook. If you cook them together, be sure to add the leaves 3-4 minutes after the stems.

A Book of Vegetables 139

TARO

[ta-ro]

earthy, nutty, starchy, sticky, sweet

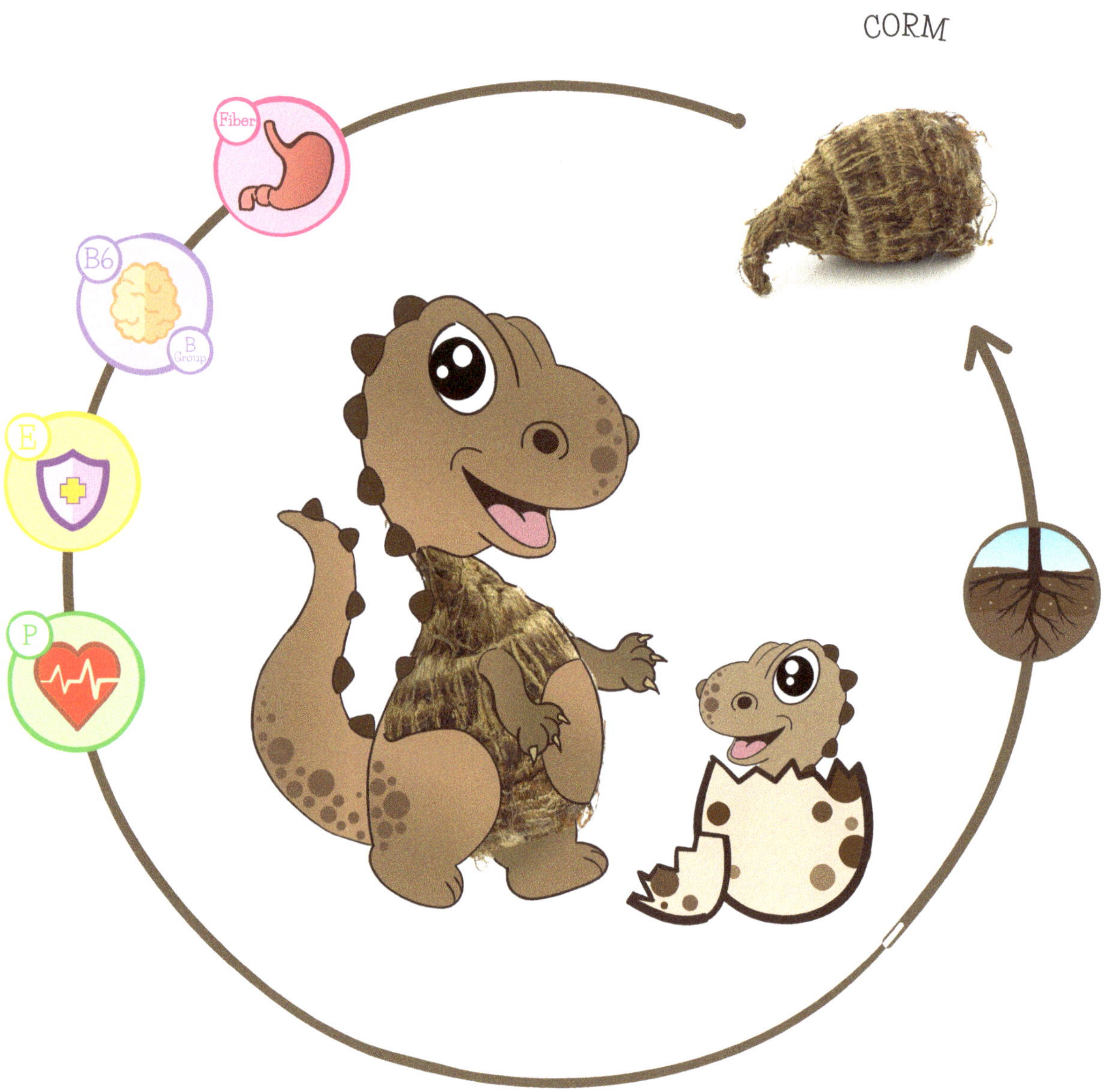

CORM

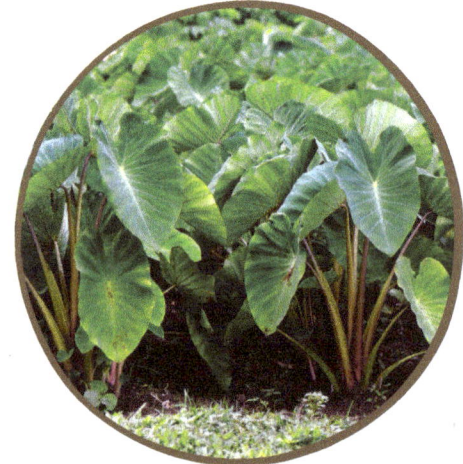

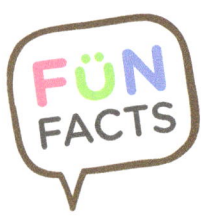

Taro is sometimes called the "potato of the tropics" because it can be **prepared** the same way as potatoes. It is also referred to as "elephant ears" because of its huge elephant ear-like **leaves**.

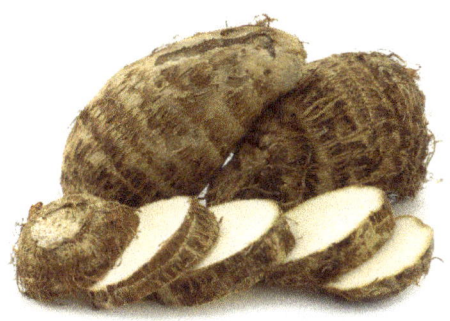

PICK
Pick firm **corms** that are heavy for their size. Avoid taro with cuts, wrinkled skin, soft spots, and **mold**.

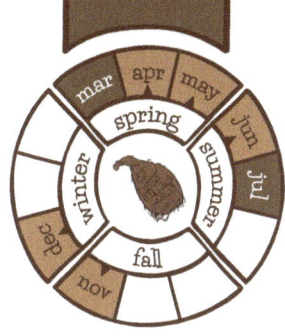

Available March to July; November to December; Imported year-round

Peak Season
April-June; November-December

STORE
Keep taro in a basket that is well-ventilated and store in a cool, dark place for up to 3 days. Refrigerate cooked taro in an air tight container for 3-5 days.

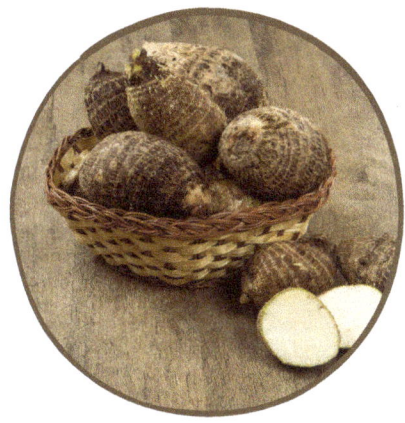

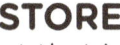
Taro is known for a Hawaiian dish called poi. Poi is a paste made from fermented and baked taro.

TARO TIDBITS

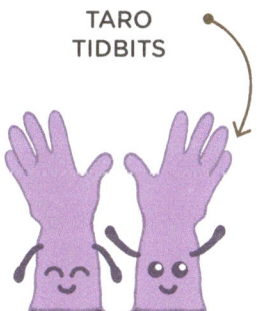

Wear gloves to peel taro because it has **oxalic acid** in the raw **flesh** that may **irritate** the skin when peeled.

EAT
Clean the skin with a vegetable brush. To peel skin, put on gloves or coat hands in oil, then chop or slice per recipe. Taro should be cooked or placed in cold water with vinegar or lemon juice immediately after peeling to prevent browning.

Baked Taro
Preheat your oven to 400 degrees F. Chop taro into fry-sized pieces, toss in a bowl with 1 tablespoon of coconut oil, coconut milk, shredded coconut, and sprinkle with salt. Then place in a single layer on a **greased**, foil-lined roasting tray in the top third of the oven for about 30 minutes, turning taro midway through baking, until it is tender and golden brown.

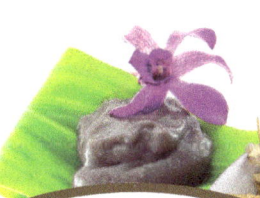

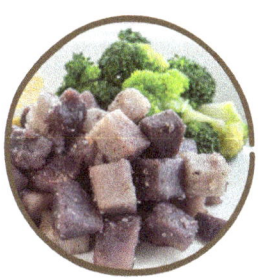

When taro is cooked the flesh turns a gray-violet color.

A Book of Vegetables 141

TIGER NUT
EARTH ALMOND

[ti-grr nuht] | [err-th all-mond]

chewy, earthy, nutty, starchy, sweet

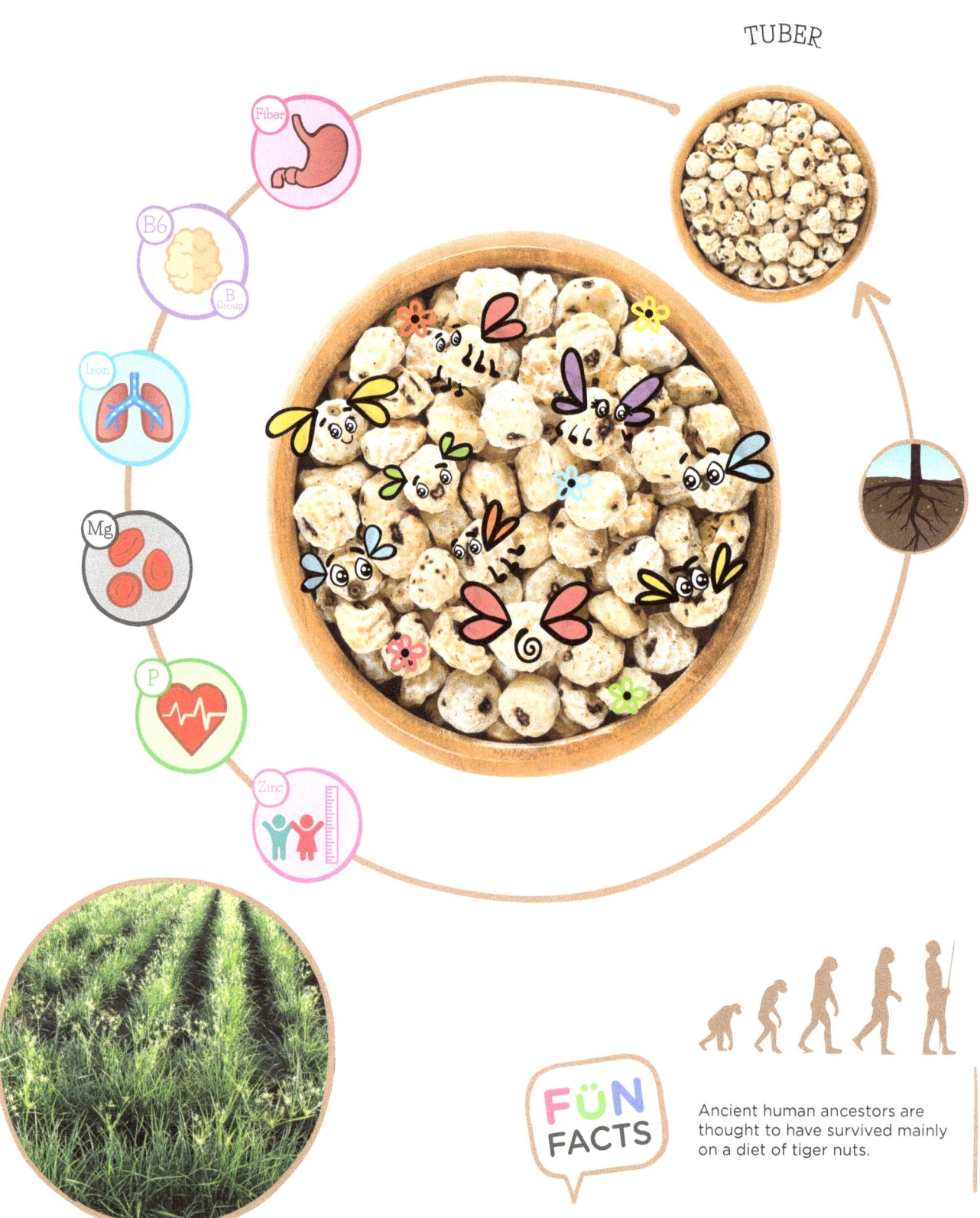

TUBER

FUN FACTS

Ancient human ancestors are thought to have survived mainly on a diet of tiger nuts.

142 | Where Does Broccoli Come From?

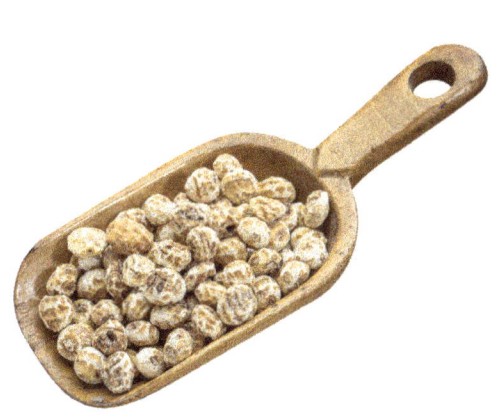

PICK
Tiger nuts are typically sold in dried form.

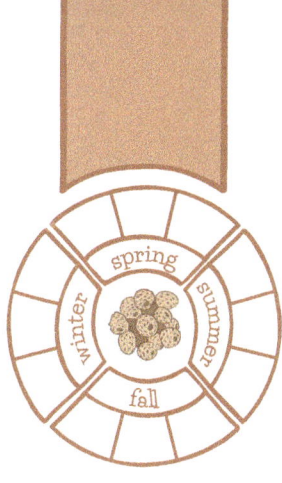

Available imported year-round

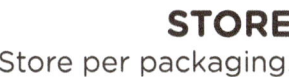

STORE
Store per packaging.

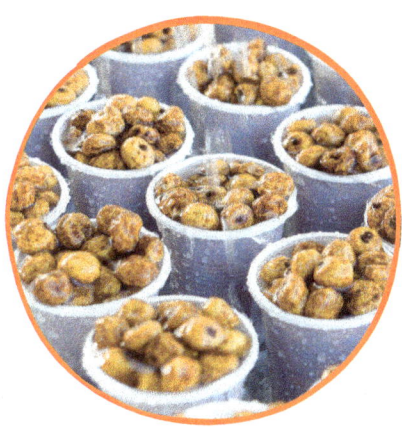

TIGER NUT TIDBITS

Tiger nuts are similar in size to a chickpea.

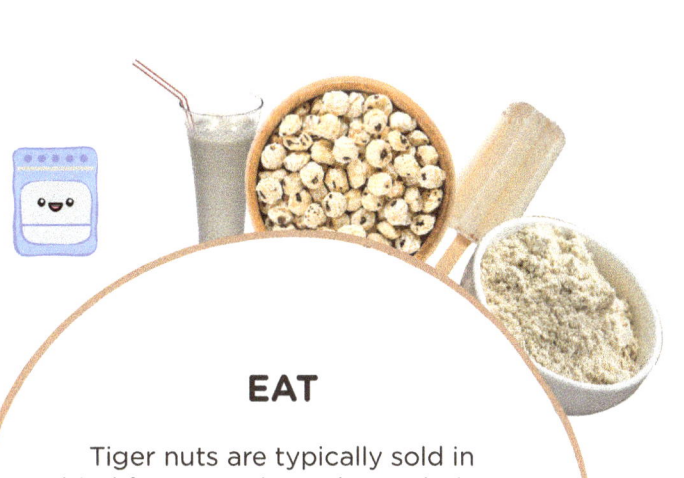

EAT

Tiger nuts are typically sold in dried form. Purchase them whole as a snack, ground into flour, pressed into an oil, or pre-made into a drink such as a smoothie or horchata, a sweetened drink made with spices.

Raw Tiger nuts
Try them as a snack on the go!

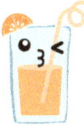

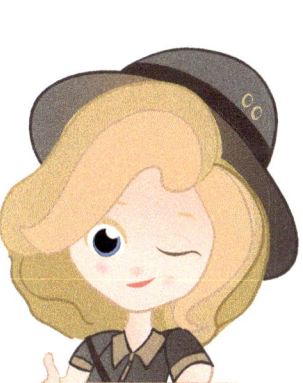

Try using flour made out of ground tiger nuts in your next baked goods recipe!

A Book of Vegetables

TOMATILLO

[to-ma-tea-oh]

acidic, bright, firm, herbal, tart

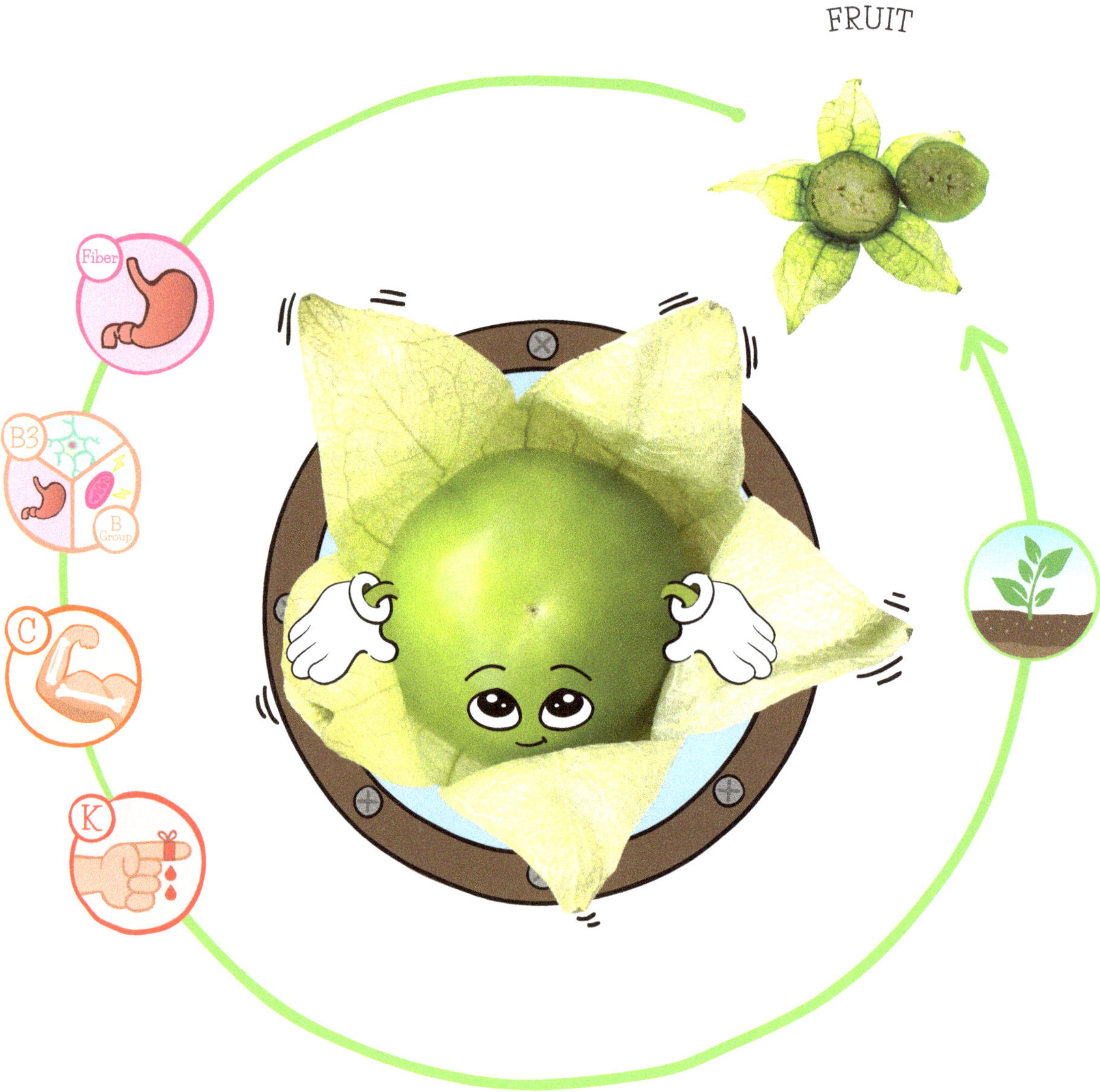

FRUIT

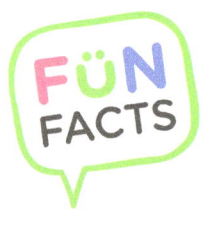

The husk of the tomatillo forms before the **fruit**. When the fruit begins to grow it fills up the husk and pops through when it is fully grown. Be sure to eat them while they are green because as they continue to **ripen** and turn yellow, they are less flavorful.

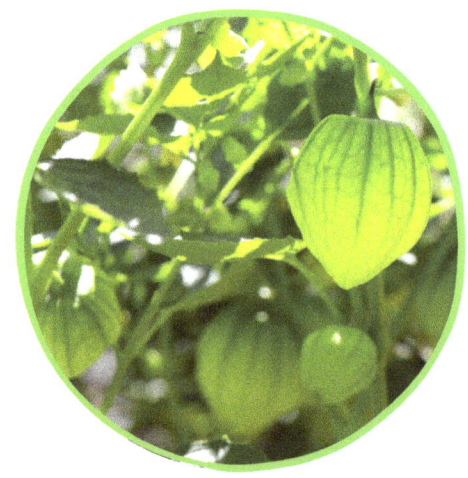

144 | Where Does Broccoli Come From?

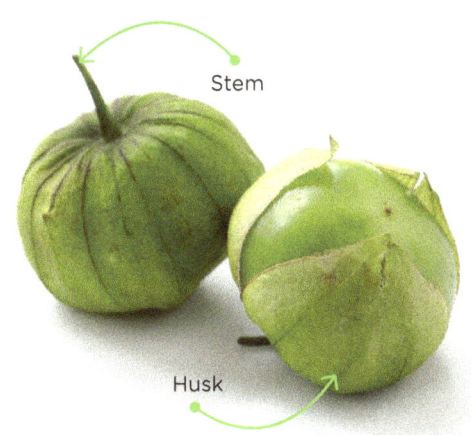
Stem
Husk

PICK
Pick bright green, firm **fruit** with crisp green **husks**. Avoid tomatillos with dry, brown, or torn husks and fruit with wrinkled skin, soft spots, and **bruises**.

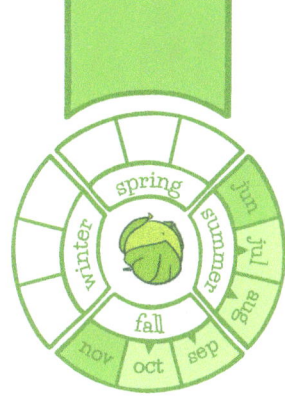

Available June to November; Imported year-round

Peak Season
July-October

STORE
Keep tomatillo in their papery husk at room **temperature** for up to 2 days. Refrigerate tomatillo without their husk in a closed paper bag for 2-3 weeks.

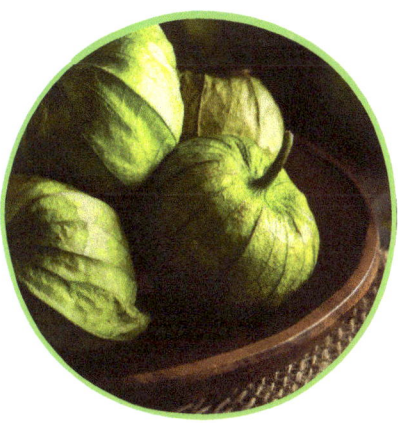

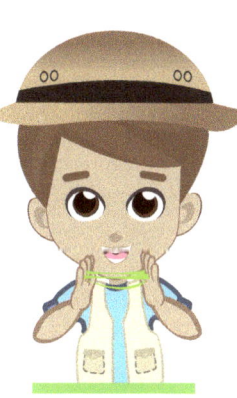

TOMATILLO TIDBITS

EAT
Remove the husk, clean the skin, slice the tomatillo in half from **stem** to tip (hotdog style), and chop or slice per recipe.

Tomatillo Sauce
Chop 1 pound of tomatillos, 1 small onion, 3 cloves of garlic, 2 tablespoons of fresh cilantro, and place into a saucepan with 2 cups of water. Then add 1 tablespoon fresh oregano, 1/2 teaspoon ground cumin, and 1 teaspoon salt. Bring to a boil and then reduce the heat to medium-low and simmer for 10-15 until tomatillos are soft and easily **pierced** with a fork. Puree in a blender until smooth and enjoy with chips or as a sauce!

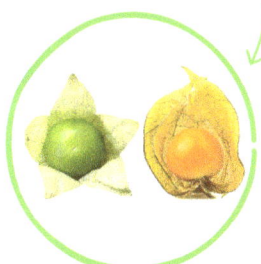

Tomatillos are closely related to the fruit physalis, also know as a cape gooseberry, which are both sticky under their papery husk.

TOMATO

[toe-may-toe]

aromatic, juicy, slimy, sweet, tangy

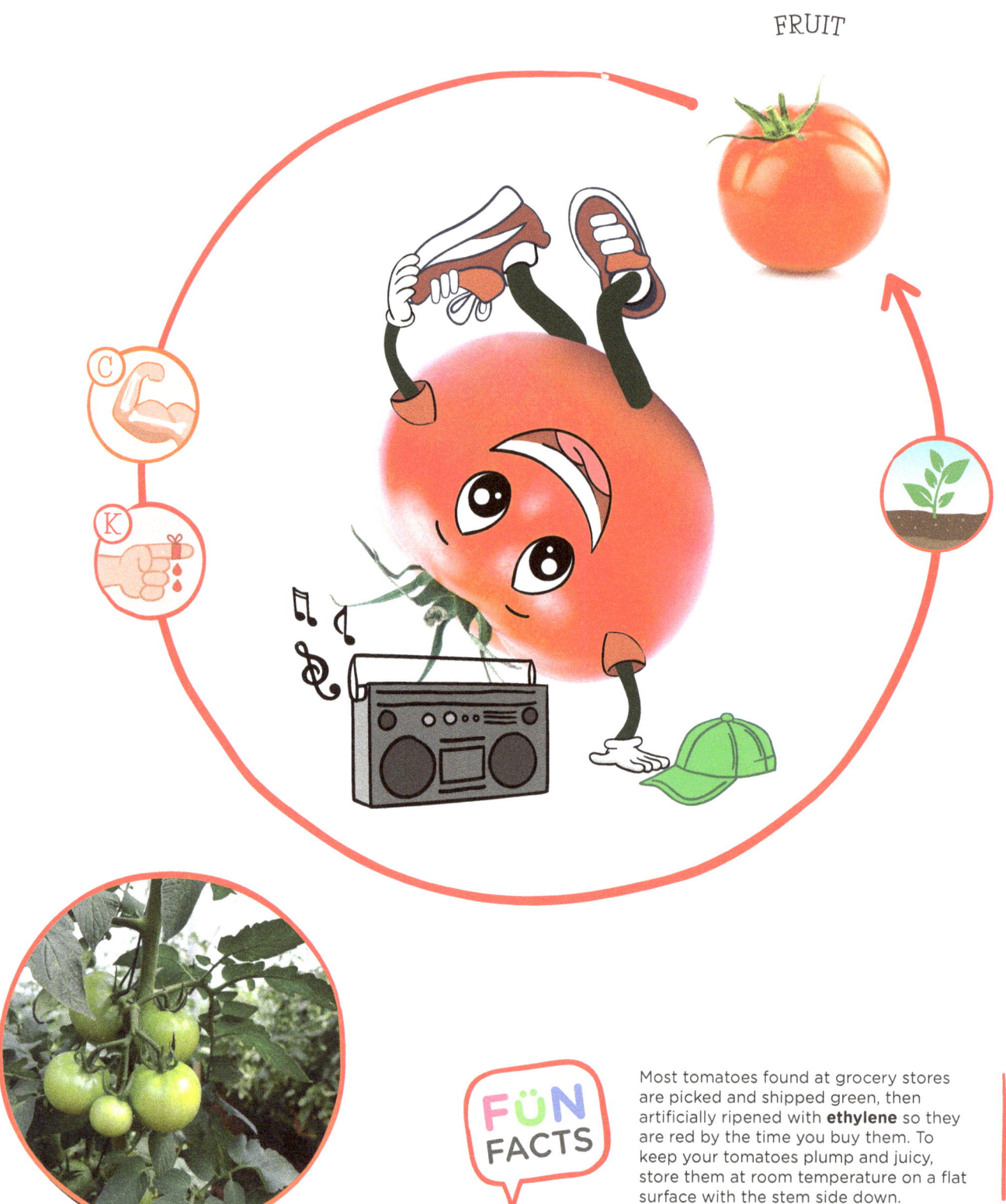

FRUIT

FUN FACTS

Most tomatoes found at grocery stores are picked and shipped green, then artificially ripened with **ethylene** so they are red by the time you buy them. To keep your tomatoes plump and juicy, store them at room temperature on a flat surface with the stem side down.

146 | Where Does Broccoli Come From?

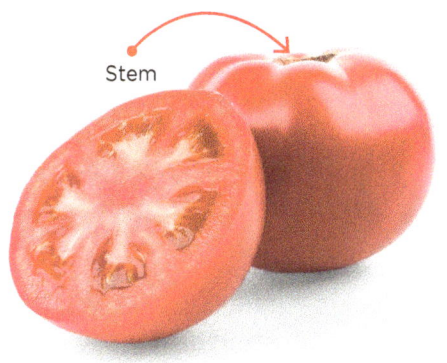

PICK
Pick deeply colored, firm, aromatic **fruit**, that are heavy for their size. Avoid tomatoes with soft spots and **bruises**.

Available May to December; Imported year-round

Peak Season
June-August

STORE
Keep **ripe** tomato at room **temperature** out of direct sunlight on the countertop for up to 3 days. Refrigerate raw sliced or chopped tomato in an airtight container for 3-4 days and cooked tomato in an airtight container for 3-5 days.

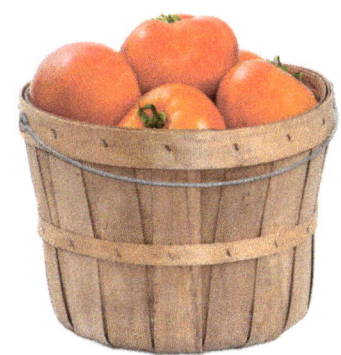

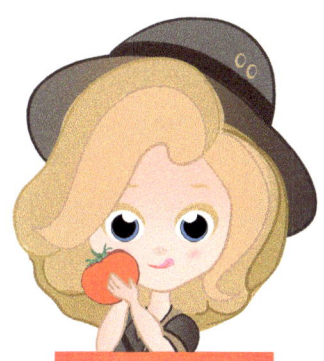

TOMATO TIDBITS

The stronger a tomato smells, the more flavor it will have.

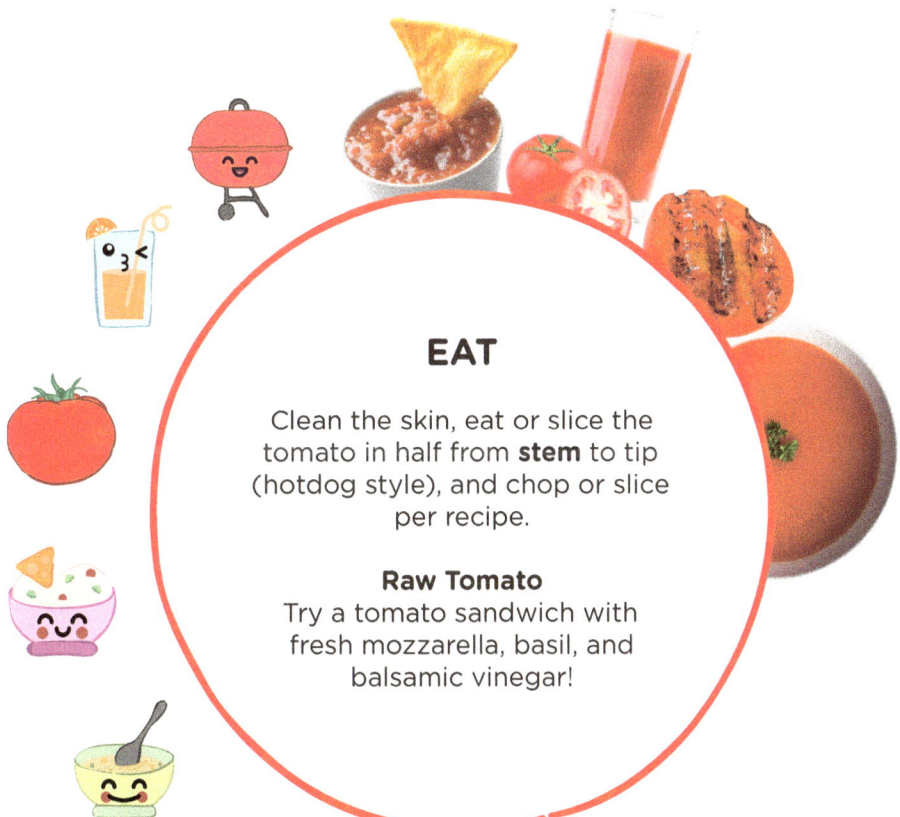

EAT
Clean the skin, eat or slice the tomato in half from **stem** to tip (hotdog style), and chop or slice per recipe.

Raw Tomato
Try a tomato sandwich with fresh mozzarella, basil, and balsamic vinegar!

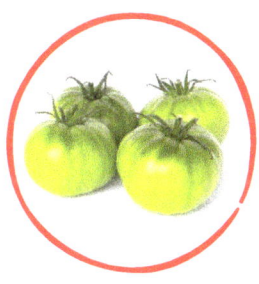

Green tomatoes are hard, unripe, astringent tomatoes that have not yet changed color and are most often fried. However, there are a few **varieties** of tomatoes that stay green when they are **ripe** such as Green Zebra and Aunt Ruby's German Green.

A Book of Vegetables

TOMATO VARIETIES

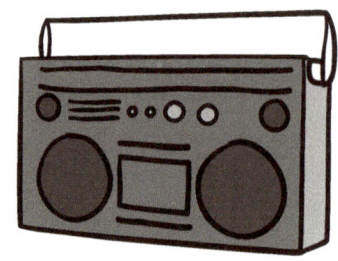

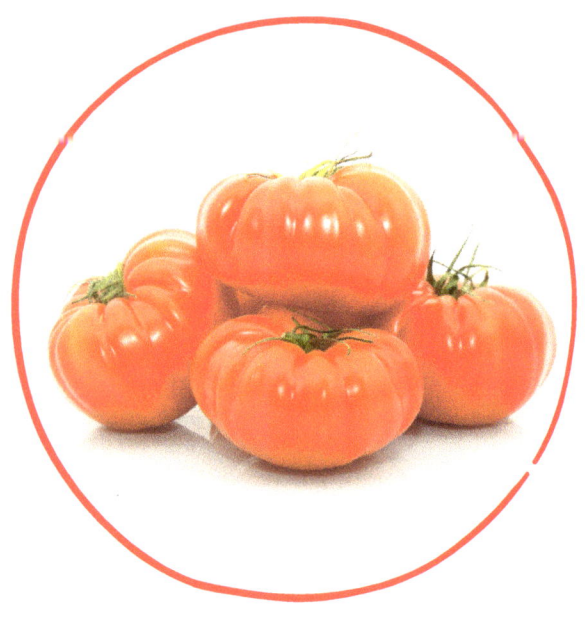

BEEFSTEAK [BEEF-STAKE]

Big, red, round, meaty, mild, and juicy, beefsteak tomatoes are perfect for burgers and sandwiches! Beefsteak tomatoes are also great roasted and added to soups or sauces.

CAMPARI [CAM-PAR-E]

Typically purchased on the vine, Campari tomatoes are smaller than a beefsteak and larger than a cherry tomato. Their sweet flavor and juicy bite make them perfect for salads and sandwiches.

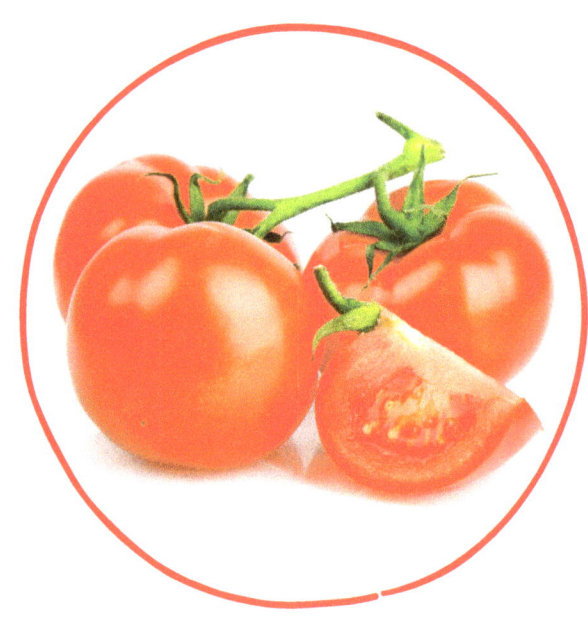

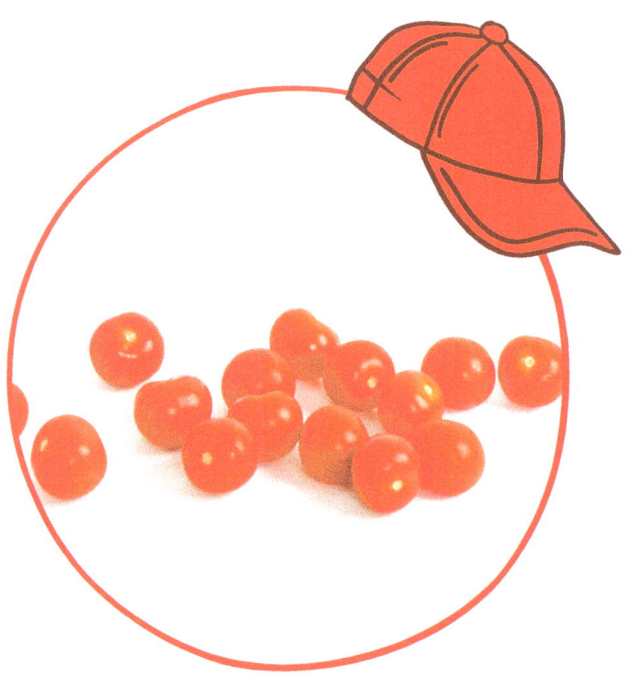

CHERRY | GRAPE
[CHER-EE] | [GREYP]

Cherry or grape tomatoes are small, sweet, and juicy. These tomatoes are easy to snack on and available in colors that range from red to orange to yellow. They are also an easy addition to salads and kabobs.

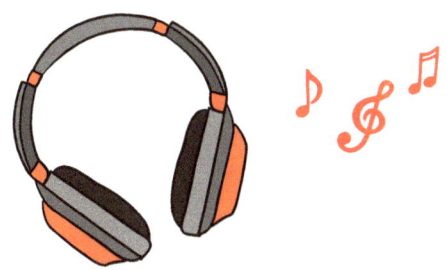

KUMATO [COO-MA-TOE]

Kumato tomatoes are sweet-tart and almost sour. They are brownish-red to green-gold in color and are firm yet juicy. Try them roasted or raw in salsas and salads.

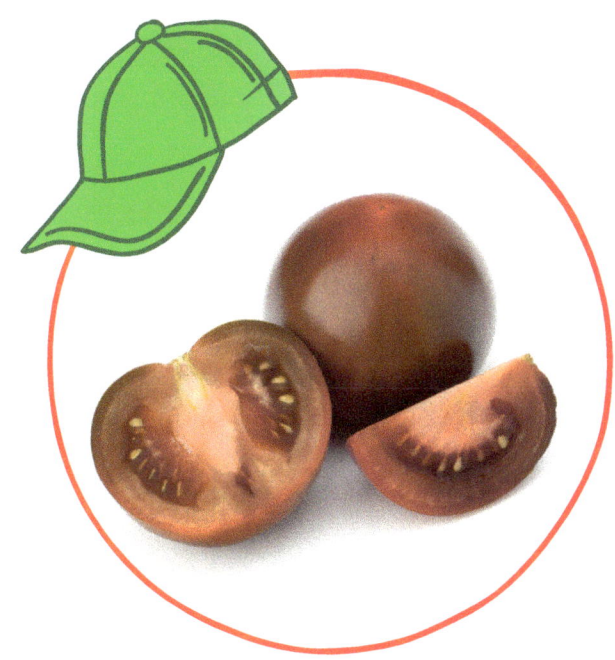

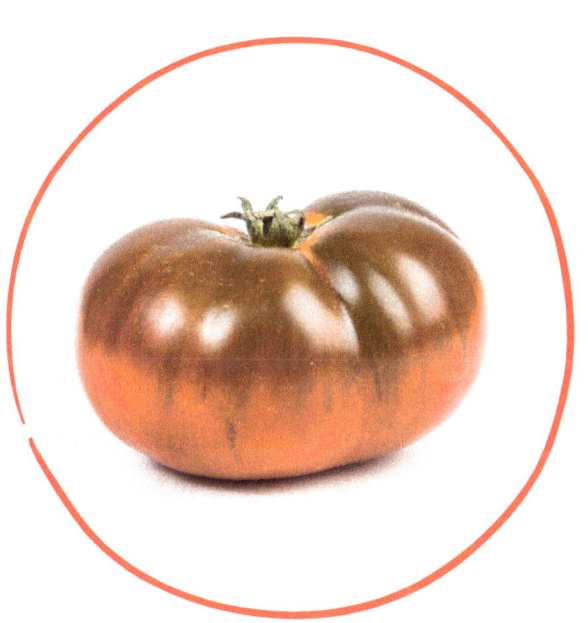

HEIRLOOM | HERITAGE [AIR-LOOM] | [HER-I-TIJ]

Heirloom or heritage tomatoes are grown from **seeds** that have been passed down through generations. They are grown outside by natural pollination and are known for their flavor. They may not be perfectly shaped, but they are considered the most flavorful **variety**. Try them fresh!

PLUM | ROMA | SAN MARZANO [RAW-MAH] | [SAN MAR-ZAN-O]

Plum tomatoes are known for their firm flesh, minimal seeds, and juice. These medium-sized tomatoes are oval in shape and perfect for sauces, salsa, sautéing, and grilling.

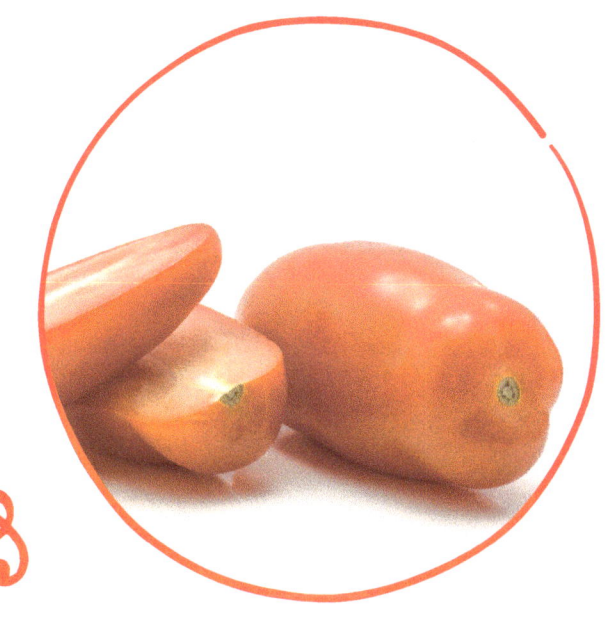

TURNIP AND GREENS

[tur-nip]

bitter, crisp, nutty, starchy, sweet

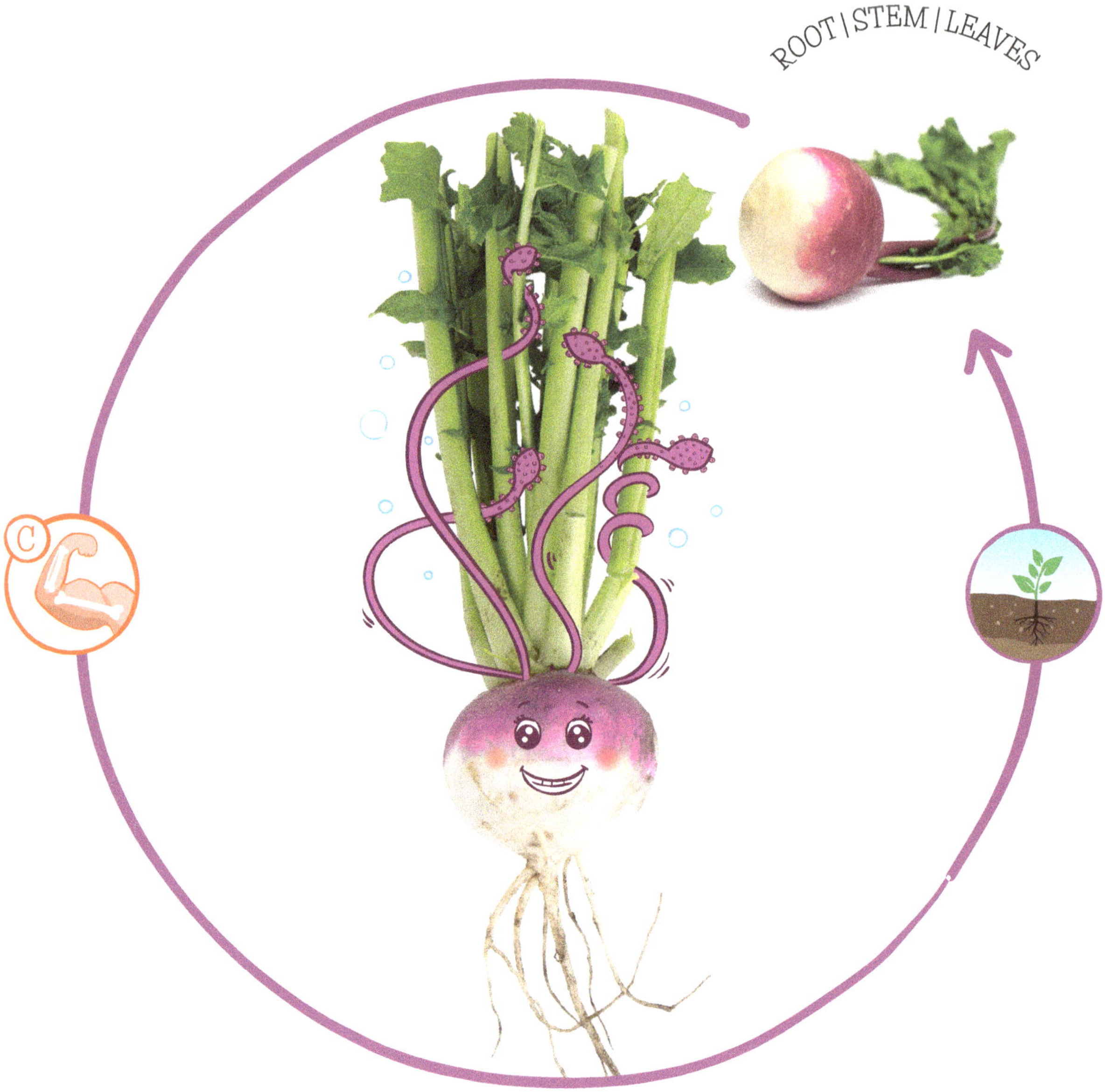

ROOT | STEM | LEAVES

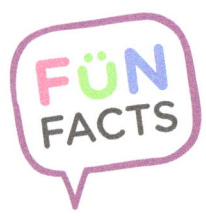

FUN FACTS — Small or young turnips are zippy, crunchy, and perfect for a vegetable tray with dip. Large or old turnips can be peppery, dense, and need to be roasted to bring out their sweet, nutty flavor.

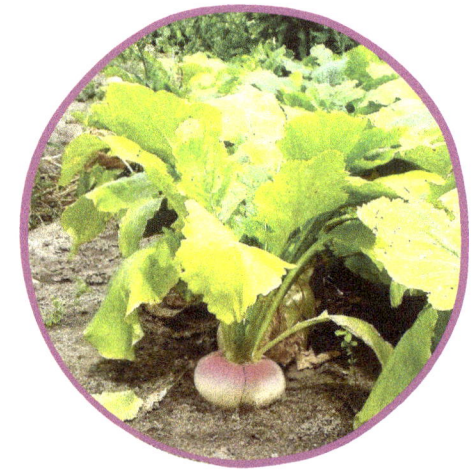

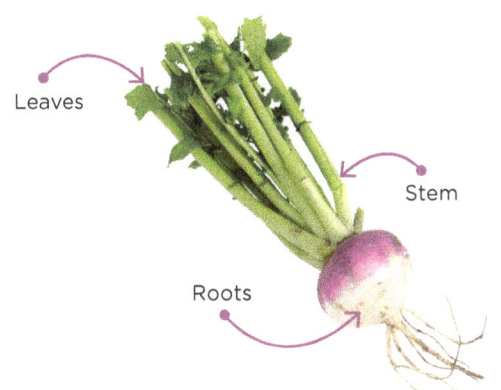

Leaves
Stem
Roots

PICK
Pick creamy white **roots** with a violet colored ring around the top that are firm, small to medium in size, with smooth skin that feel heavy for their size. Avoid turnips with soft spots and **bruises**. Attached greens should be bright green and crisp.

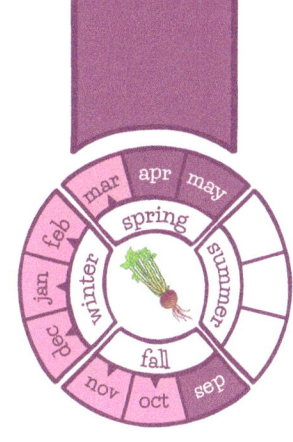

Available September to May; Imported year-round

Peak Season
October-March

STORE
Refrigerate raw turnip in an open plastic bag for up to 3 weeks and cooked turnip in an airtight container for 3-5 days. Raw turnip greens should be refrigerated separately in an airtight container for 2-3 days.

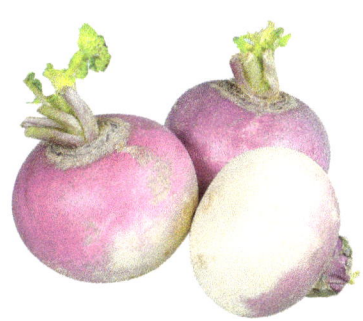

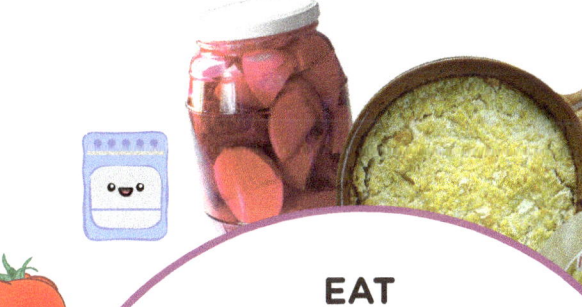

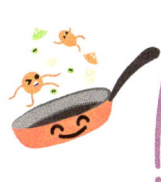
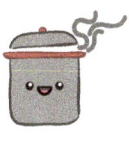
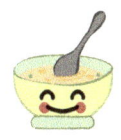

EAT
Clean the skin with a vegetable brush, slice off greens, peel if desired, then chop or slice per recipe.

Roasted Turnip
Preheat your oven to 400 degrees F. Slice turnips into wedges, toss in a bowl with olive oil, honey, salt and pepper, then place in a single layer on a **greased**, foil-lined roasting tray in the top third of the oven. Roast turnips for 30-35 minutes, turning occasionally until tender and golden brown.

TURNIP LEAVES

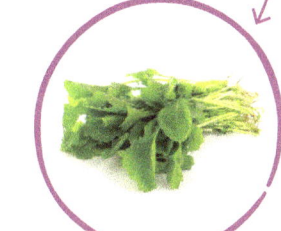

You can eat the **stem** and **leaves** of young turnips! Try them raw in a salad where you would include arugula or sauté them just as you would **prepare** beet greens.

A Book of Vegetables 151

WATER CHESTNUT

[wot-er chest-nut]

crisp, crunchy, nutty, refreshing, sweet

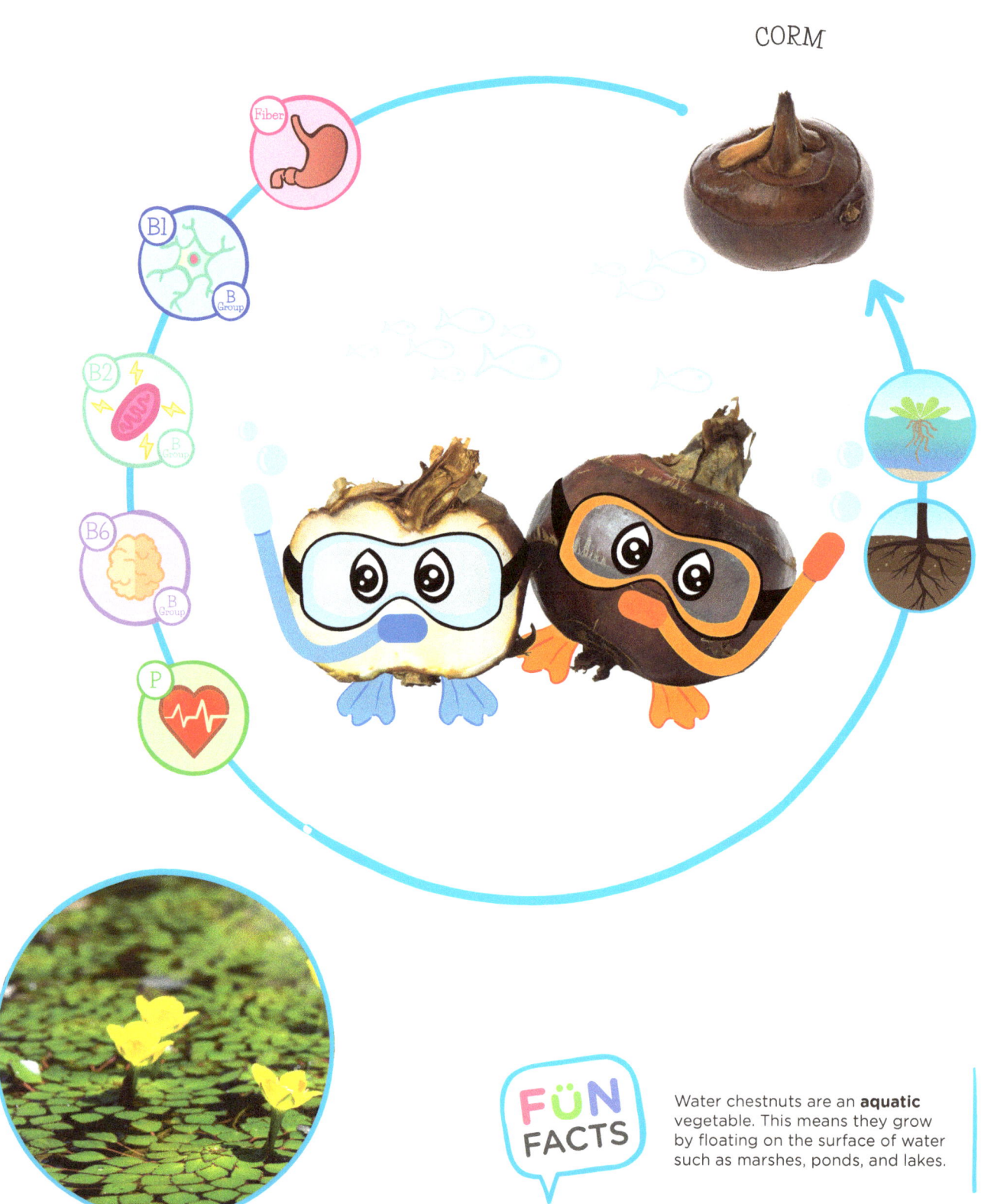

CORM

FUN FACTS

Water chestnuts are an **aquatic** vegetable. This means they grow by floating on the surface of water such as marshes, ponds, and lakes.

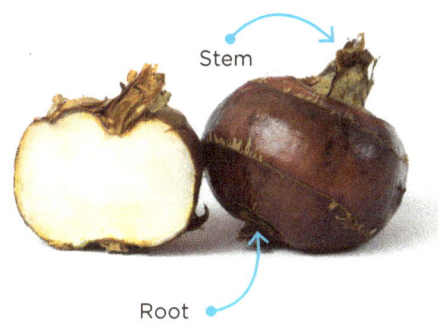

PICK
Water chestnuts are typically only sold canned outside of the countries where they grow because they **spoil** very quickly. For fresh chestnuts, pick hard **corms**. Avoid water chestnuts with wrinkled skin and soft spots.

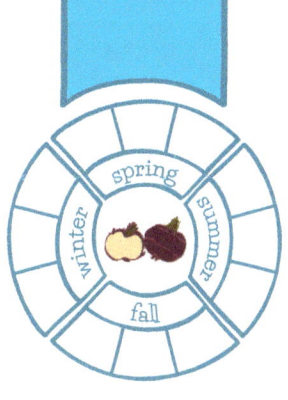

Available imported year-round

STORE
Refrigerate fresh water chestnuts unpeeled in a closed plastic bag for up to 7 days and opened, canned water chestnuts in an airtight container for 2-3 days.

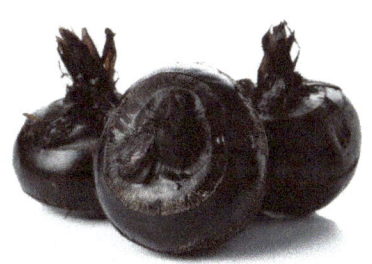

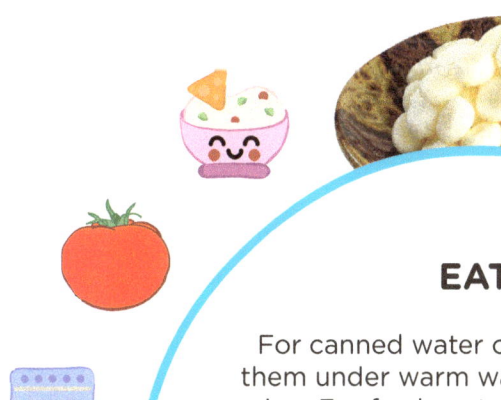

EAT
For canned water chestnuts, rinse them under warm water and use per recipe. For fresh water chestnuts, clean the skin, slice off the **stem** end and **root** end, peel, and chop or slice per recipe. Always buy a few extra fresh water chestnuts than needed as you may find some that are spoiled once peeled.

Raw Water Chestnuts
Add raw water chestnuts to your next **fruit** salad for a unique refreshing crunch!

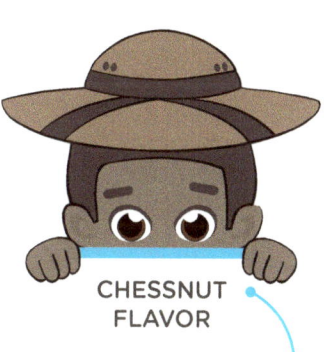

CHESSNUT FLAVOR
Some describe the flavor and **texture** of fresh water chestnuts as similar to a mildly sweet apple and fresh coconut.

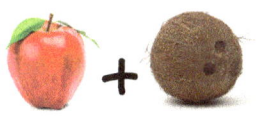
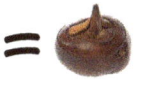

WATERCRESS

[wot-er-cress]

crunchy, peppery, pungent, refreshing, sharp

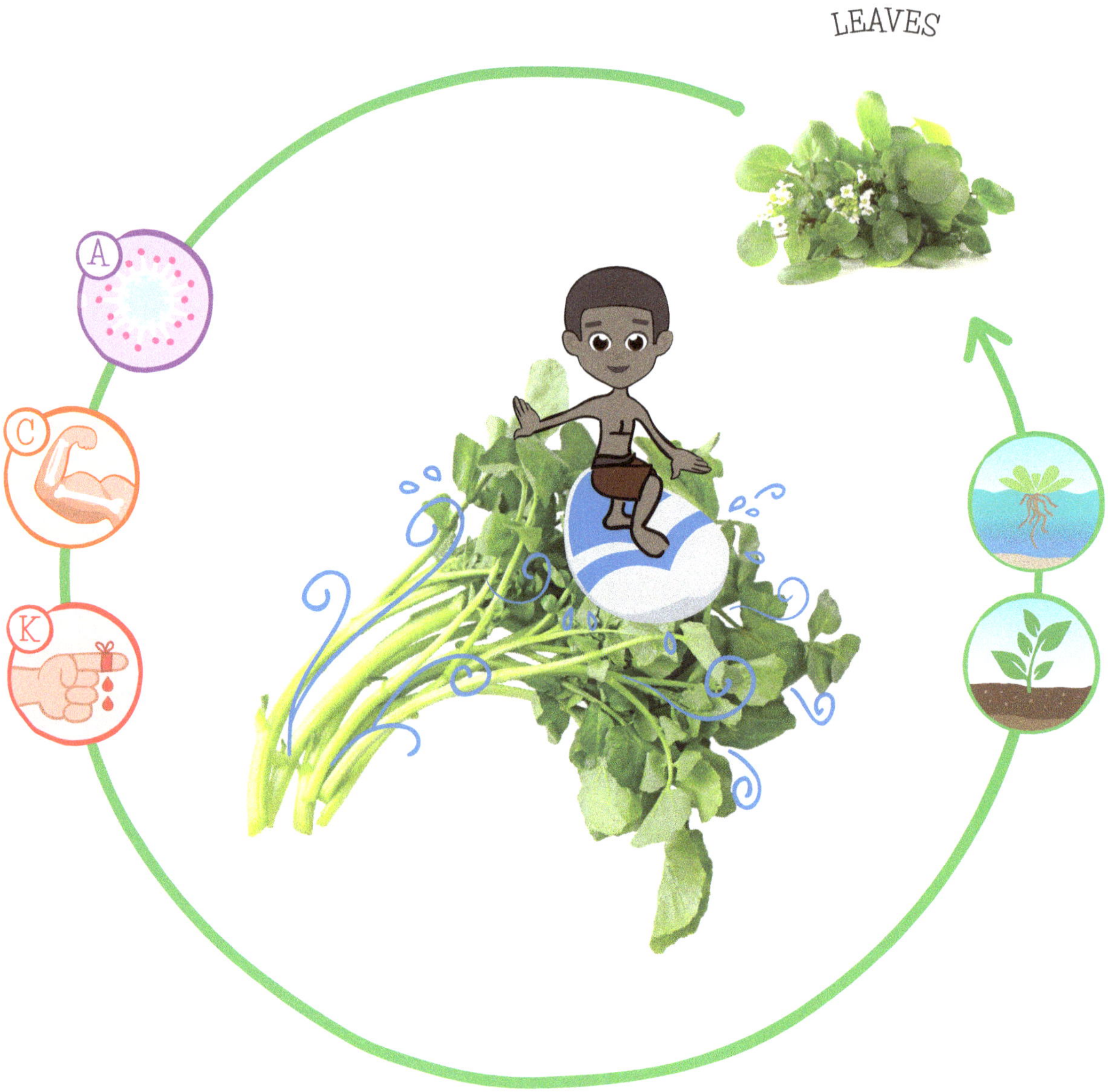

LEAVES

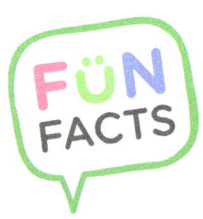

Fun Facts: Watercress is an **aquatic** or semi-aquatic leafy green related to the cabbage. It is considered a "Powerhouse **Fruit** and Vegetable" because it is an extremely nutrient dense green. This means it has a lot of Good For My Body Nutrients compared to the **energy** food will produce in the body.

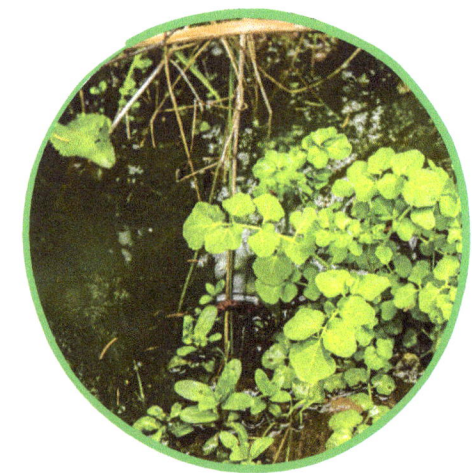

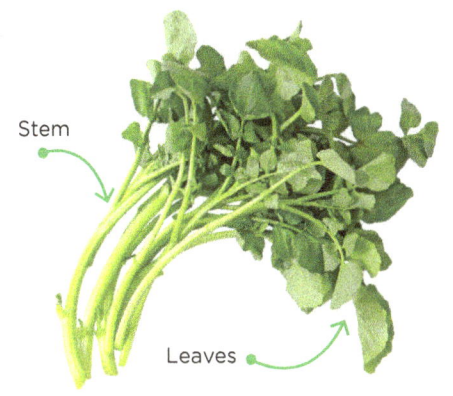

Stem

Leaves

PICK
Pick dark green, crisp **leaves**. Avoid watercress that are **wilting**, yellowing, or slimy.

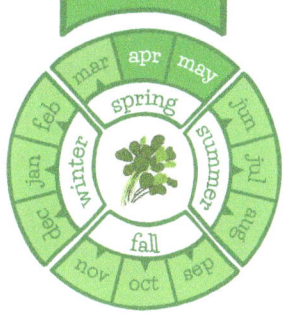

Varieties available year-round

Peak Season
June-March

STORE
Wrap unwashed watercress in a moist paper towel, place in a closed plastic bag and refrigerate up to 3 days.

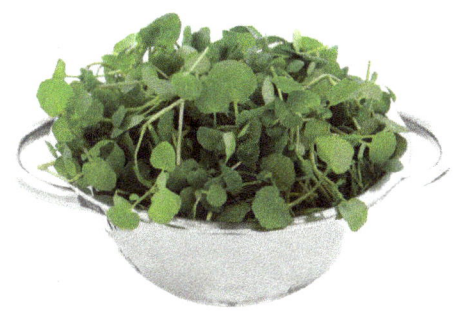

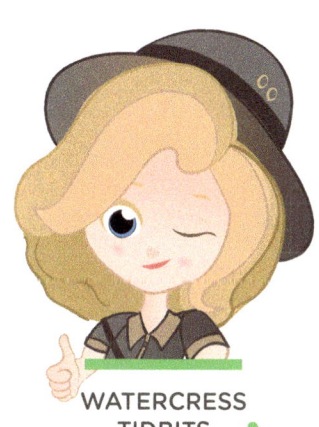

WATERCRESS TIDBITS

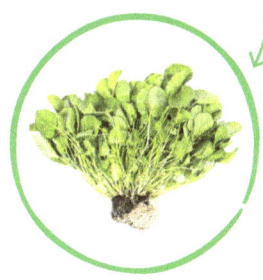

Watercress is in season year-round because it is **hydroponically** grown and can be **farmed** indoors. Peak season for wild watercress is spring and fall when their sharp flavor is the most pungent.

EAT
Clean the leaves several times to remove all dirt and shake off the excess water, slice off any tough **stems**, and use whole or chop per recipe.

Raw Watercress
Try watercress in place of lettuce on sandwiches, salads, and wraps.

A Book of Vegetables 155

YAM

[yeah-m]

bland, dry, starchy, sweet, tender

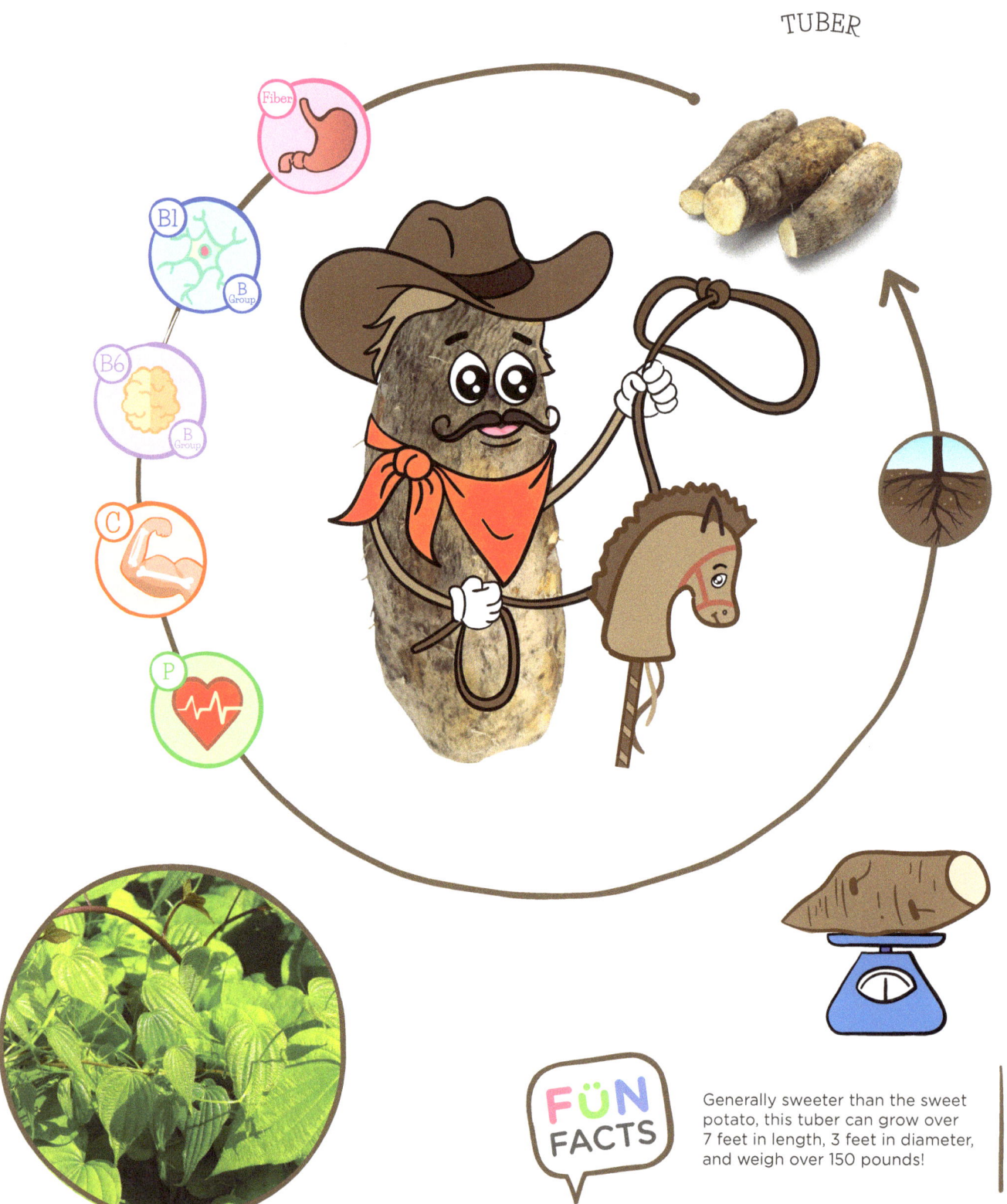

TUBER

FUN FACTS: Generally sweeter than the sweet potato, this tuber can grow over 7 feet in length, 3 feet in diameter, and weigh over 150 pounds!

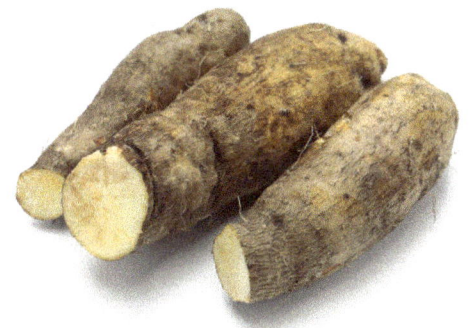

PICK
Pick brown or black firm **tubers** with rough skin. Avoid yams with wrinkled skin and soft spots. In the United States, most yams are sold in large pieces that are sealed in plastic wrap.

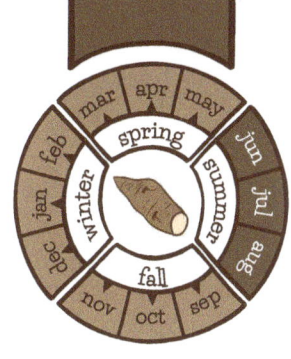

Varieties available year-round

Peak Season
September-May

STORE
Keep yam in a basket that is well-ventilated and store in a cool, dark place for up to 1 month and at room **temperature** 5-7 days. Refrigerate cooked yam in an airtight container for 3-5 days.

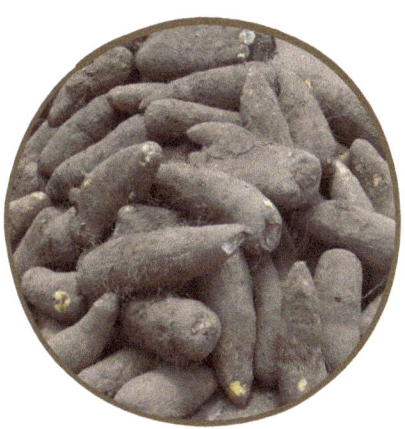

EAT
Clean the skin with a vegetable brush, peel skin, then chop or slice per recipe.

Mashed Yam
Chop yam into small chunks and boil in salted water for 10-15 minutes until tender or can be easily **pierced** with a fork. Drain water, add butter and milk, and mash or whip with an electric mixer until smooth and creamy, then season with salt and pepper.

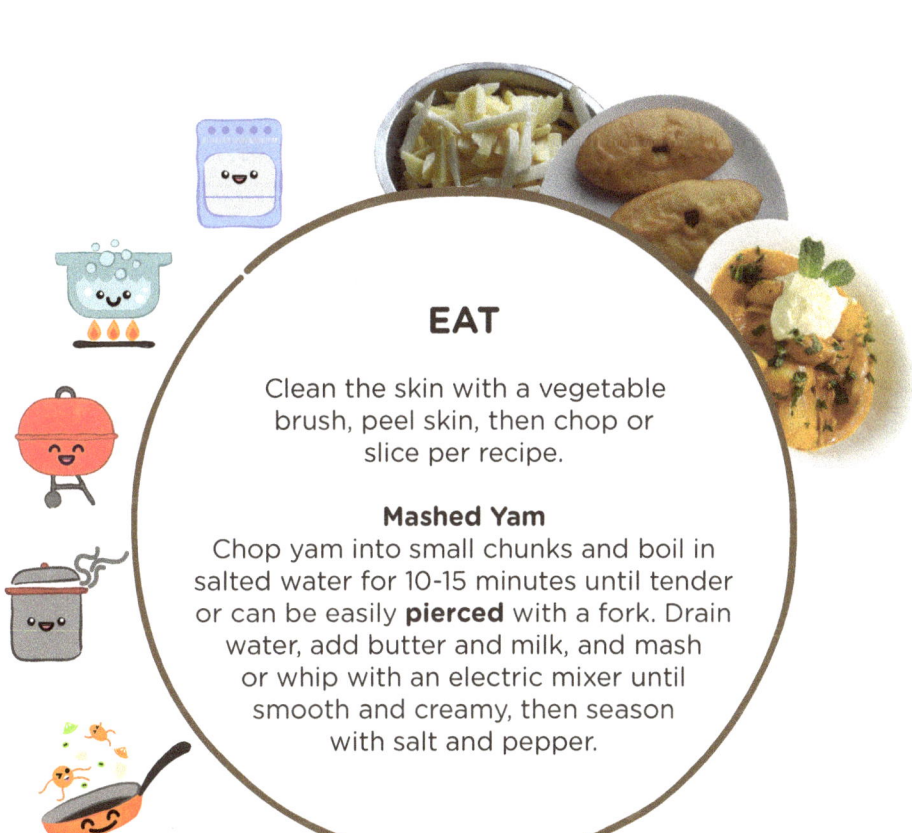

YAM SKIN

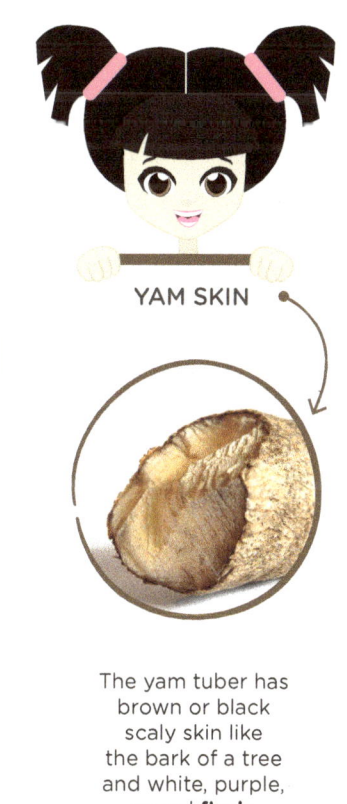

The yam tuber has brown or black scaly skin like the bark of a tree and white, purple, or red **flesh**, depending on the **variety**.

A Book of Vegetables 157

Descriptive Words

Descriptive words help us identify qualities about foods and explain what we like or dislike about something we eat.

When you sit down for a meal or snack take a moment to think about how it looks, how it smells, how it sounds, how it feels, and how it tastes using your 5 senses. It's like your very own experiment every time you eat!

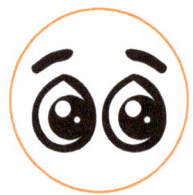

SEE
What colors or textures do you SEE?

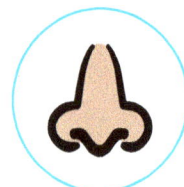

SMELL
What does it SMELL like?

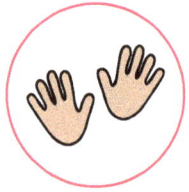

FEEL
How does it FEEL when you hold it or eat it?

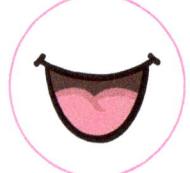

TASTE
How does the flavor TASTE?

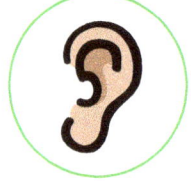

HEAR
What sound do you HEAR when you touch or take a bite?

	WORD	DESCRIPTION	SENSE(S)
1	Acidic	bitter, sharp, sour	Taste
2	Ambrosial	delicious, fragrant, sweet	Smell · Taste
3	Anise	herbal smell, sweet, tastes similar to licorice	Smell · Taste
4	Aroma; aromatic	scent, smell, odor	Smell
5	Astringent	mouth-puckering, sharp	Taste
6	Bitter	acidic, harsh, sharp, sour	Taste
7	Bland	flavorless, mild	Taste
8	Bright	acidic, sharp, tart, giving out or reflecting light, shiny appearance	See · Taste
9	Buttery	creamy, rich, smooth, velvety, feels similar to butter	Feel · Taste
10	Chewy	leathery, sticky, tough	Feel
11	Citrusy	looks, smells, or tastes similar to a citrus fruit such as lemons, oranges, or grapefruit	See · Smell · Taste
12	Complex	multiple aromas, flavors, or textures	Feel · Smell · Taste
13	Creamy	smooth, velvety	Feel
14	Crisp(y)	crunchy, firm, snappy	Feel · Hear
15	Crumbly	breaks into pieces under pressure, brittle, crisp	Feel · See
16	Crunchy	brittle, crisp, loud	Feel · Hear
17	Delicate	fine texture, tender, light or subtle taste	Feel · Taste
18	Dense	compact, heavy, thick	Feel
19	Distinctive	unlike other textures or flavors, unique qualities	Feel · Taste
20	Dry	free of liquid or moisture	Feel · See · Taste
21	Dull	having little color, smell, or taste	See · Smell · Taste
22	Earthy	feels, smell, or tastes similar to soil	Feel · Smell · Taste
23	Exotic	different, unusual, unfamiliar	See · Taste
24	Fibrous	stringy, thick, tough	Feel
25	Firm	hard, solid, stiff	Feel
26	Flavorful	having a lot of flavor	Taste
27	Flesh(y)	pulpy, soft, thick	Feel
28	Floral; flowery	smell or taste similar to a flower	Smell · Taste
29	Fluffy	airy, light	Feel · See · Taste
30	Fragrant	sweet smell or scent, perfumed	Smell
31	Fresh	new, peak of ripeness, unspoiled	Feel · See · Smell · Taste

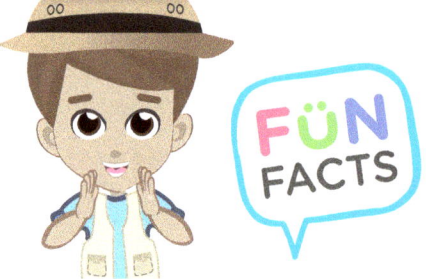

FUN FACTS

When a food feels, looks, smells, or tastes similar to another food you can say it is "like" another food or add a "y" to the end of the word. For example, foods may be described as butter-like, celery-like, or honey-like and citrusy, lemony, or watery.

	WORD	DESCRIPTION	SENSE(S)
32	Fruity	varies and can mean citrusy, sweet, or tangy	Taste · Smell
33	Fuzzy	fibrous, furry, or hairy coating	Feel · See
34	Glossy	glazed, polished, shiny	See
35	Glutinous	gluey, starchy, sticky	Feel · See · Taste
36	Grainy	coarse, granular, gritty	Feel · See
37	Grassy	smell, taste, or feel similar to grass	Feel · Smell · Taste
38	Gritty	coarse, grainy, granular, rough	Feel · See · Taste
39	Hard	firm, solid	Feel
40	Hearty	large, filling, substantial, tough	Feel · See · Taste
41	Herbal	smell or taste similar to an herb	Smell · Taste
42	Honeyed	feels, looks, smells, or tastes similar to honey	Feel · See · Smell · Taste
43	Juicy	full of juice or liquid, succulent	Feel · Hear · See
44	Knobby	lumpy surface, rounded	See
45	Light	contains air, does not make you feel full quickly, lacks a strong color, smell or taste	Feel · See · Smell · Taste
46	Limp	soft, lifeless, un-firm	Feel · See
47	Mealy	crumbly, dry, grainy	Feel · See
48	Meaty	dense, thick, taste or texture similar to meat	Feel · Taste
49	Mild	bland, free of a strong smell or taste	Smell · Taste
50	Moist	slightly damp or wet	Feel · See
51	Mushy	may feel spoiled, soft, wet	Feel
52	Mustardy	smells or tastes similar to mustard	Smell · Taste
53	Musty	bad odor, moldy, stale	Smell · Taste
54	Nutty	tastes similar to nuts	Taste
55	Odor	aroma, musk, scent	Smell
56	Peppery	hot, pungent, spicy, smells or tastes similar to pepper	Smell · Taste
57	Plump	fleshy, full, round	Feel · See
58	Pulpy	fibrous, fleshy, soft	Feel · See
59	Pungent	bitter, hot, peppery, sharp, powerful smell or taste	Smell · Taste
60	Refreshing	cool, fresh, or different	Feel · Smell · Taste
61	Rich	creamy, dense, fatty, full-flavored, heavy, strong and pleasant smell or taste	Feel · Taste · Smell
62	Rotten	bad, moldy, spoiled	Taste · See · Smell
63	Rough	bumpy, textured, uneven surface	Taste · See · Feel
64	Rubbery	elastic, flexible, tough, similar to rubber	Feel · See
65	Salty	tasting or containing salt	Taste
66	Savory	delicious smell or taste, having a salty or spicy quality without sweetness, well-seasoned	Taste · Smell
67	Seeded	having seeds	Feel · Hear · See
68	Sharp	distinct, powerful smell or taste, pungent	Taste · Smell
69	Shrivel	shrink, wither, wrinkle	Feel · See
70	Silky	glossy, smooth, soft, similar to silk	Feel · See
71	Slimy	gooey, slippery, wet, similar to slime	Feel · See
72	Smoky	smell or taste similar to smoke from a wood grill	Smell · Taste
73	Smooth	even, flat, uniform consistency	Feel · See
74	Soft	smooth, easy to press	Feel · See
75	Sour	acidic, bitter, tart, similar to lemon or vinegar	Feel · Smell · Taste
76	Spicy	aromatic, hot, peppery, pungent, strongly flavored	Smell · Taste
77	Spongy	airy, light, soft, feels similar to a sponge	Feel · See
78	Squeaky	high pitched sound	Hear
79	Stale	dry, old, musty, change in texture or appearance	Smell · Taste
80	Starchy	feel or taste similar to other high starch foods such as potatoes or rice	Feel · Taste
81	Sticky	glue-like, syrupy, tacky, viscous	Feel · See
82	Stinky	unpleasant smell	Smell
83	Stringy	fibrous, tough, similar to string-like pieces	Feel · See
84	Subtle	delicate, faint, light	Smell · Taste
85	Sugary	sweet, honeyed, similar to sugar	Feel · See · Smell · Taste
86	Sweet	smell or taste similar to sugar or honey	Smell · Taste
87	Sweet-sour	both sweet and sour	Feel · Smell · Taste
88	Sweet-tart	both sweet and tart	Feel · Smell · Taste
80	Tangy	aromatic, flavorful, sharp, strong	Smell · Taste
90	Tart	acidic, sharp, sour	Feel · Taste
91	Tender	delicate, soft	Feel
92	Tough	dense, fibrous, hard	Feel
93	Umami	meaty taste, one of the basic taste sensations along with bitter, salty, sour, and sweet	Taste
94	Velvety	delicate, smooth, soft	Feel
95	Watery	feels, looks, or tastes similar to water	Feel · See · Taste
96	Waxy	shiny, sticky, similar feel and look to wax	Feel · See
97	Woody	fibrous, feels, looks, or smells similar to wood	Feel · Smell · Taste
98	Wrinkly	bumps, creases, or folds on a surface	See
99	Zesty	pungent, seasoned, sharp, spicy, tart	Smell · Taste
100	Zippy	fresh, invigorating	Taste

A Book of Vegetables

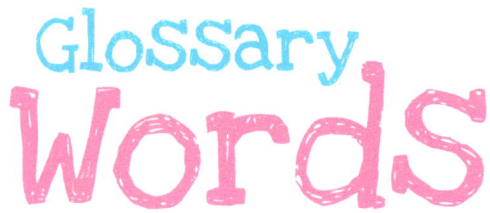
Glossary Words

A glossary helps us learn definitions of new or unusual words found in the book. Anytime you see a **bold** word throughout the book, you can find the definition here.

WORD	PHONETIC	DEFINITION
Algae	[al-gee]	a plant or plant-like form that lacks leaves or stems and grows in or near water
Anchor	[ang-ker]	provides strength and support or holds something firmly in place
Antioxidant(s)	[an-ti-ox-i-dant]	nutrients found in food that fight off sickness
Aquatic	[uh-kwot-ik]	living or growing in or near water
Asparagusic acid	[uh-spar-uh-jin-ik as-id]	a natural acid found in asparagus that changes the smell of urine after you eat it
Bacteria	[bak-teer-ee-uh]	very small living organisms that are everywhere and can either be harmful and make you sick or helpful and keep you healthy
Basal plate	[baz-al play-te]	the bottom of bulbs where roots grow (e.g., taro)
Brine	[bry-en]	a mix of salty water often used to preserve or add flavor to food
Bruise	[brewz]	a dark area on a plant, fruit, or vegetable that has been damaged
Bud	[buhd]	a part on a plant that can grow and develop into a flower, leaf, or new stem also known as eyes
Bulb	[buhlb]	layers of overlapping, fleshy leaves that surround a short stem and grow just below the surface of the ground (e.g., onion)
Calcium	[kal-see-uhm]	a mineral that helps build strong bones and teeth and keeps your heart beating strong
Carbon dioxide (CO_2)	[car-bon di-ox-eyed]	a substance or gas that is created when people and animals breathe out and is used by plants for energy
Carrageenan	[kar-uh-gee-nuhn]	a substance found in seaweed that is added to food and beauty products to thicken and provide a firmer texture
Cell	[sell]	the basic structural and functional unit of all living things or the smallest unit of life
Celsius	[sel-see-uhs]	a measurement of temperature
Chlorophyll	[klohr-uh-fil]	the green substance in plants that makes it possible for them to make food or energy from carbon dioxide and water
Classified	[klas-uh-fahyd]	arrange or organize as belonging to a specific group or category
Climate	[klahy-mit]	weather conditions in a place or region
Clot	[klot]	thickened and partly solid blood that stops bleeding when you get cuts and scrapes
Compact	[kuhm-pakt]	joined or close together with little space in-between; dense
Corm	[kawrm]	large, dense, scaly leaves, and buds or eyes that can grow new plants above ground and have underground stems with a solid basal plate
Cylindrical	[sil-in-dri-kuhl]	a shape that has straight sides and two circular ends like a straw
Cynarin	[sin-are-in]	a natural acid found in artichokes that coats the mouth and makes water taste sweet
Digestion; digestive system	[dih-jes-chuhn]	how the body breaks down food and gets nutrients and energy from food

Dissolve	[dih-zolv]	a reaction that occurs when a solid is mixed with a liquid and the solid becomes part of the liquid
Diverse	[dih-vurs]	having various kinds or forms
DNA	[d-n-a]	the instruction manual for your body on how your body works and the way you look
Drizzle	[driz-uhl]	pour a small amount of liquid onto or over something
Edible	[ed-uh-buhl]	safe to eat
Electrolyte(s)	[ih-lek-truh-lahyt]	minerals that balance the amount of fluid in your body, e.g. sodium, potassium, and chloride
Energy	[en-er-jee]	a usable source of nutrition that can come from food and enables animals and plants to function
Ethylene	[eth-uh-leen]	a gas that is naturally released when fruits ripen and helps soften fruit
Fahrenheit	[far-uhn-hahyt]	a measurement of temperature; labeled as degrees F in in this book
Farm; farming; farmed	[fahrm]	land used for growing crops such as fruits and vegetables; the process of growing crops; those who work to raise crops are known as farmers
Flavor	[fley-ver]	a characteristic or quality of how something tastes
Flesh; fleshy	[flesh]	the soft pulpy portion of a fruit or vegetable that is eaten
Floret	[floor-ets]	a group of flower buds that are part of a vegetable (e.g., cauliflower)
Flourish	[flur-ish]	to grow or develop well
Flower	[flou-er]	edible part of a plant that may also include the stems (e.g., broccoli); the part of a plant form which the seed or fruit develops
Food borne illness	[food bohrn il-ness]	any illness caused by food that includes harmful bacteria
Forage	[for-ij]	to search for food
Frond	[frond]	a large, long leaf
Fruit	[froot]	fleshy, fully-grown, and ready to eat part of a plant or flower that has seeds (e.g., eggplant)
Gas	[gas]	a substance like air that does not have fixed shape such as a solid or a liquid
Greased	[grees-ed]	a thin layer of fat or oil
Harvest	[hahr-vist]	to gather crops or the season when crops are gathered
Herb	[urb]	a plant or a part of a plant that is used to give flavor or scent to food
Horticulture	[hawr-ti-kuhl-cher]	the science of growing fruits, vegetables, and flowers
Husk	[huhsk]	a thin, dry layer that covers some seeds and fruits
Hydroponic	[hahy-druh-pon-iks]	a method of growing plants in gravel, sand, or water rather than in soil
Immune system	[im-u-n sis-tem]	the system in your body that protects your body and fights off sickness
Imported	[im-pohr-ted]	to bring a product into another country to be sold
Inulin	[in-yuh-lin]	a type of fiber that cannot be digested by the body
Iodine	[eye-Uh-Dahyn]	important mineral for growth and development
Irritate	[ir-i-teyt]	to make a body part sore or painful
Leaves	[leevz]	edible part of a plant that grows from the stem (e.g., cabbage)
Marinate	[mar-uh-neyt]	to put food in sauce for a period of time to add flavor or make food more tender
Mineral(s)	[min-er-uhl]	substances that occur naturally in certain foods and have different jobs in the body to help you grow healthy and strong
Mold; moldy; molding	[mohld]	a substance that grows on the surface of damp or rotting foods that can cause them to spoil

Mushroom	[muh-sh-room]	an organism that is a form of fungi, typically reproduces from spores, and lack seeds, roots, leaves, and flowers; not classified as vegetables but commonly eaten as vegetables
Nervous system	[nur-vuh s sis-tem]	the system of nerves in your body that sends messages for controlling movement and feeling between the brain and the other parts of your body
Nutrient(s)	[nu-tree-uhnt]	a substance found in food that our bodies use to grow, run, and play
Oxalic acid	[ox-al-ick as-id]	an acid found in many plants including fruits, vegetables, nuts, and seeds that is typically not harmful but may irritate the skin or make you sick if consumed in large amounts
Oxygen	[ok-si-juh n]	a colorless, odorless, and tasteless element that makes up the air we breathe and is vital to all living things
Photosynthesis	[foh-tuh-sin-thuh-sis]	how plants make energy or food plant + sun + water + nutrients from soil + carbon dioxide = energy or sugar and oxygen
Phytonutrient(s)	[fi-toe-new-tree-ent]	helpful parts of plants that keep us from getting sick
Pierce	[peer-sss]	to make a hole in or through something
Pigment	[pig-muhnt]	a substance that gives color to something else
Plump	[pluhmp]	well filled out or a full, rounded shape
Poisonous	[poi-zuh-nu s]	when a substance is harmful and can make you sick
Prepare	[pre-pair]	to make or create something ready to eat
Probiotic	[proh-bahy-ot-ik]	helpful bacteria
Processed	[pro-ses-ed]	to change a food from one form into another by preparing it in a special way
Prototaxites	[pro-toe-tax-eye-tz]	organisms believed to be giant mushrooms dating back more than 420 million years
Reproduce	[ree-pruh-doos]	to make new plants
Ripe	[rahyp]	fully grown and developed fruit or vegetable that is ready to be eaten
Root	[rue-et]	round, long, fleshy tissue sprouting from the base of a plant stem with a thin "tail" that grows downward (e.g., carrots)
Sea vegetable	[see vej-tuh-buhl]	edible plants grown in the sea that lack true roots, stems, or leaves and are technically classified as marine algae; not classified as vegetables but commonly eaten as vegetables
Seasonal	[see-zuh-nl]	produce that is grown during a particular time of the year due to varying climates; the four seasons are winter, spring, summer, and fall
Seed	[seed]	a small object formed by a plant from which a new plant can grow
Shoots	[shoe-ets]	the tender, first stems that develop from seeds which are grown a little longer than sprouts and have more developed stems and small leaves; not classified as vegetables but commonly eaten as vegetables
Shuck	[shuhk]	to remove the outer covering of a plant such as the husk on corn
Spine	[spahyn]	a hard or woody part on a plant
Spoil	[spoy-el]	to lose freshness and become rotten or bad and can no longer be eaten
Spore	[spohr]	a cell similar to a seed that can grow a new plant
Sprouts	[sprouts]	the tender, first stems that develop from seeds which grow with seeds and tiny leaves; not classified as vegetables but commonly eaten as vegetables
Stabilizing	[stey-buh-lahyz-ing]	a substance added to food that is used to thicken and provide a firmer texture
Stain	[stay-en]	to leave a mark on something that is not easily removed
Stalk	[stawk]	another name for a plant stem

Stem	[stem]	main part of a plant that supports leaves and flowers (e.g., asparagus)
Stock	[stok]	a broth prepared by boiling meat, poultry, fish, or vegetables that is used to make soups or sauces
Sulfoxide	[suhl-fok-sahyd]	a gas released when cutting onions that makes eyes sting and water
Symbols	[sim-buhls]	an image used to represent a word or a group of words
Temperature	[tem-per-uh-cher]	a measurement that indicates how hot or cold something is and can be measured using a thermometer in degrees Fahrenheit or degrees Celsius; Fahrenheit is labeled as degrees F in this book
Texture	[teks-cher]	visual or physical qualities of a surface that you can see and touch
Thickening	[thik-un-ing]	to make something thick or thicker like a gravy
Thrive	[thrahyv]	to grow or develop well
Tissue	[tish-oo]	a material that forms the parts in a plant or animal
Translucent	[trans-loo-cent]	when an object is not completely clear, but light can pass through
Tuber	[too-ber]	large, solid, thickened underground stems that store energy or food and can grow new plants from their buds or eyes (e.g., potato)
Uniform	[yoo-nuh-fawrm]	identical or consistent in size or shape
Variety	[vuh-rahy-i-tee]	a number or collection of different things in the same general category
Versatile	[vur-suh-tl]	having many different uses
Vinaigrette	[vin-uh-gret]	a dressing or sauce made from a mixture of oil, vinegar, and seasonings
Vitamin(s)	[vahy-tuh-min]	substances that occur naturally in certain foods and have different jobs in the body to help you grow healthy and strong
Vitamin B12	[vahy-tuh-min b12]	supports many functions in the body including making red blood cells, supporting your body's nervous system, and using energy from the food you eat
Vitamin D	[vahy-tuh-min d]	promotes healthy bones, teeth, and muscles
Wilt; wilted; wilting	[wilt]	to become limp or drooping

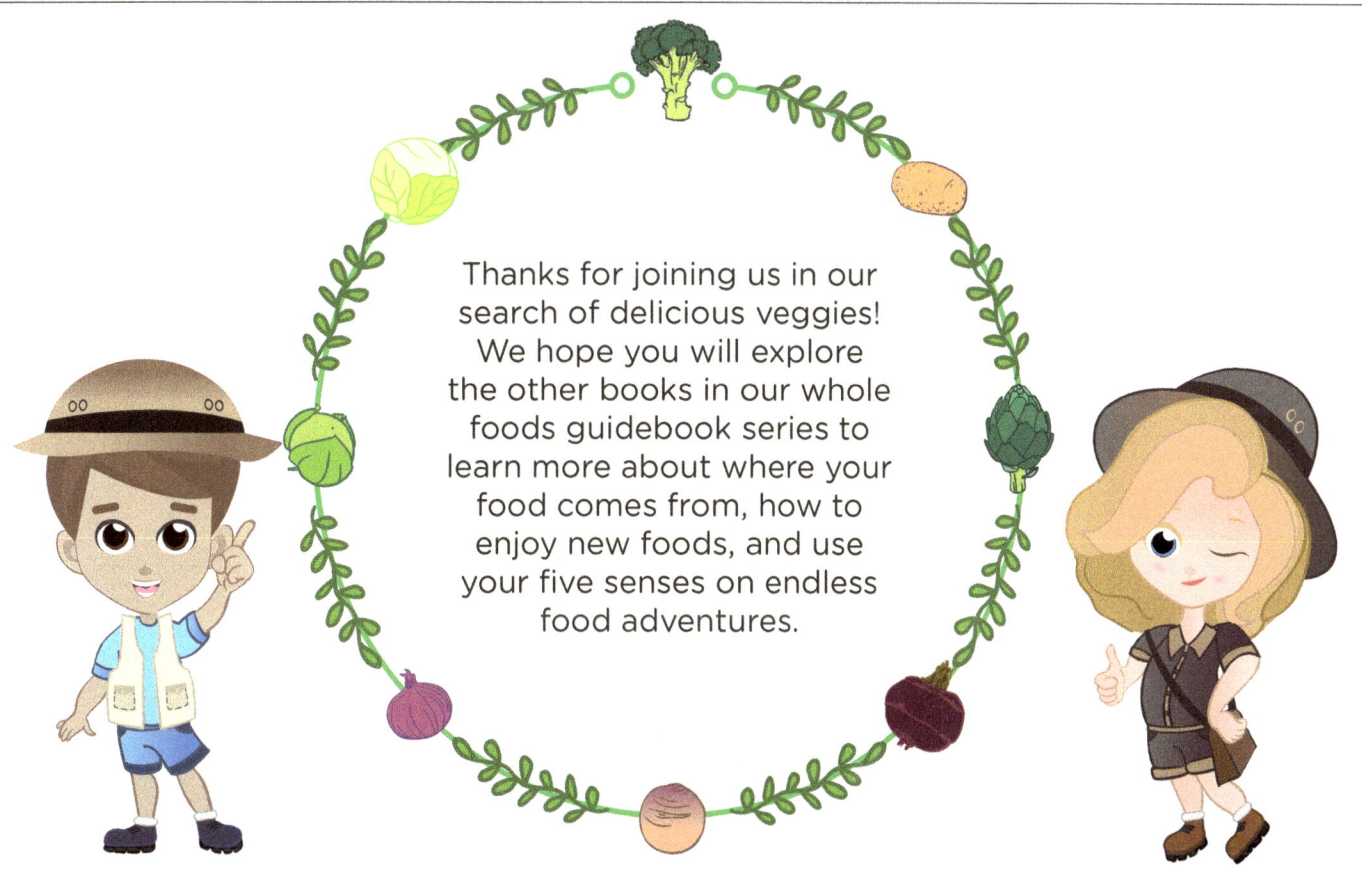

Thanks for joining us in our search of delicious veggies! We hope you will explore the other books in our whole foods guidebook series to learn more about where your food comes from, how to enjoy new foods, and use your five senses on endless food adventures.